OXFORD MEDICAL PUBLICATIONS

Paediatric Gastroenterology, Hepatology, and Nutrition

General Oxford Specialist Handbooks
A Resuscitation Room Guide (Banerjee and Hargreaves)

Oxford Specialist Handbooks in End of Life Care
Cardiology: From advanced disease to bereavement (Beattie, Connelly, and Watson eds.)
Nephrology: From advanced disease to bereavement (Brown, Chambers, and Eggeling)

Oxford Specialist Handbooks in Anaesthesia
Cardiac Anaesthesia (Barnard and Martin eds.)
Neuroanaesthesia (Nathanson and Moppett eds.)
Obstetric Anaesthesia (Clyburn, Collis, Harries, and Davies eds.)
Paediatric Anaesthesia (Doyle ed.)

Oxford Specialist Handbooks in Cardiology
Cardiac Catheterization and Coronary Angiography (Mitchell, West, Leeson, and Banning)
Pacemakers and ICDs (Timperley, Leeson, Mitchell, and Betts eds.)
Echocardiography (Leeson, Mitchell, and Becher eds.)
Heart Failure (Gardner, McDonagh, and Walker)
Nuclear Cardiology (Sabharwal, Loong, and Kelion)

Oxford Specialist Handbooks in Neurology
Epilepsy (Alarcon, Nashef, Cross, and Nightingale)
Parkinson's Disease and Other Movement Disorders (Edwards, Bhatia, and Quinn)

Oxford Specialist Handbooks in Paediatrics
Paediatric Gastroenterology, Hepatology, and Nutrition (Beattie, Dhawan, and Puntis)
Paediatric Nephrology (Rees, Webb, and Brogan)
Paediatric Neurology (Forsyth and Newton eds.)
Paediatric Oncology and Haematology (Bailey and Skinner eds.)
Paediatric Radiology (Johnson, Williams, and Foster)

Oxford Specialist Handbooks in Surgery
Cardiothoracic Surgery (Chikwe, Beddow, and Glenville)
Hand Surgery (Warwick)
Neurosurgery (Samandouras)
Operative Surgery (McLatchie and Leaper eds.)
Otolaryngology and Head and Neck Surgery (Warner and Corbridge)
Plastic and Reconstructive Surgery (Giele and Cassell eds.)
Renal Transplantation (Talbot)
Urological Surgery (Reynard, Sullivan, Turner, Feneley, Armenakas, and Mark eds.)
Vascular Surgery (Hands, Murphy, Sharp, and Ray-Chaudhuri eds.)

Oxford Specialist Handbook of
Paediatric Gastroenterology, Hepatology, and Nutrition

R. Mark Beattie
Consultant Paediatric Gastroenterologist and Honorary
Senior Lecturer in Nutrition, Paediatric Medical Unit,
Southampton General Hospital, UK

Anil Dhawan
Professor of Paediatric Hepatology,
Consultant Paediatric Hepatologist, King's College Hospital,
London, UK

John W.L. Puntis
Consultant Paediatrician, The Children's Centre,
The General Infirmary at Leeds, UK

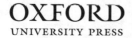

OXFORD
UNIVERSITY PRESS

OXFORD

UNIVERSITY PRESS

Great Clarendon Street, Oxford OX2 6DP

Oxford University Press is a department of the University of Oxford.
It furthers the University's objective of excellence in research, scholarship,
and education by publishing worldwide in

Oxford New York

Auckland Cape Town Dar es Salaam Hong Kong Karachi
Kuala Lumpur Madrid Melbourne Mexico City Nairobi
New Delhi Shanghai Taipei Toronto

With offices in

Argentina Austria Brazil Chile Czech Republic France Greece
Guatemala Hungary Italy Japan Poland Portugal Singapore
South Korea Switzerland Thailand Turkey Ukraine Vietnam

Oxford is a registered trade mark of Oxford University Press
in the UK and in certain other countries

Published in the United States
by Oxford University Press Inc., New York

British Library Cataloguing in Publication Data
Data available

Library of Congress Cataloguing in Publication Data
Data available

Typeset by Cepha Imaging Private Ltd., Bangalore, India
Printed in China through Asia Pacific Offset

ISBN 978-0-19-856986-2

10 9 8 7 6 5 4 3 2 1

Contents

Foreword

There is a romantic notion that paediatric gastroenterology in the UK began in a smoke-filled room in a pub somewhere in the 1970s. In fact, the truth is more prosaic. It did begin in the early 1970s, but in a seminar room in the Medical School in Birmingham, when a small group of leading exponents decided to form the British Paediatric Gastroenterology Group. Then, there were only a handful of tertiary specialists in paediatric gastroenterology, and only one in hepatology; nutrition was only incorporated twenty years later.

Since then, of course, paediatric hepatology has come of age, its growth helped enormously by progress in transplantation science and immunology. In Victorian households, feeding the children was usually left to the most junior and inexperienced housemaid. Perhaps as a consequence, the observation that malnutrition is bad for the child, has only been formally recognised somewhat belatedly in developed economies. Indeed, we now recognize that in certain disorders, nutritional therapy is a key component of the primary treatment.

The editors and their contributors are to be congratulated for having condensed a large subject into a small format and for having left nothing of importance out; the bullet point style is particularly suited to this kind of publication. It is particularly pleasing to see clinical nutrition so comprehensively dealt with; there is much here that makes this publication relevant to all paediatric specialties. One disadvantage of clinical nutrition having been championed by gastroenterologists has been the mistaken belief that nutrition is relevant only to those patients with gastrointestinal disease.

This book provides a valuable concentrate of all the clinically-relevant knowledge that we have acquired in this burgeoning field over the last thirty years. Often in paediatrics, the evidence base on which to make decisions is lacking and this specialty is no exception. The reader is therefore fortunate in having access to a pragmatic blend of evidence and clinical wisdom distilled and organised by three highly experienced specialists. The book provides a quick reference for the specialist, but is likely to be particularly useful for the non-specialist and for the trainee in paediatrics. Whatever changes may occur in the role of the doctor, they will still have to make diagnoses and initiate treatment. Moreover, all members of the large clinical team now required to look after many of these complex patients will find it helpful to have this book close to hand.

Professor Ian Booth
Dean
Leonard Parsons Professor of Paediatrics and Child Health
The Medical School,
Birmingham, UK

Preface

Paediatric gastroenterology, hepatology, and nutrition encompass a wide range of paediatric practice with conditions being managed in a wide variety of settings, dependent upon their complexity. This includes primary care, secondary services, and specialist paediatric practice. Conditions such as abdominal pain and constipation can be assessed in any of these settings. Conditions such as inflammatory bowel disease, intestinal failure, and liver failure require specialist assessment but still shared care within the wider health care environment. Nutritional problems are seen by us all in everyday practice with nutritional support being an integral part of the management of any chronic disease.

This book is intended as a practical reference for practitioners who commonly see such conditions both in training and in clinical practice. The idea is that they can dip in for information on practical management but also background information on specific conditions. The chapters reflect common situations encountered in practice.

I have been fortunate to collaborate with Dr John Puntis (nutrition) and Professor Anil Dhawan (hepatology) in the production of the book, both of whom are well recognized authorities in their respective areas. We have all had excellent support from Helen Liepman and the team at Oxford University Press.

We have included bullet points, lists, and managements guidelines where possible. We have limited the further reading as much of this is available through the internet, and websites have been listed where helpful. We have intentionally included only limited information about drug dosing and would refer the reader to the *British National Formulary for Children* for further information.

It is a source of great pride to produce an Oxford Handbook and I hope the book helps readers understand and enjoy the specialist areas of gastroenterology, hepatology, and nutrition in children

RM Beattie
Southampton
February 2009

Contributors

Dr R. Mark Beattie
Paediatric Medical Unit,
Southampton General Hospital
Chapters 21, 23–45

Professor Anil Dhawan
King's College Hospital, London
Chapters 22, 46–65

Dr John W. L. Puntis
The Children's Centre, The
General Infirmary, Leeds
Chapters 1–21

Dr Alistair Baker
Paediatric Liver Centre
King's College Hospital
London
*Chapter 51 Familial and inherited
intrahepatic cholestatic
syndromes*

Dr Sanjay Bansal
Paediatric Liver Centre
King's College Hospital
London
*Chapter 57 Hepatitis B,
Chapter 58 Hepatitis C, and
Chapter 63 Acute liver failure*

Dr Dharam Basude
Paediatric Liver Centre
King's College Hospital
London
*Chapter 61 Complications of
chronic liver disease*

Ms Carole Davidson
Paediatric Liver Centre
King's College Hospital
London
*Chapter 62 Dietary interventions
in liver disease*

**Dr Tassos
Grammatikopoulos**
Paediatric Liver Centre
King's College Hospital
London
*Chapter 54 Metabolic liver
disease*

Dr Dino Hadzic
Paediatric Liver Centre
King's College Hospital
London
*Chapter 48 Biliary atresia, and
Chapter 49 Alpha-1 antitrypsin
deficiency*

Mrs Nicky Heather
Paediatric Medical Unit
Southampton General Hospital
*Chapter 34 Nutritional
management of coeliac disease,
and Chapter 43 Nutritional
management of Crohn's disease
(co-authored with Dr Mark
Beattie)*

Dr Jonathan Hind
Paediatric Liver Centre
King's College Hospital
London
Chapter 64 Portal hypertension

Dr Lucy Howarth
Paediatric Medical Unit
Southampton General Hospital
*Chapter 30 Gastrointestinal
bleeding (co-authored with
Dr Mark Beattie)*

Dr Fevronia Kiparissi
Paediatric Liver Centre
King's College Hospital
London
*Chapter 52 Drug-induced liver
injury*

Professor Giorgina Mieli-Vergani
Paediatric Liver Centre
King's College Hospital
London
Chapter 53 Autoimmune liver disease (co-authored with Dr Marianne Samyn)

Dr Stephen Mouat
Paediatric Liver Centre
King's College Hospital
London
Chapter 65 Paediatric liver transplantation

Dr Marianne Samyn
Paediatric Liver Centre
King's College Hospital
London
Chapter 53 Autoimmune liver disease, and Chapter 60 Liver tumours

Dr Pushpa Subramaniam
Paediatric Liver Centre
King's College Hospital
London
Chapter 50 Alagille syndrome

Dr Nancy Tan
Paediatric Liver Centre
King's College Hospital
London
Chapter 47 Neonatal jaundice

Professor Stuart Tanner
Sheffield Children's Hospital
Sheffield
Co-author of Chapter 56 Wilson's Disease

Dr Roshni Vara
Paediatric Liver Centre
King's College Hospital
London
Chapter 55 Fatty liver disease in children

Dr Anita Verma
Paediatric Liver Centre
King's College Hospital
London
Chapter 59 Bacterial, fungal, and parasitic infections of the liver

Dr A.E. Wiskin
Paediatric Medical Unit
Southampton General Hospital
Chapter 24 Acute Gastroenteritis, and Chapter 32 Chronic diarrhoea (co-authored with Dr Mark Beattie)

Nutritional assessment and requirements

Nutritional assessment

Nutritional status reflects the balance between supply and demand and the consequences of any imbalance. Nutritional assessment is therefore the foundation of nutritional care for children. When judging the need for nutritional support an assessment must be made both of the underlying reasons for any feeding difficulties, and of current nutritional status. This process includes a detailed dietary history, physical examination, anthropometry (weight, length; head circumference in younger children) with reference to standard growth charts, and basic laboratory indices when possible. In addition, skin fold thickness and mid-upper arm circumference measurements provide a simple method for estimating body composition.

The multisystem consequences of protein–energy malnutrition include:
- Growth failure
- Impaired gastrointestinal function
  - hypochlorhydria
  - reduced mucosal function
  - pancreatic exocrine impairment
- Immunodeficiency
  - impaired cell-mediated immunity
  - anergy
- Respiratory dysfunction
  - reduced respiratory force and minute volume
- Myocardial dysfunction
- Reduced muscle mass
- Increased operative morbidity/mortality
- Delayed wound healing
- Impaired intellectual development
- Altered behaviour
  - apathy
  - depression.

Risk factors for undernutrition

Factors which may decrease food intake
- Age-inappropriate food being offered
- Inadequate amount of food being offered
- Unappetizing food
- Too much food
- 'Forced' feeding
- Reduced appetite resulting from illness
- Symptoms associated with disease or treatments, e.g. nausea, vomiting, sore mouth, pain, diarrhoea, breathlessness
- Repeated fasting for treatments or procedures
- Swallowing or chewing difficulties
- Difficulty self-feeding
- Poor child–carer interaction at meal times
- Impaired conscious level.

Increased nutritional requirements
- Illness/metabolic stress
- Wound or fistula losses.

Impaired ability to absorb or utilize nutrients due to
- Disease or treatment, e.g. coeliac disease, short bowel, pancreatic exocrine insufficiency
- Intraluminal factors, e.g. high/low pH
- Abnormal gut motility
- Infection, e.g. gastroenteritis, parasites; chronic suppuration.

Nutritional intake

Questions regarding mealtimes, food intake and difficulties with eating should be part of routine history taking. This gives a qualitative impression of nutritional intake. For a more quantitative assessment a detailed dietary history may need to be taken and can involve recording a food diary or (less commonly) weighing food intake. Use of compositional food tables or computer software allows these data to be analysed so that a more accurate assessment of intake of energy and specific nutrients can be made.

When considering if such intakes are sufficient, reference can be made to **dietary reference values** (DRV) which provide estimates of the range of energy and nutrient requirements in groups of individuals. Comparison of reported or measured average intakes against the **reference nutrient intake** (RNI), **estimated average requirement** (EAR), or **lower reference nutrient intake** (LRNI) provides an indication of whether intake is likely to satisfy demands. In a particular individual, intakes above the RNI are almost certainly adequate and those below the LRNI almost certainly inadequate (see p 19 for definitions).

Taking a feeding history

A careful history is an important component of nutritional assessment. Listed below are some of the questions and 'cross checks' that are integral to an accurate feeding/diet history.

Infant
- Is the baby taking breast-feeds or formula?

For breast-fed infants
- How often is the baby being fed and for how long on each breast? (check positioning and technique—see section on breast-feeding)
- Are supplementary bottles or other foods offered?

For formula-fed infants
- What type of formula?
- How do you make up the feed? (what is final energy concentration/ 100 mL?)
- Is each feed freshly prepared?
- How many feeds are taken over 24 hours?
- How often are feeds offered—2, 3, 4 hourly?
- What is the volume of feed offered each time?
- How much feed is taken?
- How long does this take?
- Are you adding anything else to the bottle?

Older children
- How many meals and snacks are eaten each day?
- What does your child eat at each meal and snack (obtain 1 or 2 days' sample meal pattern)
- How would you describe your child's appetite?
- Where does your child eat meals?
- Do you have family mealtimes?
- Are these happy and enjoyable situations?
- How much milk does your child drink?
- How much juice does your child drink?
- How often are snacks/snack foods eaten?

Basic anthropometry: the assessment of body form

Accurate measurement and charting of weight and height (length in children <85 cm, or unable to stand) is essential if malnutrition in the hospital and community is not to be missed; clinical examination without charting anthropometric measurements ('eyeballing') has been shown to be very inaccurate. For those infants born prematurely it is important to deduct the number of weeks born early from actual ('chronological age') in order to derive the 'corrected age' for plotting on growth charts. This correction is usually made up to the age of 2 years. Head circumference should be routinely measured and plotted in children <2 years.

Measuring weight
- Weigh infants <2 years naked
- Weigh older children in light clothing only
- Use self-calibrating or regularly calibrated scales.

Measuring length
- When possible, use an infant measuring board, measuring mat (easily rolled and transported), or measuring rod
- Two people are required to use the measuring board: one person holds the head against the headboard, the other straightens the knees and holds the feet flat against the moveable footboard.

Measuring height
- Use a stadiometer if possible (a device for standing height measurement comprising a vertical scale with a sliding horizontal board or arm that is adjusted to rest on top of the head)
- Remove the child's shoes
- Ask the child to look straight ahead
- Ensure that the heels, buttocks, and shoulder blades make contact with the wall.

Measuring head circumference
- Use a tape measure that does not stretch
- Find the largest measurement around the mid-forehead and occipital prominence.

Mid-upper arm circumference
- Mark the mid-upper arm (half way between the acromion of the shoulder and the olecranon of the elbow) then, using a non-stretch tape measure, take the average of three readings at the mid point of the upper arm.

Measuring triceps and sub-scapular skinfold thickness

- Pinch the skin between two fingers and apply specialized skinfold callipers; experience is needed to produce accurate and repeatable measurements; take triceps skinfold thickness readings at the mid-upper arm using the relaxed non-dominant arm; the layer of skin and subcutaneous tissue is pulled away from the underlying muscle, and readings taken to 0.5 mm, 3 seconds after application of the callipers; measurements can also be taken at other sites.

Measuring waist circumference

- Waist defined as mid-way point between the lowest ribcage and the iliac crest
- Measure with special tension tape.

References and resources

Further information on anthropometry:

www.cdc.gov/nchs/data/nhanes/nhanes3/cdrom/nchs/manuals/anthro.pdf

Measuring devices:

http://healthsciences.qmuc.ac.uk/labweb/Equipment/skin_fold_calipers.htm

www.miami-med.com/Height_Measuring_Devices.htm

Growth

Growth rate in infancy is a continuation of the intrauterine growth curve, and is rapidly decelerating up to 3 years. Growth rate in childhood is a steady and slowly decelerating growth curve that continues until puberty, a phase of growth lasting from adolescence onwards. During puberty, the major sex differences in height are established, with a final height difference of ~12.5 cm between males and females. Growth charts are derived from measurements of many different children at different ages (cross-sectional data). Data for growth of children are distributed 'normally' (i.e. form a bell-shaped curve). These data can be expressed mathematically as mean and standard deviations from the mean. The centile lines delineate data into percentages: the 50th centile represents the mean (average); 25% of children are below the 25th centile. The 0.4th, 2nd, 9th, 25th, 50th, 75th, 91st, 98th, and 99.6th centiles are each 2/3 of a standard deviation away from the adjacent line.

Anthropometric indices

Weight-for-height compares a child's weight with the average weight for children of the same height, i.e. actual weight/weight-for-height at the 50th centile. For example, for a 2.5 year old girl:

height = 88 cm

weight = 9 kg

50th centile weight for a child who, at 88 cm, is on the 50th centile for height = 12 kg

weight-for-height = 9/12 = 75% (moderate malnutrition).

- Weight-for-height can be expressed either as % expected weight, or as z score (i.e. the number of standard deviations from the mean).
- Mid-upper-arm circumference (MUAC) is used for children aged 1–5 years and provides a quick population screening tool for malnutrition (i.e. more detailed assessment required if <13.5 cm).
- Skin fold thickness is measured with callipers and gives an assessment of fat stores.
- Body mass index (BMI) is derived from weight in kg divided by square of the height in metres; it is an alternative to weight-for-height as an assessment of nutritional status.
- Growth velocity evaluates change in rate of height growth over a specified period of time (generally cm/yr); it is helpful in early identification of undernutrition and standard reference charts are available.

Assessment of growth potential

- Plot height of both parents at 18 year old end of centile chart.
- Add together parental heights and divide by 2.
- Add 7 cm (male child), subtract 7 cm (female) = midparental height (MPH); MPH ± 8.5 cm (girl), or ± 10 cm (boy) = target height centile range.

Normal growth—simple rules of thumb

Approximate average expected weight gain for a healthy term infant

- 200 g/week in the first 3 months
- 130 g/week in the second 3 months
- 85 g/week in the third 3 months
- 75 g/week in the fourth 3 months
- Birth weight usually doubles by 4 months and triples by 12 months.

Length

- Increases by 25 cm in the first year
- Increases by 12 cm in the second year
- By 3 years roughly half adult height is attained.

Head circumference

- Increases by 1 cm/month in the first year
- Increases by 2 cm in the whole of the second year
- Will be 80% of adult size by 2 years.

N.B. growth rates vary considerably between children; these figures should be used in conjunction with growth charts (Fig. 1.1a–f).

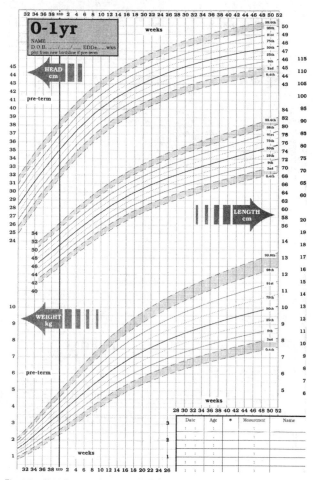

Fig. 1.1a Child Growth Foundation 9-centile growth chart for boys 0–1 years. Reproduced with permission from the Royal College of Paediatrics and Child Health (www.rcpch.ac.uk).

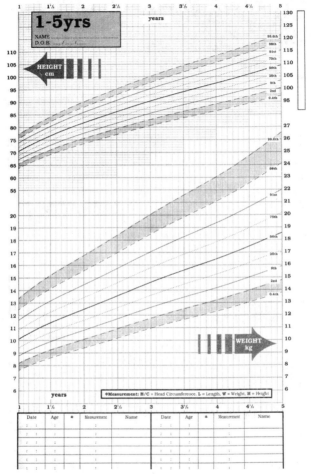

Fig. 1.1b Child Growth Foundation 9-centile growth chart for boys 1–5 years. Reproduced with permission from the Royal College of Paediatrics and Child Health (www.rcpch.ac.uk).

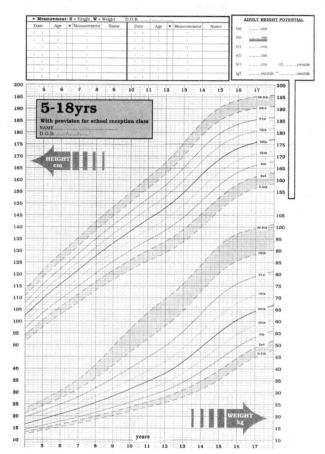

Fig. 1.1c Child Growth Foundation 9-centile growth chart for boys 5–18 years. Reproduced with permission from the Royal College of Paediatrics and Child Health (www.rcpch.ac.uk).

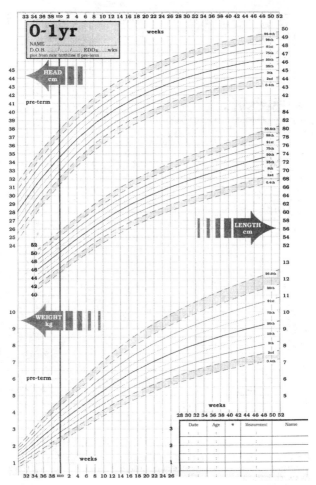

Fig. 1.1d Child Growth Foundation 9-centile growth chart for girls 0–1 year. Reproduced with permission from the Royal College of Paediatrics and Child Health (www.rcpch.ac.uk).

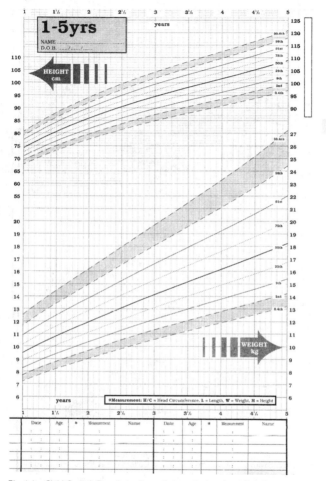

Fig. 1.1e Child Growth Foundation 9-centile growth chart for girls 1–5 years. Reproduced with permission from the Royal College of Paediatrics and Child Health (www.rcpch.ac.uk).

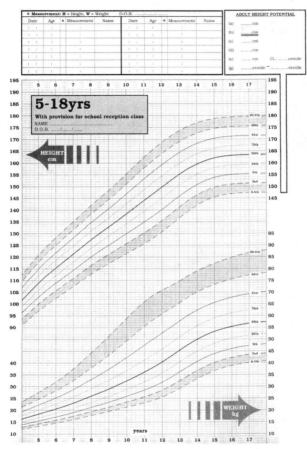

Fig. 1.1f Child Growth Foundation 9-centile growth chart for girls 5–18 years. Reproduced with permission from the Royal College of Paediatrics and Child Health (www.rcpch.ac.uk).

Patterns of growth

- Birth weight/centile is not always a good guide to genetic potential; some infants cross centile lines in the first few months of life ('catch-down'), but from then on continue to follow along a lower centile.
- The maximum weight centile achieved between 4–8 weeks is the best predictor of weight centile at 12 months.
- Infants born <10th centile for gestational age may either have intrauterine growth retardation (IUGR), or be within the normal 10% of the population who fall below the line.
- Long-standing IUGR results in low weight, head circumference, and length; catch-up growth is unlikely.
- Infants with late IUGR are thin, but may have head circumference and length on higher centile, and subsequently show catch-up in weight centile.
- Rates of growth vary in young children, and assessments should be based on a number of serial measurements.

Abnormal growth

- Short-term energy deficit will make a child thin (low weight for height; wasting).
- Long-term energy deficit limits height gain (and head/brain growth) causing stunting (and reduced head circumference).
- Chronically undernourished children may be both thin and short.

Puberty

Growth accelerates during puberty (the sequence of physical and physiological changes occurring at adolescence culminating in full sexual maturity; Table 1.1). Average age at onset is 10–12 years in girls, and 12–13 years in boys. Age at onset is partly familial. Afro-Caribbean girls tend to have earlier puberty than whites. Earlier puberty is seen in girls who are overweight and may be delayed in girls who are thin.

Table 1.1 Stages of puberty

Boys			
Stage	Genitalia	Pubic hair	Other events
I	Prepubertal	Vellus not thicker than on abdomen	TV <4 mL
II	Enlargement of testes and scrotum	Sparse long pigmented strands at base of penis	TV 4–8 mL
III	Lengthening of penis	Darker, curlier and spreads over pubes; axillary hair	TV 8–10 mL
IV	Increase in penis length and breadth	Adult type hair but covering a smaller upper lip hair area	TV 10–15 mL; Peak height velocity
V	Adult shape and size	Spread to medial thighs (Stage 6: spread up linea alba)	TV 15–25 mL Facial hair spreads to cheeks; adult voice

Girls			
Stage	Breast	Pubic hair	Other events
I	Elevation of papilla only	Vellus not thicker than on abdomen	
II	Breast bud stage: elevation of breast and papilla	Sparse long pigmented strands along labia	Peak height velocity
III	Further elevation of breast and areola together	Darker, curlier, and spreads over pubes	
IV	Areola forms a second mound on top of breast	Adult type hair but covering a smaller area	Menarche
V	Mature stage: areola recedes and only papilla projects	Spread to medial thighs (stage 6: spreads up linea alba)	

TV, testicular volume; measure by comparing with orchidometer.

From: Tanner JM. Growth at adolescence, 2nd edn, Blackwell, Oxford, 1962.

Malnutrition

Classification

There is no universally agreed definition of malnutrition in children, but the criteria shown in Table 1.2 are commonly used. Classification does not define a specific disease, but rather clinical signs that may have different aetiologies. Other nutrients such as iron, zinc, and copper may be deficient in addition to protein and energy.

The Wellcome classification of malnutrition (Table 1.3) is based on the presence or absence of oedema and the body weight deficit.

When to intervene

Malnutrition is difficult to define and quantify because of insensitive assessment tools and the challenges of separating the impact of malnutrition from that of the underlying disease on markers of malnutrition (e.g. hypoalbuminaemia is a marker of both malnutrition and severe inflammation) and on outcome.

Nutritional intervention may be indicated both to prevent and to reverse malnutrition. In general the simplest intervention should come first, followed if necessary by those of increasing complexity: for example, give energy-dense foods and energy supplements before progressing to tube feeding. Parenteral nutrition should be reserved for children with impairment of gastrointestinal function to a degree that precludes maintaining growth and homeostasis using enteral feeding. If simple measures aimed at increasing energy intake by mouth are ineffective, tube feeding should be considered according to the criteria shown in Table 1.4.

Table 1.2 Classification of malnutrition

	Obese	Overweight	Normal	Mild	Moderate	Severe
Height for age %				90–95	85–90	<85
Weight for height %	>120	110–120	90–100	80–90	70–80	<70
BMI	>30 (>98th centile)	>25 (>91st centile)				

Table 1.3 Wellcome classification of malnutrition

Marasmus	<60% expected weight for age No oedema
Marasmic kwashiorkor	<60% expected weight for age Oedema present
Kwashiorkor	60–80% expected weight for age Oedema present
Underweight	60–80% expected weight for age No oedema

Table 1.4 Criteria for tube feeding

Impaired energy consumption	Usually 50–60% recommended daily amount despite high energy supplements
plus	
Severe and deteriorating wasting	Weight for height >2 SD below the mean
plus	
Skin fold thickness <3rd centile	
and/or	
Depressed linear growth	Fall in height of >0.3 SD/yr *or* In early to mid puberty, height velocity <5cm/yr *or* Decrease in height velocity of >2 cm from previous year

Nutritional requirements

Energy metabolism

In order to maintain body weight, energy intake must equal energy expenditure. For growth to occur in children, energy intake must be greater than energy expenditure. Conversely, weight loss is achieved by increasing energy expenditure or decreasing energy intake. The energy content of food is usually expressed in kilojoules (kJ) or kilocalories (kcal). A calorie is defined as the energy needed to heat 1 g water by 1 °C; 1 kcal is equivalent to 4.184 kJ.

Energy balance

- Total energy expenditure (TEE) is made up of:
  - basal metabolic rate (BMR) 50–75%
  - physical activity 20–40%
  - diet-induced thermogenesis (DIT) 10%.
- Growth, injury, and fever will increase energy expenditure.
- BMR is the amount of energy expended by the body to maintain normal physiological functions.
- Energy metabolism is sustained by the oxidation of fatty acids, carbohydrate, and amino acids to carbon dioxide and water, with the release of some heat.
- An individual's metabolic rate can therefore be measured from either oxygen consumption and carbon dioxide production, or from the amount of heat produced.
- For clinical purposes, **indirect calorimetery** (measurement of oxygen consumption and carbon dioxide production) is used to determine metabolic rate.

Nutrient requirements for healthy children

- The Department of Health publishes recommendations regarding nutrient intakes at different ages (DHSS 1979). These can be used as a baseline for the individual child, although reference values are intended to relate to healthy groups rather than the sick (Table 1.5).
- Dietary reference value (DRV) is a term used to cover LRNI, EAR, RNI, and safe intake.
- Recommended daily amount (RDA)—the average amount of the nutrient which should be provided per head in a group of people if needs of practically all members of the group are to be met.
- Requirement—the amount of a nutrient that needs to be consumed in order to maintain normal nutritional status.
- EAR—the mean requirement of a nutrient for a population or group of people; on average 50% will consume more and 50% less than the EAR.
- LRNI—two standard deviations below the EAR; only 2.5% of the population likely to be meeting their requirements at this level of intake.
- RNI—two standard deviations above EAR; at this level intake will be adequate for 97.5% of the group
- Safe level—is given when insufficient information is available to derive requirements; it is believed to be adequate for most people's needs.

Table 1.5 Some nutrient requirements in childhood

Age	Weight (kg)	Fluid (mL/kg)	Energy (kcal/d)	Protein (g/d)	Na (mmol/d)	K (mmol/d)	Vitamin C (mg)	Ca (mmol/d)	Fe (µmol/d)
			EAR	RNI	RNI	RNI	RNI	RNI	RNI
Males									
0.3 m	5.1	150	545	12.5	9	20	25	13.1	30
4.6 m	7.2	130	690	12.7	12	22	25	13.1	80
7–9 m	8.9	120	825	13.7	14	18	25	13.1	140
10–12 m	9.6	110	920	14.9	15	18	25	13.1	140
1–3 y	12.9	95	1230	14.5	22	20	30	8.8	120
4–6 y	19	85	1715	19.7	30	28	30	11.3	110
7–10 y	–	75	1970	28.3	50	50	30	13.8	160
11–14 y	–	55	2220	42.1	70	80	30	25	200
15–18 y	–	50	2755	55.2	70	90	40	25	200

Females									
0–3 m	4.8	150	515	12.5	9	20	25	13.1	30
4–6 m	6.8	130	645	12.7	12	22	25	13.1	80
7–9 m	8.1	120	765	13.7	14	18	25	13.1	140
10–12 m	9.1	110	865	14.9	15	18	25	13.1	140
1–3 y	12.3	95	1165	14.5	22	20	30	8.8	120
4–6 y	17–2	85	1545	19.7	30	28	30	11.3	110
7–10 y	-	75	1740	28.3	50	50	30	13.8	160
11–14 y	-	55	1845	42.1	70	70	35	20	260
15–18 y	-	50	2110	45.4	70	70	40	20	260

- Saturated fatty acids should be 11% of total dietary energy.
- Essential fatty acids: linoleic acid should be a minimum of 1% total dietary energy and α-linolenic acid a minimum of 0.2% total dietary energy.
- There are no specific recommendations for non-starch polysaccharides (NSP) or fibre in children, but the 'age + 5' rule is commonly used, e.g. a 4 year old child should have a daily intake of 4 + 5 = 9 g of NSP.
- A rough estimate of energy requirement from one year of age is '1000 + 100 for each year of life, e.g. a 7 year old requires 1000 + 700 = 1700 kcal/day.
- Nutritional needs of sick children will vary, and increased demands from infection, sepsis, inflammation etc. may be offset by decreased energy expenditure.

References and resources

Aggett PR, Bresson J, Haschke F. Recommended dietary allowances (RDAs), recommended dietary intakes (RDIs), recommended nutrient intakes (RNIs) and population reference intakes (PRIs) are not 'recommended intakes'. J Pediatr Gastroenterol Nutr 1997;25:236–241 (www.jpgn.org; enter 'archive' and go to reference)

Department of Health and Social Security. Recommended daily amounts of food, energy and nutrients for groups of people in the UK. Reports on Health and Social Subjects No.15, HMSO, London, 1979

Growth and its measurement. Factsheet and interactive tutorial available from www.infantandtoddlerforum.org

Olsen IE, Mascarenhas MR, Stallings VA. Clinical assessment of nutritional status. In: Walker WA, Watkins JB, Duggan C (eds), Nutrition in paediatrics, BC Decker, London, 2005, pp. 6–16

Scientific Advisory Committee on Nutrition. Application of WHO Growth Standards in the UK. www.sacn.gov.uk/pdfs/report_growth_standards_2007_08_10.pdf

Breast-feeding

Breast milk is the ideal food for infants. The World Health Organization recommends exclusive breast-feeding for at least the first 6 months of life. Until March 2001, the WHO recommended exclusive breast-feeding only for the first 4–6 months of life. This change in policy was based on a systematic review of the published scientific literature which highlighted a protective effect of prolonged breast-feeding against gastrointestinal disease, and confirmed health benefits to mothers. The applicability of these findings to developed countries has been questioned.

The Department of Health in the UK promotes exclusive breast-feeding for the first 6 months of life. This ideal is currently achieved for only about 10% of infants in the UK, where although 2/3 of women begin breast-feeding, within four months half have moved to formula feeding. Around 1/5 of women who begin breast-feeding discontinue in the first 2 weeks; breast-feeding is more likely to occur with higher socio-economic status. Nearly all mothers have the potential to successfully breast-feed their newborn infants. Healthcare professionals play an important role in providing consistent advice and support (Table 2.1), and in ensuring that parents are aware of the potential benefits.

Benefits of breast-feeding

For the baby
- Ideal nutrient composition, including whey casein ratio (70:30); protein of high biological value; fat 40–50% of calories; essential fatty acids; long chain fatty acids (docosahexaenoic acid and arachidonic acid) may improve vision and cognition; cholesterol, important for CNS development and may influence later cholesterol metabolism.
- Low renal solute load.
- Breast milk contains beneficial immunological, antimicrobial, and anti-inflammatory agents: secretory IgA; lactoferrin; lysozyme; macrophages and lymphocytes.
- Breast milk also contains digestive enzymes: lipase and amylase.
- Reduced risk of gastroenteritis, otitis, respiratory tract infection, and in preterm, necrotizing enterocolitis.
- Long-term-effects include a reduction in blood pressure, cholesterol, overweight/obesity, type 2 diabetes, improvement in IQ.
- Lower risk of atopy in those with a family history.
- May prevent or delay onset of coeliac disease.

For the mother
- Uterus contracts faster postpartum.
- Inexpensive and convenient compared with formula.
- Promotes bonding between mother and infant.
- More rapid return to pre-pregnant weight.
- Possible decreased risk of osteoporosis.
- Lactation amenorrhoea (and so infertility) and conservation of iron stores with less anaemia.
- Possible reduced risk of ovarian cancer and premenopausal breast cancer.

Breast-feeding basics

The following are important for successful breast-feeding:

- Infant needs to be sufficiently awake and alert for feeding.
- Coordinated suck and swallow.
- Baby needs to be correctly positioned on the breast (Fig. 2.1).
- Adequate time at the breast to provide stimulation (5–15 minutes).
- Adequate feeding frequency, usually 8–12 times a day for the first 2–3 months.
- Extra water and juice are not necessary until after weaning.
- Avoid introduction of bottle until breast-feeding well established.
- Good nutritional health of mother.
- Relaxed, positive attitude of mother and other family members.
- Social and emotional support for mother.
- Support from health professionals.

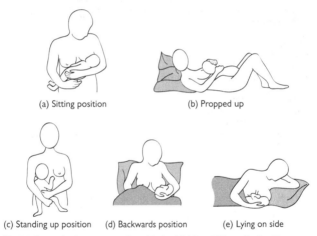

(a) Sitting position   (b) Propped up

(c) Standing up position   (d) Backwards position   (e) Lying on side

Fig. 2.1 Breast-feeding positions. From Vinther T, Helsing E. Breastfeeding: How to support success. A practical guide for health workers. World Health Organization, Geneva, 1997. Reproduced with permission.

Contraindications to breast-feeding

It is important to note that there are very few reasons not to breast-feed a baby.

Maternal illness

- Infection with human immunodeficiency virus, provided that formula feeding is a safe and feasible option.
- Active tuberculosis; mother can maintain milk with breast pump until treatment renders non-infectious.
- Drug abuse, e.g. amphetamine, cocaine, heroin, marijuana, phencyclidine.
- Excessive alcohol intake.

NB: Hepatitis B and C are **not** contraindications to breast-feeding.

Illness in baby

- Galactosaemia (use lactose-free infant formula).
- Phenylketonuria (PKU infants may alternate breast-feeds with phenyla-lanine free formula).

Medications taken by breast-feeding mothers

Comprehensive information on drugs in breast milk is provided in the appendix to the British National Formulary. Sometimes alternative drugs can be substituted to allow continuation of breast-feeding, and few drugs constitute an absolute contraindication. Discuss with pharmacist before advising against continuing feeding.

Promotion of breast-feeding

Maternity hospitals may seek baby-friendly accreditation once they have adopted the 'ten steps to successful beast feeding':
- Have a written breast-feeding policy that is routinely communicated to all healthcare staff.
- Train all healthcare staff in skills necessary to implement this policy.
- Inform all pregnant women about the benefits and management of breast-feeding.
- Help mothers to initiate breast-feeding within 1 hour of birth.
- Show mothers how to breast-feed, and how to maintain lactation even if they are separated from their infants.
- Give newborn infants no food and drink other than breast milk unless medically indicated.
- Practice rooming in, allowing mother and infant to remain together 24 hours a day.
- Encourage breast-feeding on demand.
- Give no artificial teats or dummies to breast-feeding infants.
- Foster the establishment of breast-feeding support groups and refer mothers to them on discharge from hospital.

WHO International Code of Marketing

The WHO International Code of Marketing of Breastmilk Substitutes is summarized below and was published in 1981 following discussions on promotion of breast-feeding and the marketing of infant formula:
- No advertising to the public.
- No promotion of products in healthcare facilities, including no free supplies.
- No company mothercraft nurses to advise mothers.
- No gifts or personal samples to healthcare workers.
- No words or pictures idealizing artificial feeding including pictures of infants on labels of products.
- Information to health workers should be scientific and factual.
- All information on artificial infant feeding, including the labels, should explain the benefits of breast-feeding and the costs and hazards associated with artificial feeding.
- Unsuitable products such as sweetened condensed milk should not be promoted for babies.
- All products should be of a high quality and take account of the climatic and storage conditions of the country in which they are used.

Table 2.1 Common problems during breast-feeding

Concern	Action
Engorgement	Often occurs when milk first comes in or when feedings are missed. Use warm compresses or warm shower before feeding. Hand express before feed to make it easier for baby to suck. Breast-feed frequently, every 1–2 hours; encourage baby to suck from each breast. If unable to breast-feed, use breast pump to relieve pressure. Apply ice pack to breast and underarm after feeding until swelling decreases
Inadequate supply	Offer frequent breast-feeds. Check mother's diet and fluid intake; ensure getting adequate rest; check medications
Is baby getting enough milk?	Check for 6–8 wet nappies a day, sleeping between feeds but not for excessively long time. Good weight gain (up to 8% of birth weight lost in first week is acceptable). Frequency of bowel movements very variable, and can be after every feed or every few days
Jaundice	Feed every 2–3 hours around the clock. If breast-feeding is stopped, express to maintain supply
Leaking	It is a normal sign of 'let down', especially in the early weeks of breast-feeding. Breast pads can be worn between feeds
Mastitis	Rest, frequent breast-feeds; mother should drink plenty of fluids. Antibiotics may be needed; use one that is safe for breast-feeding. Do not stop breast-feeding
Flat or inverted nipples	Frequent breast-feeds to avoid engorgement. Use nipple rolling or stretching before breast-feeds. Express for a short period before each breast-feed
Sore nipples	Some tenderness can be normal but breast-feeding should not be painful. Check for correct latch on and positioning. Vary baby's position at breast, air dry nipples after feeding, avoid soap, alcohol wipes and nipple creams. Shorter, more frequent feedings. Rub a little breast milk on nipples after each feed.
Poor weight gain in infant	Check adequate number of feeds. Increase to 2 hourly during the day. Check position and feeding technique. Ensure baby fully completes feeding at one breast before switching to the other breast; hind milk is high in fat. Alternate breast-feeds at each feeding. If formula feeding is necessary, give bottle at the end of each breast-feed to encourage stimulation of breast milk, with a goal to fully resume breast-feeding. Reassure mother; encourage relaxation. Seek specialist advice (e.g. lactation advisor) early

References and resources

British National Formulary for Children. http://bnfc.org/bnfc/bnfc/current/129132.htm

Department of Health guidelines. www.dh.gov.uk/en/Policyandguidance/index.htm

Horta BL, Bahl R, Martines JC, Victora CG. Evidence on the long-term defects of breast-feeding. Systematic reviews and meta-analysis. World Health Organization, Geneva, 2007.

Vinther T, Helsing E. Breast-feeding: how to support success. A practical guide for health workers. WHO Regional Office for Europe, Copenhagen, 1997. www.euro.who.int/document/e557592.pdf

World Health Organization. Protecting, promoting and supporting breast-feeding: the special role of maternity services, a joint WHO/UNICEF statement. World Health Organization, Geneva, 1989.

World Health Organization. The optimal duration of exclusive breast-feeding. Report of the expert consultation. Geneva, Switzerland, March 28–30 2001. Document WHO/NHD/0.1.09.

Formula and complementary feeding

Bottle-feeding

Although the WHO recommends exclusive breast-feeding for 6 months and partial breast-feeding thereafter, it was recognized that some mothers would be unable, or would choose not to breast-feed, and that these mothers also deserved support to optimize their infant's nutrition. It is important that formula feeds are made up according to instructions and that both formula milk and expressed breast milk is handled in a way that minimizes the risk of bacterial proliferation in the feed. Some simple guidelines are given below:

- If using milk formula, use a modified infant formula that meets manufacturing standards.
- Clean the bottle and teat in hot soapy water as soon as possible after a feed using a bottle brush
- Rinse before sterilizing.
- Cold water or steam sterilizing apparatus may be used; follow the manufacturer's instructions.
- Before making up a feed, clean the work surface and wash your hands.
- If using a cold-water sterilizer, shake off any fluid from the teat and bottle before rinsing in cooled, boiled water.
- Boil tap water in the kettle and allow to cool for half an hour.
- Put the water in the bottle before the milk powder, filling it just up to the desired level.
- Loosely fill the scoop with powder then level without compacting the powder.
- Only use 1 scoop of powder to 30 mL (1 oz) water; too much powder can cause dehydration through high renal solute load; too little powder can lead to undernutrition.
- Add the powder to the water in the bottle, put the teat in place, and shake gently until the powder is dissolved.
- It is best to make up a fresh feed each time one is required, rather than to store made up feeds in the fridge, in order to prevent bacterial proliferation.
- Bottles of infant formula should not be heated in a microwave oven as high temperatures reached in the feed can cause severe burns.
- The feed can be cooled by holding the bottle under cold running water from the tap (keep the teat under a cap and away from the water).
- The temperature of the feed can be tested by allowing a few drops to fall on the inside of the wrist; these should be warm and not hot.
- When feeding, the baby should lie comfortably in the crook of the arm, and the bottle be held at an angle so that the teat is always full of milk; this stops excessive ingestion of air during the feed.

Guidance on the average number and volume of feeds in given in Table 3.1.

Type of formula feed

The composition of infant formula is closely regulated in terms of the acceptable range of nutrient content. There are two main types of infant formula that differ mainly in their protein composition. These are whey-dominant formula (60% whey, 40% casein) and casein-dominant formula (20% whey, 80% casein). Whey proteins are quickly eliminated from the stomach whereas casein forms curds which are more slowly digested. Full-term normal infants readily digest both types of formula. Although casein-based formulas are promoted as being more satisfying for hungry babies, there is little evidence to support this.

- Some formula feeds have long-chain polyunsaturated fatty acids added as these are important for development of the brain and retina.
- Prebiotics (oligosaccharides) are now added to some milks in order to influence gut flora; there is little convincing clinical evidence of benefit.
- Follow-on formula are designed for infants over the age of 6 months; they contain less protein, calcium, and phosphorus than cow's milk but more than standard infant formulae.
- Most follow-on milks contain almost twice as much iron as standard infant formula and 45% more vitamin C.
- Follow-on formula can be used for older infants if breast-feeding has been stopped, and may have a role in the prevention of iron-deficiency anaemia.
- Other 'special' formula feeds include those containing a thickener (anti-regurgitation milk) for infants with gastro-esophageal reflux, or those for infants with colic (these have not been shown to be beneficial).
- Changing from one type of milk to another is seldom helpful in resolving feeding difficulties or symptoms, and should be avoided.

Table 3.1 Average number and volume of feeds for the formula-fed infant

Age	Approximate volume of a single feed (mL)	Number of feeds per 24 hours
1–2 weeks	50–70	7–8
2–6 weeks	75–110	6–7
2 months	110–180	5–6
3 months	170–220	5
6 months	220–240	4

These figures are for guidance; many babies will vary the volumes ingested from day to day and feed to feed. Total volume of formula milk will be around 150 mL/kg/24 h.

Complementary feeding

Complementary feeding embraces all solid and liquid food other than breast milk and infant formula. There is considerable variation between different countries with regard to introduction of complementary food, reflecting the absence of scientific data regarding optimal practice. In general, complementary foods should not be introduced before 17 weeks of age, and should not be delayed beyond 26 weeks. Cultural and economic factors influence timing of introduction of solid foods. For example, in the 2005 UK Infant Feeding Study 51% of infants had received complementary foods before 4 months, and earlier introduction was associated with formula feeding, lower maternal age, and maternal smoking. The following points are relevant to weaning practices:

• Kidneys and gastrointestinal tract are sufficiently physiologically mature by 4 months to metabolize nutrients from complementary food.

• From around 6 months most infants can sit with support and can 'sweep' food off a spoon with their upper lip; by around 8 months they can chew and swallow more lumpy foods; from 9–12 months they have developed the manual skills to feed themselves.

• Continued breast-feeding is recommended along with the introduction of complementary feeding; infant formula or follow-on formula may be used in addition to or instead of breast milk.

• Unmodified cow's milk should not be used as the main drink before 12 months as it may be associated with iron deficiency; during complementary feeding more than 90% of iron requirements in a breast-fed infant may be met by complementary food.

• There is little evidence that delaying or avoiding the introduction of allergenic foods (e.g. egg, fish, nuts, seafood) prevents or delays the development of allergy.

• The most effective measure for the prevention of allergic diseases is exclusive breast-feeding for 4–6 months.

• Although there is evidence for an adverse effect of rapid infant growth on later cardiovascular outcomes, little is known about diet in the complementary feeding period as a mediator of these effects; given the effect of salt intake on blood pressure, additional salt should not be added to foods during infancy.

• Both breast-feeding during the introduction of dietary gluten and increasing duration of breast-feeding are associated with a reduced risk of developing coeliac disease; it is not clear whether breast-feeding delays the onset or permanently reduces the risk.

• There is an innate preference for sweet-tasting food at birth; this can subsequently be modified by dietary experience; offering complementary foods without added sugars and salt may therefore have long lasting effects on taste preferences.

References and resources

Agostoni, C, Decsi T, Fewtrell M et al. ESPGHAN Committee on Nutrition:Complementary Feeding: a commentary by the ESPGHAN Committee on Nutrition. J Pediatr Gastroenterology Nutr 2008;**46**:99–110 http://www.espghan.med.up.pt/position_papers/con_28.pdf

Bolling K, Grant C, Hamlyn B, Thornton A. Infant Feeding Survey 2005. The Information Centre, London, 2007. www.ic.nhs.uk

Infant and Dietetic Foods Association. Infant feeding in the UK. May 2005. www.idfa.org.uk/inform.position.aspx

The premature newborn

Developments in care for the premature newborn have lead to increasing survival (50% of infants born at 24 weeks gestation) and an increased awareness of the importance of nutritional support. Many have difficulty tolerating enteral nutrition in the early weeks of life until gastrointestinal motility has matured. Some develop necrotizing enterocolitis (NEC) which carries a high risk of morbidity and mortality, and may be regarded as a failure of adaptation to postnatal life. Optimum nutrition should allow adequate growth in the short term, free of metabolic and other complications, with long-term fulfilment of both genetic growth and developmental potential.

General principles

- Low nutritional reserve and high energy requirements underlie the importance of providing timely and effective nutritional support (particularly in infants <1500 g) (Table 4.1).
- Ideally, *in utero* growth and nutrient accretion would be replicated, but in practice this is difficult to achieve and early temporary growth cessation is common, with variable degree of later catch-up.
- Undernutrition in the early weeks of life may have a lasting adverse effect on neurodevelopment and increase risk of chronic disease in adulthood.
- Parenteral nutrition (PN) is used more widely in the premature newborn than in any other group of paediatric patients.
- The principal indication for PN is immaturity of gastrointestinal function since gastric stasis, abdominal distension, and infrequent stooling impede advancement of enteral feeding.
- Rapid incrementation of milk feeds (>25 mL/kg/24 h) is associated with the development of NEC in case–control studies.
- In terms of enteral feeding regimen, the most appropriate strategy for prevention of NEC remains undefined, but breast milk appears to be more protective than formula feeds, and volumes should be increased cautiously over the first 10 days of life.
- There is considerable variation in the practice of neonatal nutritional support, reflecting lack of evidence base; however, there has been a trend towards providing the best possible nutrition as soon after delivery as feasible (sometimes referred to as 'aggressive nutritional support').

Parenteral nutrition

- Significant risks of PN include glucose intolerance (with osmotic diuresis), blood-stream infection related to a central venous catheter, cholestasis, and hypertriglyceridaemia.
- Variable fluid and electrolyte requirements mean that individualized PN prescriptions are often desirable, although there is an increasing role for standard bags driven both by increasing demand and by the need to have PN readily available.
- Aim to begin PN within the first 24 h of life if possible; also begin 'minimal enteral feeding' (use mother's or banked breast milk if available); start at 0.5 mL/h in infants <1 kg, and 1 mL/h in those >1 kg.
- Parenteral nutrient intake may be built up over a number of days; glucose and fat tolerance needs to be monitored carefully with blood glucose and plasma triglyceride measurements.

Enteral feeding

- Respiratory disease or immaturity of suck and swallow mechanisms mean that most premature infants (<37 weeks gestation) will be tube fed, usually nasogastrically.
- In some units orogastric tubes are favoured for infants with respiratory distress.
- When fully established, daily milk feeds are of the order of 150–180 mL/kg.
- Continuous feeds may be better tolerated in infants with immature gastrointestinal motor function, and are associated with a lower energy expenditure than bolus feeds, and possibly improved weight gain.
- Bolus feeds are thought by some to be more 'physiological' and may be better than continuous feeds at stimulating gut hormone release, promoting motor development, and stimulating bile flow.
- Mother's milk appears to be protective against NEC and tolerated better than formula feed in sick infants; it may be expressed breast milk from the infant's own mother (maternal EBM) or donor breast milk, expressed by feeding mothers in the community and given to a milk bank.
- Breast milk is associated with neurodevelopmental advantage, possibly because of its n–3 fatty acid content, or through an effect of its various biologically active peptides.
- Enthusiasm for milk banking waned in the late 1980s because of concerns regarding nutritional adequacy (low energy and mineral content) and the potential for viral transmission; there has been a recent resurgence of interest in part related to the availability of breast milk fortifiers that can be used to make up the nutritional deficiencies.
- Breast milk fortification with human milk or bovine proteins, minerals, and vitamins has been shown to influence short-term outcomes including growth, nutrient retention, and bone mineralization.
- Fortified human milk may not produce as much weight gain as preterm formula milk, but is associated with a reduction in late-onset sepsis and NEC.
- Breast milk fortifiers include Nutriprem® (Cow & Gate), Eoprotin® (Milupa), Enfamil® (Mead Johnson), SMA® (SMA Nutrition).
- When breast milk is not available, a preterm formula milk should be used; this has a higher energy, protein and mineral content than a term formula.
- Preterm formula include Nutriprem 1® (Cow & Gate), Osterprem® (Farley's), SMA Low Birthweight® (SMA Nutrition), Prematil® (Milupa).
- Infants are often discharged from the neonatal unit a little before their expected date of delivery; they often weigh much less than a term infant, and their nutritional requirements for catch-up growth are now being taken into account through provision of nutrient-enriched post-discharge formula such as Nutriprem 2® (Cow & Gate) and Premcare® (Farley's).
- Recent evidence suggests that either low birthweight or rapid early weight gain (or the combination) may predispose to adverse long-term effects, including increased risk of hypertension, cardiovascular disease, type 2 diabetes, and osteoporosis.

- Poorer neurodevelopmental outcomes have been documented both in infants small for gestational age who remained small at 9 months of age, and in those appropriately grown infants who had crossed down weight centiles.
- So far, nutrient-enriched post-discharge formula have been shown to improve growth but not to enhance neurodevelopment; in the formula-fed infant, these should be used until a post-conceptional age of 40 weeks, and possibly up to 3 months post-term.
- Careful growth monitoring must be part of routine follow-up of all premature infants, and both over- and under-feeding avoided.

Table 4.1 Estimated nutrient intake needed to achieve fetal weight gain (from Ziegler et al. 2002)

Body weight (g)	500–700	700–900	900–1200	1200–1500	1500–1800
Fetal weight gain					
g/day	13	16	20	24	26
g/kg/day	21	20	19	18	16
Protein (g)					
Urinary/skin loss	1.0	1.0	1.0	1.0	1.0
Growth (accretion)[a]	2.5	2.5	2.5	2.4	2.2
Required intake					
parenteral:	3.5	3.5	3.5	3.4	3.2
enteral[b]:	4.0	4.0	4.0	3.9	3.6
Energy (kcal)					
Loss	60	60	60	60	60
Resting expenditure	45	45	50	50	50
Misc. expenditure	15	15	15	20	20
Growth (accretion)[c]	29	32	36	38	39
Required intake					
parenteral:	89	92	101	108	109
enteral:	105	108	119	127	128
Protein/energy (g/100 kcal)					
parenteral:	3.9	4.1	3.5	3.1	2.9
enteral[d]:	3.8	3.7	3.4	3.1	2.8

[a] includes correction for 90% efficiency of conversion from dietary to body protein.

[b] same as parenteral but assuming 88% absorption of dietary protein.

[c] energy accretion plus 10 kcal/kg/day cost of growth.

[d] assuming 85% absorption of dietary protein.

References and resources

Cooke RJ, Embleton ND. Feeding issues in preterm infants. *Arch Dis Child Fetal Neonatal Ed* 2000;**83**:F215–218

Jones E, Spencer SA. Optimising the provision of human milk for preterm infants. *Arch Dis Child Fetal Neonatal Ed* 2007;**92**:F236–F238

Klein CJ, Heird WC. Summary and comparison of recommendations for nutrient content of low-birth-weigh infant formulas. Life Sciences Research Office http://www.lsro.org/articles/lowbirthweight_rpt.pdf

Ziegler EE, Thureen PJ, Carlson SJ. Aggressive nutrition in the very low birthweight infant. *Clin Perinatol* 2002;**29**:225–244

Reference and resources

Necrotizing enterocolitis

Necrotizing enterocolitis (NEC) is the most common gastroenterological emergency in the neonatal intensive care unit (NICU) and the major cause of death for all newborns undergoing surgery. The mortality is greater than that from all the congenital disorders of the gastrointestinal tract combined. Survivors may be left with short-bowel syndrome as well as other long-term gastrointestinal, growth and neurodevelopmental sequelae. NEC frequently presents as feed intolerance with bile-stained gastric residuals, abdominal distension, blood in the stools, apnoea, and acidosis. It may develop insidiously, or be a rapidly progressive illness culminating in shock followed by death. The characteristic finding on abdominal radiograph is intramural gas (pneumatosis), produced by bacteria that have invaded the bowel wall. Other radiographic findings include portal gas, persistently dilated loops of bowel and pneumoperitoneum. Immediate management involves stopping enteral feeding, and giving intravenous fluids with broad-spectrum antibiotics. Blood and platelet transfusion may be required. Hypotheses regarding aetiology include the possibility that enteric bacteria ferment maldigested carbohydrate creating an acidic intraluminal environment that adversely affects mucosal blood flow. Immaturity of gastrointestinal motor function, digestion, immunity, and circulation are all implicated in the pathogenesis.

Diagnosis and classification of severity of NEC is by Bell's criteria:
- Stage 1: abdominal distension, vomiting, feed intolerance, ileus on plain abdominal radiograph
- Stage 2: all of stage 1 findings, plus gastrointestinal bleeding and either portal venous gas or intestinal pneumatosis on radiograph
- Stage 3: pneumoperitoneum with septic shock.

A survey in the UK recorded 300 cases of NEC over one year, 65% of whom were <1500 g birth weight; almost 1/3 required surgical intervention and overall mortality was 22%.
- Nearly 90% were preterm (median gestational age 29 weeks) with presentation most commonly in the second week of life.
- Cases of NEC in term infants were usually in children with a predisposing condition such as congenital cyanotic heart disease.
- The estimated incidence of NEC was 0.23/1000 live births, or around 2/1000 NICU admissions; in the USA, prevalence has been reported to vary from 4 to 20% between units.
- Recognized risk factors in addition to prematurity include early introduction and rapid incrementation of enteral feed (>25 mL/kg/day) and hyperosmolar feeds or medication.
- Delaying introduction of enteral feed probably has no impact on prevention, but merely delays clinical presentation.
- In one study, the risk of NEC was 6–10 × higher in preterm infants fed formula milk than those fed breast milk; a systematic review of the limited available literature also suggests a protective effect of breast milk.
- Merely the standardization of enteral feeding management in a NICU appears to have some impact on reducing risk.
- Probiotics may have a role in prevention, but conflicting study results and unresolved safety issues mean that they cannot be recommended at present.

- Parenteral nutrition coupled with minimal enteral feeding for the first week of life is the approach commonly advocated for the initial management of high-risk infants.
- Intestinal perforation is an absolute indication for surgical intervention; relative indications include deteriorating clinical condition despite medical management, abdominal mass, erythema of the abdominal wall, persistently dilated loops of bowel.
- The most important factor influencing mortality rate is the extent of bowel involvement.
- Intestinal strictures develop in 12–35% of patients managed medically, most commonly affecting the left colon; presentation is usually with abdominal distension and vomiting with radiographic signs suggestive of partial bowel obstruction.

Case study

A male infant with a birth weight of 800 g was delivered vaginally at 30 weeks gestation following spontaneous onset of premature labour. He required ventilatory support, and an umbilical artery catheter was inserted for blood sampling and pressure monitoring His condition remained stable over the next few days, and small volumes of enteral feed were introduced. Weaning from the ventilator occurred on day 8 of life, from which time enteral feed volumes were further advanced. On day 11 he had a sudden collapse requiring re-intubation; aspiration of the NGT showed large gastric residuals, and this was followed by some abdominal distension, leading to the discontinuation of milk feeds. An increasing metabolic acidosis was noted on blood gas analysis, and widespread pneumatosis seen on abdominal radiograph. Initial treatment was with intravenous fluids and broad spectrum antibiotics. Despite this, his clinical condition continued to deteriorate and a laparotomy was performed. This confirmed NEC with extensive involvement of the small bowel. Non-viable bowel was resected and a jejunostomy fashioned; 40–50 cm of potentially viable small bowel was left behind, including the last few centimetres of ileum together with the ileocaecal valve. Parenteral nutrition was commenced and after 10 days 1 mL/kg per hour of formula milk was introduced. Over the following 3 months feed volumes were slowly advanced unless unacceptably high stoma losses (>20 mL/kg per day) were provoked. Subsequently, the jejunostomy was closed and after 4 months of parenteral nutrition, full enteral feeding was established.

See also Chapter 13, Short-bowel syndrome (p. 98).

References and resources

Henry MCW, Moss RL. Necrotizing enterocolitis. In: Stringer MD, Oldham KT, Mouriquand PDE (eds.) *Paediatric surgery and urology. long-term outcomes*, 2nd ed. Cambridge University Press, Cambridge, 2006, pp. 329–350

Lin PW, Stoll BJ. Necrotising enterocolitis. *Lancet* 2006:**368**:1271–1283

Patole S, de Klerk M. Impact of standardized feeding regimens on incidence of neonatal necrotizing enterocolitis: a systematic review and meta analysis of observational studies. *Arch Dis Child Fetal Neonatal Ed* 2005;**90**:192–193

Growth faltering (failure to thrive)

Growth faltering or failure to thrive (FTT) is a descriptive term implying failure not only of growth, but also impairment of other aspects of a child's well-being. It is a dynamic process involving a failure to meet expected potential, and there is no universally accepted definition. Weight crossing down two major centile lines is often taken as an indicator of need for referral to a paediatrician. In the absence both of symptoms suggesting specific organ dysfunction (e.g. vomiting, diarrhoea, breathlessness, etc.) and physical findings other than poor growth, an underlying illness is unlikely. It is important to bear in mind common factors influencing growth, such as parental size and *in utero* growth retardation.

Epidemiological work has demonstrated associations between poor early growth and several adult diseases such as stroke, coronary heart disease, and type 2 diabetes. More recently, attention has also focused on the role of childhood growth patterns in this association. Rather than small size itself predisposing to later disease, there is increasing evidence that it is the disparity between early and later size that is important. Growth faltering may result from a combination of dietary, organic, and social factors leading to undernutrition; the aetiology includes:

- Unintentional inadequate energy intake
- Inappropriate feeding, e.g. failure to progress with solids, force feeding, dietary restriction
- Subtle oromotor problems impairing food intake
- Behavioural feeding difficulties/food refusal
- Disturbed parent–child interaction
- Neglect by parents or carers
- Abuse by parents or carers
- Chronic illness or disability adversely affecting nutritional status (the minority, ~5%).

Factors influencing growth

- Familial height (familial short stature)
- Genetic abnormality (e.g. Turner syndrome, Down syndrome)
- Birth size (intrauterine growth retardation)
- Chronic illness (e.g. cystic fibrosis, heart failure, inflammatory bowel disease)
- Psychological factors (psychosocial deprivation)
- Environmental factors (poverty)
- Endocrine factors (e.g. growth hormone deficiency, hypothyroidism).

Investigations should generally be determined by symptomatology or abnormal physical findings (e.g. chromosome analysis if dysmorphic features). In attempting to rule out or confirm underlying disease it is reasonable to perform some basic investigations, although the precise choice will depend upon the individual clinical circumstances; initial investigations might include:

- inflammatory markers (platelets, CRP, albumin)
- Liver, renal, and thyroid function
- Full blood count
- Calcium, phosphate
- Sodium, potassium, chloride, bicarbonate
- Ferritin
- Albumin
- Urine culture, pH and test for blood and protein
- IgA anti-tissue transglutaminase (coeliac disease) if eating gluten-containing food
- Wrist radiograph for bone age if >18 months

Pitfalls

Coeliac disease can cause growth faltering without associated symptoms; the IgA anti-tissue transglutaminase antibody test may be negative in children who are IgA deficient. Infants with renal tubular acidosis may present with growth faltering; there will be a hyperchloraemic metabolic acidosis on investigation, with a urine pH <5.8.

Management

Multidisciplinary assessment including paediatrician, psychologist, social worker, speech and language therapist, specialist nurse, etc., is often required to fully assess growth faltering and coordinate effective intervention. Accurate monitoring of growth parameters including length is vital (see Chapter 1).

Visits to the home and video recording of interactions at mealtimes can be extremely enlightening.

References and resources

Growth and its measurement. Factsheet and interactive tutorial available from www.infantandtoddlerforum.org

Raynor P, Rudolf MCJ. Anthropometric indices of failure to thrive. *Arch Dis Child* 2000;**82**:364–365

Raynor P, Rudolf MCJ, Cooper K, Marchant P, Cottrell D, Blair M. A randomised controlled trial of specialist health visitor intervention for failure to thrive. *Arch Dis Child* 1999;**80**:500–506

Rudolf MCJ, Logan S. What is the long term outcome for children who fail to thrive? A systematic review. *Arch Dis Child* 2005;**90**:925–931

Iron deficiency

Iron deficiency is the most common nutritional deficiency in the world, affecting around 5 billion people, most of them from developing countries. The prevalence of iron deficiency anaemia in UK preschool children is ~8%, increasing considerably in inner city children; ~9% of under 5s in the USA are thought to be iron deficient. Depletion of iron stores is followed by the development of anaemia, initially with a normal mean cell volume (MCV). Continuing deficiency leads to impairment of erythropoiesis, with hypochromia and microcytosis apparent on blood film. Iron is essential in haemoglobin for oxygen transport, and is also found in myoglobin, and some enzymes (peroxidase, catalase, and cytochromes). Iron from red blood cell breakdown is recycled and excess iron stored as ferritin and haemosiderin.

Iron deficiency may cause:
- Pallor, koilonychia, angular stomatitis, glossitis
- Tiredness; irritability
- Poor appetite
- Impaired exercise tolerance
- Increased risk of infections (impaired lymphocyte and polymorph function)
- Developmental delay
- Poor educational achievement
- Dysphagia (pharyngeal web)
- Breath holding attacks
- Pica (e.g. licking newspapers, eating soil, carpet underlay, wood, etc.).

Diagnosis

- Anaemia (haemoglobin <110 g/L in children 1–2 years, <112 g/L older children)
- Microcytic red cells, hypochromia, anisocytosis, occasional target cells
- Increased red cell distribution width (>20%)
- Low MCV and mean cell haemoglobin
- Low plasma ferritin concentration (<10 µg/L)
- Other causes of anaemia excluded (e.g. β-thalassaemia trait)
- Rise in haemoglobin with therapy.

Other indices of iron status

- Serum iron; unreliable as a measure of iron deficiency, can be depressed as part of the acute phase response
- Total iron binding capacity (TIBC); a measure of total transferrin; as serum iron decreases TIBC increases
- Transferrin saturation—ratio of serum iron:TIBC × 100; low percentage suggestive of iron deficiency
- Transferrin receptor; bound to transferrin in circulation and relates to concentration of cellular transferrin receptor, increases with iron deficiency
- Erythrocyte protoporphyrin, increased
- Zinc protoporphyrin, increased.

Management

Prevention

- Breast-feed: high bioavailability of iron in breast milk.
- If breast milk not available use an iron-fortified formula (12 mg Fe/L).
- Use iron-fortified weaning foods.
- Encourage iron-rich foods, e.g. red meat, egg yolk, iron-fortified breakfast cereals, beans and pulses, dark green vegetables, dried fruit.
- Give vitamin C-rich fruit/fortified juices with meals to promote iron absorption.
- Avoid whole cow's milk during the first year of life, and then restrict intake to <750 mL/day.

Treatment

- 3–6 mg/kg body weight (max. 200 mg) of elemental iron daily in 2–3 divided doses (1 mg elemental iron = 0.3 mg ferrous sulfate or 9 mg ferrous gluconate).
- Increase in reticulocytes 5–10 days after starting treatment.
- Haemoglobin should rise by 10–20 g/L over 3–4 weeks; continue treatment for further three months once anaemia corrected to replenish iron stores.
- Poor compliance is the most likely cause of non-response in children (but consider other pathology such as coeliac disease, blood loss, malignancy, inflammation, etc.).
- Parenteral iron rarely needed unless severe intolerance to oral iron, gastrointestinal disease preventing absorption or exacerbated by oral iron, chronic bleeding, refractory non-compliance; (rare risk of anaphylaxis).

NB: Side effects of oral iron medication include nausea, epigastric pain (gastric irritation—try lowering dose), constipation or diarrhoea, and turning stools black; accidental overdose is a medical emergency.

References and resources

Booth IW, Aukett MA. Iron deficiency anaemia in infancy and early childhood. *Arch Dis Child* 1997;**76**:549–554

Micronutrients and minerals

The term 'micronutrients' includes two main classes of nutrient substances required in the diet in very small amounts: the essential organic micronutrients (vitamins) and the essential inorganic micronutrients (trace elements). Vitamin and mineral deficiencies may complicate malnutrition arising from underlying disease or inadequate diet. Key features are given below. However, micronutrients have wide-ranging effects, far beyond the simple prevention of deficiency states.

In children with restricted diets, a detailed dietary assessment by an experienced dietitian may help identify likely vitamin or mineral deficiencies. Children with cow's milk allergy maintained on a strict dairy-free diet, for example, are likely to require calcium supplements unless they are drinking adequate volumes of calcium-containing milk substitute. Fat-soluble vitamin supplementation may be necessary in any chronic condition where there is impairment of fat digestion or absorption.

Plasma concentrations of vitamins and trace elements do not always accurately reflect tissue stores and should be interpreted with caution, particularly when paediatric reference ranges are not well defined (e.g. selenium). Plasma zinc falls during an acute phase response, whereas plasma copper increases.

Vitamin deficiency

Vitamin A
- Xerophthalmia; cornea becomes dry and hazy and may progress to necrosis and scarring (keratomalacia), occasionally to perforation
- Major cause of preventable childhood blindness worldwide
- Subclinical deficiency associated with increased mortality
- Sources: vegetables (carrots); fish oils; liver
- Assessment: plasma retinol; retinol binding protein.

Vitamin B$_1$ (thiamine)
- The deficiency syndrome (beriberi) is mainly seen in South-east Asia, and associated with polished rice diet
- Acute cardiomyopathy at a few months of age
- Hoarseness, aphonia, encephalopathy, apathy, drowsiness, convulsions, death in older children
- Sources: germ of cereals, pulses, yeast
- Assessment: red cell transketolase, blood thiamine.

Vitamin B$_2$ (riboflavin)
- Usually associated with other nutritional defects, rather than occurring by itself
- Angular stomatitis, fissuring of lips, nasolabial seborrhoea, magenta-coloured tongue
- Sources: liver, milk, eggs, vegetables
- Assessment: red cell glutathione reductase.

Folic acid

- Nutritional deficiency mainly in developing countries; may occur in prematurity, malignant disease and its treatment, chronic haemolytic anaemia; malabsorption; drugs (e.g. methotrexate; anticonvulsants); B_{12} deficiency
- Megaloblastic anaemia on blood film, macrocytosis, neutropenia with hypersegmentation of polymorph nuclei, thrombocytopenia
- Supplementation in pregnancy reduces risk of neural tube defects
- Sources: green vegetables, liver
- Assessment: serum folate, red cell folate.

Vitamin B_6 (pyridoxine)

- Deficiency rare; reported in association with use of infant formula deficient in pyridoxine
- Convulsions; abnormal EEG
- Consider in any newborn with persistent seizures
- Features in children include weakness, depression, stomatitis, diarrhoea, and dermatitis
- Sources: animal products, milk
- Assessment: red cell transaminase, blood pyridoxal phosphate.

Nicotinic acid (niacin)

- Deficiency causes pellagra (children eating maize diet; toddlers with kwashiorkor)
- Child usually of school age; symmetrical, desquamating pigmented dermatitis affecting exposed areas of skin
- Dementia and diarrhoea (more common in adults)
- Sources: meat, fish, cereals, yeast, tryptophan
- Assessment: urine *N*-methyl nicotinamide, blood niacin.

Vitamin B_{12}

- Deficiency may occur in infants of strict vegetarians, B_{12}-deficient mothers, feeding with unfortified artificial milks
- Pernicious anaemia (intrinsic factor deficiency associated with autoantibodies against gastric parietal cells causing B_{12} malabsorption) may occur in older children
- Complication of ileal resection; may take years to become apparent
- Pallor, fatigue, glossitis
- Subacute combined degeneration of spinal cord (diminished tendon reflexes, loss of vibration sense, ataxia, extensor plantar response)
- Megaloblastic anaemia on blood film; neutropenia, hypersegmentation of neutrophil nuclei, thrombocytopenia
- Sources: animal products, milk
- Assessment: serum vitamin B_{12}.

Biotin

- Scaly dermatitis and hair loss
- Sources: most foods, intestinal bacteria
- Assessment: serum biotin, urine biotin.

Vitamin C

- Scurvy; rarely before 6 months of life
- Associated with extremely limited dietary intake (e.g. in a child with severe neurological handicap) or tube feeding with special formula
- Petechial haemorrhage into the skin, impaired growth, irritability; painful joints with 'pseudoparalysis'
- Radiologically may be mistaken for rickets; long bones show thinning of cortex; 'eggshell' calcification around epiphysis; periosteal elevation; occasionally epiphyseal separation
- Sources: fresh fruit and vegetables, particularly citrus fruits
- Assessment: leucocyte vitamin C, plasma vitamin C.

Vitamin D

- Rickets; impaired bone formation and growth
- Decreased calcium absorption, low plasma calcium; raised alkaline phosphatase
- Raised parathyroid hormone (PTH) mobilizes calcium from bone, but also leads to phosphaturia and hypophosphataemia; ultimately, PTH effect on bone is impaired and plasma calcium falls
- Hypotonia and impaired linear growth in infancy, delayed closure of anterior fontanelle; prominent forehead
- Rarely, symptomatic hypocalcaemia (e.g. stridor, seizures)
- Swelling of costochondral junctions ('rachitic rosary')
- Bowing of tibia in weight bearing children; swelling over growing end of long bones (e.g. wrists)
- Enamel hypoplasia and delayed appearance of teeth
- Coxa vara, kyphoscoliosis, pelvic deformity in long standing cases
- Radiologically: poor mineralization, delayed development of epiphyses; cupping, fraying and splaying of metaphyses; radiolucent transverse bands (Looser's zones)
- Sources: fish oil; vegetable oil; skin synthesis
- Assessment: serum Ca, PO_4, alkaline phosphatase, serum 25OH-vitamin D

Vitamin E

- Deficiency may be seen in preterm infants and children with malabsorption
- Haemolytic anaemia in the preterm
- Progressive neuropathy and retinopathy in severe, prolonged deficiency
- Sources: vegetable oils
- Assessment: plasma tocopherol/cholesterol.

Vitamin K

- Haemorrhagic disease of newborn (breast-fed infants at increased risk)
- Gastrointestinal haemorrhage or bleeding from cord; intracranial haemorrhage
- Prevented by routine prophylactic vitamin K administration after birth (usually multiple oral doses)
- Sources: green vegetables, gut flora
- Assessment: prothrombin time.

Mineral deficiency

Calcium
- Absorbed from proximal small bowel
- Nutritional deficiency in isolation very unusual
- Absorption affected by other nutrients, e.g. fat malabsorption.

Phosphorus
- Isolated deficiency very unlikely
- Prolonged treatment with aluminium or magnesium hydroxide: bind to phosphorus resulting in non-absorption
- Deficiency leads to osteoporosis or rickets.

Magnesium
- Deficiency may be encountered in protein-energy malnutrition, after small-bowel resection or with protracted diarrhoea
- Rare selective inability to absorb magnesium managed by magnesium supplementation.

Trace element deficiency

Iron
- Deficiency from poor intake (common), impaired absorption or excessive losses
- Anaemia, pallor, tiredness, loss of appetite, increased infection, impaired development, pica
- Assessment: serum iron/iron binding capacity; serum ferritin.

Zinc
- Growth retardation, hypogonadism, hepatosplenomegaly, and anaemia
- Delayed wound healing, pica, diminished taste
- Symmetrical, peri-orificial erythematous rash
- May occur in preterm newborn receiving parenteral nutrition (particularly after bowel resection)
- Assessment: plasma zinc, leucocyte zinc, alkaline phosphatase.

Copper
- May occur in infants with protein–energy malnutrition or malabsorption (or during parenteral nutrition with inadvertent omission of trace elements)
- Hypochromic anaemia unresponsive to iron; neutropenia
- Skeletal changes can resemble scurvy or non-accidental injury
- Assessment: plasma copper, caeruloplasmin.

Fluoride
- Important for reducing risk of dental caries
- Assessment: urine excretion.

Iodine
- Hypothyroidism with poor growth and development
- Assessment: serum T_4, T_3, TSH.

Chromium
- Deficiency may impair glucose tolerance; weight loss
- Assessment: plasma chromium; glucose tolerance.

Cobalt
- Essential component of vitamin B_{12}.

Manganese
- Role in human metabolism uncertain
- Deficiency in animals results in growth impairment, neonatal ataxia, chondrodystrophy, impaired fertility
- Assessment: plasma manganese.

Molybdenum
- Essential component of xanthine oxidase
- Assessment: urine xanthine, plasma molybdenum.

Selenium
- Deficiency implicated in Keshan disease (cardiomyoapthy, China) and Kashin–Beck disease (osteoarthropathy, Siberia), but other environmental factors likely to be important
- Skeletal myopathy and pseudo-albinism described during parenteral nutrition without selenium
- Assessment: plasma selenium, red cell glutathione peroxidase

Vitamin supplementation for infants and young children

Precise daily requirements for vitamins are not well established (Table 8.1) but supplementation is regarded as important in early life (children <4 yr).

- The fetus acquires vitamins from its mother, with fat-soluble vitamins being transferred towards the end of pregnancy.
- Breast milk from mothers with adequate nutritional status supplies sufficient amounts of all vitamins other than K and D.
- The UK Department of Health recommends either a single intramuscular dose of 1 mg vitamin K at birth to newborn babies, or an alternative oral regimen of three 2 mg doses during the first 6–8 weeks.
- Infant formula is fortified with vitamin K.
- Dark skin and low sunlight exposure increase the risk of vitamin D deficiency.

Risk factors for vitamin deficiency should be identified in the child and in the diet.

- In the UK there is strong evidence that vitamin D deficiency exists.
- In addition, large surveys have suggested that ~50% of children may have a suboptimal vitamin A intake, although clinical deficiency is not seen.
- The key steps in ensuring adequate vitamin status in children are giving vitamin K at birth, promoting a healthy, balanced diet in early life, and maintaining a low threshold for giving supplementary vitamin D (5 µg/day; 200 IU).

Use of vitamin and mineral supplements

This may also be required in children with a poor diet, those on therapeutic diets, and to replace increased losses. Expert dietetic assessment is appropriate and vitamin and mineral supplementation should go together with dietary advice.

- Children with eating difficulties, or those on vegan or vegetarian diets, may be short of iron and zinc.
- Children on exclusion diets for food allergy, and low-protein diets for inborn errors of metabolism or renal disease, may need comprehensive supplementation.
- Diets excluding or reducing specific items such as milk or fructose or sucrose may need supplementation with calcium or vitamin C respectively.
- Low-fat diets should routinely be supplemented with fat-soluble vitamins.
- A complete trace element and vitamin supplement is needed for children being fed a modular feed.

References and resources

Leaf AA. Vitamins for babies and young children. *Arch Dis Child* 2007;**93**:160–164

Table 8.1 Nutrient intakes for vitamins (units/day)

Vitamin	RNI	RNI	RNI	Tolerable upper intake
	0–6 months	7–12 months	1–3 years	
A (µg)[a]	350	350	400	800 µg/day (1–3 yr)
D (µg)[b]	8.5	7	7	25 µg/day (0–24 m)
E (mg)[c]	0.4 mg/g PUFA[d]	0.4 mg/g PUFA	0.4 mg/g PUFA	10 mg/100 kcal formula
K (µg)	10	10	10	not given
B$_1$ (thiamine) (mg)	0.2	0.2/0.3	0.5	not given
B$_2$ (riboflavin) (mg)	0.4	0.4	0.6	not given
Niacin (equivalents mg)	3	4/5	8	2 mg/day (1–3 yr)
B$_6$ (pyridoxine) (mg)	0.2	0.3/0.4	0.5	not given
B$_{12}$ (µg)	0.3	0.4	0.5	not given
Biotin (µg)[e]	not given	not given	not given	7.5/100 kcal
Pantothenate (mg)	1.7	1.7	1.7	1.2/100kcal
Folic acid (µg)	50	50	70	200 µg/day (1–3 yr)
C (mg)[f]	25	25	30	30 mg/100 kcal

[a] 1 µg Vitamin A retinol equivalent (RE) = 3.33 IU

[b] Vitamin D (calciferol); 1 µg = 40 IU.

[c] Vitamin E, α-tocopherol equivalent, 1 mg = 1 IU

[d] PUFA, polyunsaturated fatty acids

[e] No daily reference value given for biotin; an intake between 10 and 200 µg/day considered safe and sufficient.

[f] Vitamin C as ascorbic acid.

Nutrition support teams

There has been a considerable increase in the use of intensive nutritional support (both parenteral and enteral) in the management of children with chronic disorders. In addition, awareness of overt or potential malnutrition among hospital inpatients has increased. The identification of those with (or at risk from) malnutrition, and provision of effective nutritional intervention requires a multidisciplinary team approach since the skills required to deal with the details of assessment, prescription, administration, and monitoring of treatment frequently fall outside the remit of a single practitioner.

Malnutrition is common among hospitalized children with a reported prevalence of 15–30%. An expert report from the Council of Europe published in 2002 highlighted shortcomings in nutritional care throughout European hospitals, and provided recommendations for improving the situation, including the implementation of nutrition support teams (NST). The main goals of NST should be to provide optimal nutrition to all patients, including those who do not require parenteral nutrition or enteral tube feeding.

Malnutrition

- Is a continuum that starts with a nutrient intake inadequate to meet physiological requirements, followed by metabolic and functional alterations and later by changes in body composition.
- Is associated with an increase in morbidity and mortality in hospitalized children.
- Is a consequence of imbalance between low nutrient supplies and high substrate needs.
- In childhood, especially during infancy and adolescence, an increase in nutritional demands imposed by illness will compete with the specific needs of growth, however, increased energy requirements during acute illness may be balanced by a decrease in energy expenditure.
- Careful measurements and use of appropriate growth charts are essential for the diagnosis of malnutrition in children and for nutritional monitoring.

Suggested core composition of the NST

- Paediatrician with special interest in clinical nutrition
- Nutrition nurse specialist
- Dietician
- Pharmacist.

For managing problems associated with central venous access, impaired oromotor function, feeding difficulties, and ongoing need for parenteral nutrition the team should develop close working links with:

- Paediatric surgeon
- Microbiologist
- Interventional radiologist
- Cardiologist
- Speech and language therapist
- Occupational therapist
- Clinical psychologist
- Radiologist
- Clinical biochemist.

Roles of the NST

- To implement patient screening for nutritional risk
- To identify patients who require nutritional support
- To ensure effective nutritional management
- To plan home nutritional support following discharge when required
- To liaise with community staff and sources of social support
- To teach parents and carers how to undertake home nutritional support (enteral and parenteral)
- To educate hospital staff with respect to identification and management of nutritional problems
- To audit practice.

References and resources

Agostoni C, Axelson I, Colomb V et al. The need for nutrition support teams in pediatric units: a commentary by the ESPGHAN committee on nutrition. *J Pediat Gastroent Nutr* 2005;**41**:8–11

Beck AM, Balknäs UN, Camilo ME, et al. Practice in relation to nutritional care and support: report from the Council of Europe. *Clin Nutr* 2002;**21**:351–354

Enteral nutritional support

Assessment of a patient needing nutritional support will include a decision regarding the most appropriate method of feeding. The enteral route is preferred for children who have an adequately functioning gastrointestinal tract. Oral intake can simply be increased by use of food fortification, sip feeds, or energy supplements. If oral intake is poor or contraindicated, tube feeding may be used.

Tube feeding is used to prevent or correct malnutrition in the following groups of conditions:

- Impaired suck, chew and swallow:
  - prematurity
  - cerebral palsy
  - neurodegenerative disorders
  - orofacial malformations
  - intensive care/impaired conscious level.
- Breathlessness on feeding:
  - respiratory disease
  - congenital heart disease.
- Disordered appetite:
  - cachexia associated with chronic disease/malignancy
  - primary appetite disorder.
- Increased energy requirements:
  - cystic fibrosis
  - advanced liver disease
  - AIDS.
- Continuous supply of nutrients needed:
  - short-bowel syndrome
  - protracted diarrhoea
  - glycogen storage disease.
- Unpalatable liquid diet used as primary therapy:
  - Crohn's disease
  - multiple food intolerance/allergy.

Access routes for enteral tube feeding

Short-term feeding (<6 weeks)

- Fine-bore nasoenteral tubes (e.g. Silk tube):
  - nasogastric
  - nasojejunal (e.g. if vomiting from severe gastro-oesophageal reflux).
- Double lumen nasoenteral tubes:
  - gastric aspiration + jejunal feeding (e.g. in gastroparesis).

Longer-term feeding (>6 weeks)

Gastrostomies:

- Percutaneous endoscopic gastrostomy (PEG; most common)
- Surgical gastrostomy (e.g. when PEG technically not feasible/ contraindicated)
- Fluoroscopic percutaneous gastrostomy (interventional radiologist)
- Laparoscopic gastrostomy.

Jejunostomies

- Surgical jejunostomy (e.g. Roux-en-Y)
- Jejunal tube inserted via PEG
- Percutaneous endoscopic jejunostomy
- Subcutaneous jejunostomy.

NB. Jejunal feeding is used in particular when there is risk of aspiration, e.g. severe gastro-oesophageal reflux disease, but the patient is unsuitable for major antireflux surgery, or in severe gastroparesis.

For details of gastrostomy care, replacement of a PEG button, management of a leaking stoma and treatment of over-granulation, see Chapter 19.

How to place a nasogastric tube (NGT)

Use a tape measure to determine the length of NGT to be inserted (see Figs 10.1 and 10.2 and Table 10.1). For gastric placement in children, measure from ear to nose, then to tip of xiphisternum (Fig. 10.1). For newborns and infants, measure from ear to nose, then to the mid point between the xiphisternum and umbilicus (Fig. 10.2). The tube can be marked with a small piece of tape or permanent marker pen. Remember to record the external length of the tube

When to check the safe positioning of NGT
- After initial insertion
- Before a bolus feed
- After a bout of vomiting
- After paroxysm of coughing
- If symptoms suggest feed aspiration (coughing, choking, tachypnoea, wheezing, etc.)
- When receiving a child moving from another clinical area
- 12 hourly for children on continuous NG feeds
- 4 hourly in infants and newborns on continuous feeds.

For placement of a naso-jejunal tube (NJT) at the bedside in paediatric intensive care patients, without the need for routine radiographic confirmation, follow the steps below:

1. Select an appropriately sized NJT (≤8 kg, 6Fg; ≥8 kg, 8Fg), sterile water; tape measure, permanent marker pen, 50 mL syringe; tape; pH paper.
2. Consider appropriate sedation.
3. Open packaging and remove the guide wire from within the tube; flush the tube with 10 mL of sterile water, then lubricate the guide wire with sterile water and reinsert into the tube (NB: Do not use a gel lubricant as this may affect the accuracy of the pH paper response).
4. Using a tape measure, determine the length of the tube that needs to be inserted: for an infant <1 yr, measure from the nose to the ear to the mid-point between the xiphisternum and umbilicus, continuing to the right iliac crest, and mark the tube at this length; for a child >1 yr measure from the nose to the ear to the sternum, continuing to the right iliac crest.
5. Elevate the bed to 15–30° and if clinical condition allows turn patient on their side with left side up; aspirate the NGT already in situ.
6. Use sterile water to lubricate the tip of tube; it is often easier and more comfortable to insert the NJT through the same nostril as the NGT.
7. After aspirating gastric contents, ensure the tube is flushed with sufficient sterile water to eliminate any gastric residue in the lumen
8. Whilst advancing the NJT slowly rotate it by holding close to the nostril; a small amount of resistance may be felt as the tube advances to the pylorus.
9. Aspirate the NJT using a 50 mL syringe; if clear, bright yellow fluid is obtained with a pH >6, placement is satisfactory; alternatively, if 2–10 mL air can be injected via the tube but not aspirated back, the tip of the tube is likely to be beyond the pylorus.
10. Remove the guide wire with care so as not to dislodge the tube.
11. Give domperidone (250 µg/kg) via the NGT and wait 30 min.
12. Commence NJ feed at 5–10 mL/h and then cautiously increase, observing for misplacement of tube (feed in mouth, nostrils, or draining from NGT).

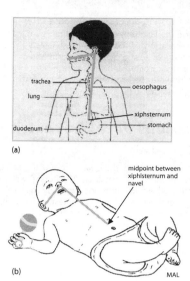

(a)

(b)   MAL

Fig 10.1 Measuring an NGT: (a) for children; (b) for infants and newborns.

Table 10.1 How to confirm correct NGT position

Confirmatory test result	Action
Positive aspiration of gastric contents (pH <5.5 using pH paper) *and* correct length of tube	Accept placement as correct
Unable to obtain aspirate of gastric contents despite correct external length of tube	1 If possible, offer drink to child and re-aspirate 2 Inject 2–5 mL of air and re-aspirate 3 Inject 2–5 mL 0.9% saline, position child on their side and re-aspirate
Unable to obtain aspirate of gastric contents *and* incorrect external length of tube	Reposition tube to correct length and re-aspirate; if no aspirate, follow steps 1–3 above
Unable to obtain aspirate of gastric contents *and* correct external length of tube	Confirm satisfactory placement by chest/abdominal x-ray *or* Remove tube and re-site, then repeat confirmatory tests

Giving medicines via an enteral feeding tube
- If possible, give medicines by mouth or other route than tube.
- Use liquid preparation, or thoroughly crush tablets and mix with water.
- Dissolve contents of gelatin capsules in warm water.
- Do not give enteric coated and slow release tablets via the tube.
- Flush tube with water before and after each medication.
- Avoid adding medication directly to liquid feed.

Complications of enteral nutritional support

It is important to consider and regularly review the objectives of nutritional support in individual patients. Monitoring will include regular review of nutritional intake, anthropometry, biochemical and haematological status, general clinical state, gastrointestinal function, tube integrity. Potential complications are shown in Table 10.2.

Table 10.2 Complications associated with tube feeding

Cause	Possible solution
Diarrhoea	
Unsuitable feed in a child with impaired gut function	Change to hydrolysed formula or modular feed
Excessive infusion rate	Slow rate and increase as tolerated
Intolerance of bolus feeds	Frequent, smaller feeds, or change to continuous feeds
High feed osmolarity	Build up strength of feed slowly and give by continuous infusion
Microbial contamination of feed	Use sterile, commercially produced feeds when possible; prepare other feeds in clean environment
Drugs (e.g. antibiotics, laxatives)	Review drug prescription
Nausea/vomiting	
Excessive infusion rate	Slowly build up feed infusion
Slow gastric emptying	Encourage lying on right side; prokinetics
Constipation	Maintain regular bowel habit with adequate fluid intake, fibre containing feed and/or laxatives
Medicines given at the same time as feed	Allow time between giving medicines and giving feed, or stop continuous feed for a short time
Psychological factors	Review feeding behaviour; consider referral to psychologist
Regurgitation/aspiration	
Gastro-oesophageal reflux	Correct positioning; feed thickener; drugs; continuous feeds; jejunal tube; fundoplication
Dislodged tube	Secure tube adequately and regularly review position
Excessive infusion rate	Slow infusion rate
Intolerance of bolus feeds	Smaller, more frequent feeds, or continuous infusion

Liquid feed composition and choice of feed

- Carbohydrates in enteral formula are derived from different starches, including corn and tapioca; maltodextrin and hydrolysed cornstarch, glucose-derived saccharides, and corn syrup are most commonly used.
- Formula for children usually contain little or no lactose.
- Protein is often derived from casein, soy, or whey protein, with a nitrogen:non-nitrogen energy ratio of approximately 1:150.
- Lipids are supplied predominantly as triglycerides, either as long-chain (LCT) or medium-chain triglycerides (MCT).
- MCT come mainly from coconut oil, and are rapidly hydrolysed and effectively absorbed even at low concentrations of pancreatic enzymes or bile acids.
- A high intake of MCT may cause osmotic diarrhoea; essential fatty acids need to be added to the feed.
- LCT promote intestinal motility and stimulate biliary and pancreatic secretions; however, when there is maldigestion, hydroxylation by bacteria can induce secretion into the bowel, worsening diarrhoea.
- Some enteral formula contain fibre, which may be useful to prevent constipation; fibre is also a substrate for bacterial production of short-chain fatty acids that are trophic to colonic mucosa and a source of energy.
- Most enteral formula contain sufficient micronutrients to meet increased needs associated with stress and wound healing; L-carnitine, taurine and inositol are commonly added.

Nutrient density and osmolarity

- The nutrient density of an enteral feed clearly depends on fluid content; at standard dilution, the energy content of infant formula is usually 0.67 kcal/mL, and standard paediatric enteral formula 1 kcal/mL
- More concentrated enteral formula are also available (1.3–2.0 kcal/mL) for patients with increased energy requirements or with restricted fluid intake.
- Osmolality refers to the concentration of osmotically active particles per litre of a liquid formula, expressed as mOsm/L; the osmolality is affected by the concentration of all constituents such as amino acids, carbohydrates, lipids, and electrolytes.
- Formula with a higher osmolality than normal body fluids may produces an osmotic diarrhoea; this is particularly important in children with severe small intestinal disease, or with jejunal feeds; isotonic formula with an osmolality of around 300 mOsm/L are preferred.

Selection of enteral formula

Enteral formula feeding must result in delivery of an adequate nutrient intake in a form and volume that the child can tolerate. In selecting an appropriate formula, the following factors are relevant to choice:

- Nutrient and energy requirements suitable for the age and clinical condition of the child
- History of food intolerance or allergy

- Intestinal function
- Site and route of delivery
- Osmolality
- Taste
- Cost.

For the great majority of paediatric patients, a standard paediatric polypeptide-based enteral formula will be appropriate. There are, however, many specialized and disease specific products designed for those with particular needs (see the British National Formulary for Children). In some children, a ready-made formula is not suitable and a 'modular' feed must be made up in the diet kitchen, or by parents at home once suitably trained. This allows flexibility with type and concentration of macronutrients so that the feed can be adjusted to suit individual requirements. A modular feed is most commonly used in severe enteropathy (for example post-gastroenteritis syndrome) or short-bowel syndrome complicating necrotizing enterocolitis.

References and resources

British National Formulary for Children: http://bnfc.org/bnfc/bnfc/current/129132.htm

ESPEN Guidelines on adult enteral nutrition. *Clin Nutr* 2006;**25**:177–360 www.espen.org/education/guidelines.htm

NGT insertion: www.npsa.nhs.uk/site/media/documents/857_Insert-finalWeb.pdf

NICE guidelines. Nutritional support in adults: http://guidance.nice.org.uk/CG32

Stroud M, Duncan H, Nightingale J. Guidelines for enteral feeding in adult hospital patients. *Gut* 2003;**52**:1–12 http://gut.bmj.com/cgi/reprint/52/suppl_7/vii1

Refeeding syndrome

Refeeding syndrome is a term used to describe the various metabolic complications that can arise as a result of instituting nutritional support (enteral or parenteral) in malnourished patients.

- Such patients are catabolic and their major sources of energy are fat and muscle; total body stores of nitrogen, phosphate, magnesium, and potassium are depleted.
- If this catabolic state is suddenly reversed by providing nutritional support (particularly excessive carbohydrate), there is a surge of insulin secretion which causes massive intracellular shift of phosphate, magnesium, and potassium with a subsequent fall in serum concentrations.
- The clinical consequences of hypophosphataemia include haemolytic anaemia, muscle weakness, and impaired cardiac function.
- This can lead to cardiac failure, fluid overload, arrhythmia, and death.
- Children at highest risk are those with severe chronic weight loss (e.g. anorexia nervosa; cancer cachexia).
- Routine phosphate supplementation may be given to anorexia nervosa patients being treated in an inpatient setting.

Guidelines for the prevention of refeeding syndrome

Refeeding syndrome is a potential complication of nutritional support in any malnourished patient. The greatest vigilance is required during the first week of feeding.

Monitoring

- Before feeding assess nutritional status and hydration, serum electrolytes, magnesium, and phosphate.
- Daily electrolytes, phosphate, magnesium, calcium, urea, and creatinine.
- Cardiac status (pulse, heart failure, ECG, ECHO).

Oral feeding regimen

- Initial volume and energy intake: start with 75% of requirements in severe cases
  - <7 y, 80–100 kcal/kg per day
  - 70–10 y, 75 kcal/kg per day
  - 11–14 y, 60 kcal/kg per day
  - 15–18 y, 50 kcal/kg per day.
- If tolerated, initial intakes may be increased over 3–5 days; use frequent small feeds with an energy density of 1 kcal/mL to minimize fluid load.
- Protein intake of 0.6–1 g/kg per day, increasing to 1.2–1.5 g/kg per day.
- Supplements: Na^+ 1 mmol/kg per day, K^+ 4 mmol/kg per day, Mg^{2+} 0.6 mmol/kg per day, phosphate up to 1 mmol/kg per day intravenously and up to 100 mmol orally for children over 5 years of age; monitor for hypocalcaemia.
- Thiamine, riboflavin folic acid, ascorbic acid, pyridoxine, and fat-soluble vitamins should be supplemented; trace elements may also be deficient.

References and resources

Afzal NA, Addai S, Fagbemi A, Murch S, Thomson M, Heuschkel R. Refeeding syndrome with enteral nutrition in children; a case report, literature review and clinical guidelines. *Clin Nutr* 2002;**21**:515–520

Kraft MD, Btaiche IF, Sacks GS. Review of the refeeding syndrome. *Nutr Clin Pract* 2005;**20**: 625–633

Parenteral nutrition

Parenteral nutrition (PN) is the supply of nutrients directly into a vein. The first case report of successful long-term PN (in an infant with small-bowel atresia) was published in 1968; since that time products for PN have been developed and refined with the result that metabolic complications are less common, and use in clinical practice has become widespread. For children with short-bowel syndrome, protracted diarrhoea, or pseudo-obstruction PN has become a life-saving intervention. Although it is also widely used in the premature infant with immaturity of gastrointestinal function, the benefit in these patients is less well defined. This is reflected by wide variation in the approach to PN support on different neonatal units. The main indication for PN is when nutritional status cannot be maintained or restored to normal using enteral feeding.

Comprehensive evidence-based guidelines on parenteral nutrition (the ESPGHAN guidelines) were published in November 2005 by the European Society of Paediatric Gastroenterology, Hepatology and Nutrition (ESPGHAN) and the European Society for Clinical Nutrition and Metabolism (ESPEN), supported by the European Society of Paediatric Research (ESPR); see References and resources, p. 96.

- PN fluids contain dextrose solution, synthetic crystalline amino acids, fat emulsion (usually derived from soya bean oil, but sometimes including olive oil in addition), electrolytes, minerals, vitamins, and trace elements.
- Details of regimens appropriate for different age groups are readily available (e.g. see ESPGHAN guidelines).
- PN fluids are usually hyperosmolar and cause phlebitis as well as tissue injury if extravasation occurs. For long-term use administration is usually via a central venous catheter (CVC) inserted surgically and with the tip just outside the right atrium.
- For children needing long term PN (>1 month), fluids are usually administered on a cyclical basis, with infusion over 12 h during the night; this allows freedom from equipment during the day when the CVC can be 'locked' with heparin, and also helps avoid hepatic complications.
- For children expected to be dependent on PN for many months, home care is a possibility. This is organized in conjunction with commercial home care companies who provide equipment and regular supplies including the PN fluids, made up according to the hospital prescription.
- PN is generally safe in that sudden unexpected serious metabolic disturbance is rare; however, blood must be monitored regularly.
- Pharmacists play a key role in ensuring the safety and efficacy of PN, and organization both in hospital and at home is best under the supervision of a multidisciplinary nutritional care team including gastroenterologist, pharmacist, dietitian and nutrition nurse specialist (see Chapter 8).
- Surgical expertise is essential for maintaining long-term venous access and minimizing risks associated with CVC insertion.
- The principal unsolved problems associated with PN are CVC-related blood stream infection (CRBSI), and intestinal failure associated liver disease (IFALD), both of which are life threatening.
- Prevention of CRBSI relies principally on accessing the CVC as little as possible, and scrupulous aseptic technique.
- Mechanical CVC-related problems such as blockage and fracture are also relatively common, and may sometimes be resolved without removal of the catheter.

Indications for parenteral nutrition

- The decision to commence PN will be based on an assessment of nutritional reserve, and the nature of the underlying illness; in tiny premature infants death from starvation may occur in under a week, and nutritional support is an urgent necessity; in a much older child with a postoperative ileus, PN may be unnecessary.
- The principle indication for PN is 'intestinal failure' (see Chapter 13), i.e. normal growth, nutritional status, and homoeostasis cannot be maintained using enteral nutrition.
- The most common causes of intestinal failure are extreme prematurity with immaturity of gastrointestinal motor function; necrotizing enterocolitis (see Chapter 5); short-bowel syndrome (e.g. ileal atresia, neonatal volvulus, extensive bowel resection for NEC); chronic intestinal pseudo-obstruction; severe, persistent diarrhoea (e.g. congenital enteropathy; immunodeficiency).

Parenteral nutrition regimens

- Suggested regimens at different ages are summarized in Tables 12.1 and 12.2 (taken from the ESPGHAN guidelines). Carbohydrate intake is usually built up gradually over the first few days in order to avoid glucose intolerance. Traditionally, nitrogen and lipid intakes have also been increased in a stepwise manner, although there seems to be no strong justification for this approach.

Table 12.1 Parenteral nutrition regimens

Age group	Water (mL/kg)	Energy (kcal/kg)	Amino acid (g/kg)	Glucose (g/kg)	Lipid (g/kg)	Na$^+$ (mmol/kg)	K$^+$ (mmol/kg)	Ca^{2+} (mmol/kg)	PO$_4{}^{2-}$ (mmol/kg)
Preterm	140–160	110–120	1.5–4	10–18	3–4	3–5	2–5	1.3–3	1–2.3
Newborn (first month)	140–160	90–100	1.5–3	8–18	3–4	2–3	1.5–3	1.3–3	0.5
1m–1 y	120–150	90–100	1–2.5	8–18	3–4	2–3	1–3	<6 m 0.8>6 m 0.5	<6 m 0.8>6 m 0.5
1–2 y	80–120	75–90	1–2	6–14	1–3	1–3	1–3	0.2	0.2
3–6 y	80–100	75–90	1–2	4–12	1–3	1–3	1–3	0.2	0.2
7–12 y	60–80	60–75	1–2	4–10	1–3	1–3	1–3	0.2	0.2
13–18 y	50–70	30–60	1–2	3–8	1–3	1–3	1–3	0.2	0.2

Table 12.2 Example of a parenteral nutrition regimen for a 12 kg infant (values given per kg body weight per day)

Day	Fluid (mL)	Amino acids (g)	Carbohydrate (g)	Lipid (g)	Na$^+$ (mmol)	K$^+$ (mmol)	Ca^{2+} (mmol)	PO$_4{}^{2-}$ (mmol)	Peditrace (mL)	Solivito (mL)	Vitlipid N infant (mL)
1	90	1	6	1.5	3	2.5	0.2	0.2	1	1	4
2	90	2	8	1.5	3	2.5	0.2	0.2	1	1	4
3	90	2	10	2	3	2.5	0.2	0.2	1	1	4
4	90	2	12	2	3	2.5	0.2	0.2	1	1	4

Parenteral nutrition products

A variety of PN products are available, as indicated in Tables 12.3 and 12.4. Further information is available in the *British National Formulary for Children.*

Table 12.3 Parenteral nutrition products

Preparation	N (g/L)	Energy[a] (kJ/L)	K+ (mmol/L)	Mg2+ (mmol/L)	Na+ (mmol/L)	Acetate (mmol/L)	Cl- (mmol/L)	Other components (L-1)
Clinoleic® (Baxter)		8360						Olive oil and soya oil 200 g, glycerol 22.5 g, egg phosphatides 12 g
Glamin® (Fresenius Kabi)	22.4					62		
Intralipid 10% (Fresenius Kabi)		4600						Soya oil 100 g, glycerol 22 g, egg phospholipids 12 g, phosphate 15 mmol
Intralipid 20% (Fresenius Kabi)		8400						Soya oil 200 g, glycerol 22 g, egg phospholipids 12 g, phosphate 15 mmol
Intralipid 30% (Fresenius Kabi)		12600						Soya oil 300 g, glycerol 16.7 g, egg phospholipids 12 g, phosphate 15 mmol
Ivelip 10% (Baxter)		4600						Soya oil, glycerol 25 g
Ivelip 20% (Baxter)		8400						Soya oil, glycerol 25 g
Lipofundin MCT/LCT 10%® (Braun)		4430						Soya oil 50 g, medium chain triglyceride 5 g
Lipofundin MCT/LCT 20%® (Braun)		8000						Soya oil 100 g, medium chain triglyceride 100 g
Lipofundin N 10%® (Braun)		4470						Soya oil 100 g, glycerol 25 g, egg lecithin 8 g
Lipofundin N 20%® (Braun)		8520						Soya oil 200 g, glycerol 25 g, egg lecithin 12 g

Primene 10%® (Baxter)[b]	15								
Synthamin 9® (Baxter)	9.1	60	5	70	100			19	70	Acid phosphate 30 mmol
Synthamin 9 EF® (electrolyte free) (Baxter	9.1				44			22	
Vamin 9® (Fresenius Kabi)	9.4	20	1.5	50				50	Ca2+ 2.5 mmol,
Vamin 9 Glucose® (Fresenius Kabi)	9.4	1700	20	1.5	50			50	Ca2+ 2.5 mmol, anhydrous glucose 100 g
Vaminolact® (Fresenius Kabi)	9.3								

[a] Excludes protein or amino acid derived energy. NB, 1000 kcal = 4200 kJ, 1000 kJ = 238.8 kcal.

[b] For use in newborns and children only.

Table 12.4 Other preparations used in parenteral nutrition

Addiphos® (Fresenius Kabi)	Solution: phosphate 40 mmol, K^+ 30mmol, Na^+ 30mmol/20mL
Additrace® (Fresenius Kabi)	Solution: trace elements for addition to Vamin® solutions and intravenous infusions, traces of Fe^{3+}, Zn^{2+}, Mn^{2+}, Cu^{2+}, Cr^{3+}, Se^{4+}, Mo^{6+}, F^-, I^-. For children over 40 kg
Cernevit® (Baxter)	Solution : dl-α-tocopherol 11.2 units, ascorbic acid 125 mg, biotin 69 micrograms, colecalciferol 220 units, cyanocobalamin 6 micrograms, folic acid 414 micrograms, glycine 250 mg, nicotinamide 46 mg, pantothenic acid (as dexpanthenol) 17.25 mg, pyridoxine hydrochloride 5.5 mg, retinol (as palmitate) 3500 units, riboflavin (as dihdrated sodium phosphate) 4.14 mg, thiamine (as cocarboxylase tetrahydrate) 3.51 mg. Dissolve in 5 mL water for injection
Decan® (Baxter)	Solution: trace elements for addition to infusion solutions, Fe^{2+}, Zn^{2+}, Mn^{2+}, Cu^{2+}, Co^{2+}, Cr^{3+}, Se^{4+}, Mo^{6+}, F^-, I^-. For children>40 kg
Dipeptiven® (Fresenius Kabit)	Solution: N(2)-L-alanyl-L-glutamine 200mg/mL (providing L-alanine 82 mg and L-glutamine 134.6 mg.) For addition to infusion solutions containing amino acids
Glycophos Sterile Concentrate® (Fresenius Kabi)	Solution: phosphate 20 mmol, Na+ 40 mmol/20 mL. For addition to Vamin® and Vaminolact® solutions, and glucose intravenous infusions
Peditrace® (Fresenius Kabi)	Solution: trace elements for addition to Vamin® and Vaminolact® traces of Zn^{2+}, Mn^{2+}, Cu^{2+}, Se^{4+}, F^-, I^- for newborns, infants, and children
Solivito N® (Fresenius Kabi)	Solution: powder for reconstitution, biotin 60 micrograms, cyanocobalamin 5 micrograms, folic acid 400 micrograms, glycine 300 mg, nicotinamide 40 mg, pyridoxine hydrochloride 4.9 mg, riboflavin sodium phosphate 4.9 mg, sodium ascorbate 113 mg, sodium pantothenate 16.5 mg, thiamine mononitrate 3.1 mg
Vitlipid N® (Fresenius Kabi)	Emulsion, adult: vitamin A 330 units, ergocalciferol 20 units, dl-α-tocopherol 1 unit, phytomenadione 15 micrograms/mL. For addition to Intralipid; for children >11 years. Emulsion, infant: vitamin A 230 units, ergocalciferol 40 unit, dl-α-tocopherol 0.7 units, phytomenadione 20 micrograms/mL. For addition to Intralipid®

Monitoring of parenteral nutrition

Serious and unexpected biochemical side effects of PN are uncommon, although particular care must be taken with children who are poorly nourished and may be at risk of refeeding syndrome. Table 12.5 provides a suggested schema for monitoring (see also Chapter 11).

Table 12.5. Suggested monitoring protocol during PN in clinically stable patients

	Before PN	Daily	Twice weekly	Once weekly	Monthly	Six monthly
Plasma						
Na	■		■			
K	■		■			
Bilirubin	■			■		
Ca				■		
PO$_4$	■			■		
Alk phos				■		
Glucose		■ week 1		■		
Cu, Zn, Se, Mn					■	
Cholesterol triglyceride			if fat >3 g			■
Full blood count; ferritin; PT/PTT						■
Al, Cr						■
Folate; Vitamins A, E, D						■
Urine						
Na	■					
K	■					
Glucose		■				
Other						
CXR						■
ECG						■
Cardiac echo						■

Complications and their management

Diagnosis and management of catheter-related bloodstream infections (CRBSI)

One of the most common unsolved problems associated with PN is CVC infection, and a high index of suspicion is required at all times. Minimizing risk is crucial and based upon faultless sterile technique being employed at all times by those carers who access the infusion system.

- Suspect in any child with indwelling CVC who develops fever/signs of sepsis.
- Additional features may include hyperglycaemia, diarrhoea, vomiting.
- Exclude tunnel/exit site, wound, urine, respiratory infection, and meningitis.
- Take 'through CVC' and/or peripheral blood samples for microbial culture.
- Start antibiotic treatment through the CVC as soon as possible if temperature >38.5 °C or other strong indication of sepsis.
- First line antibiotics should provide broad-spectrum cover against likely organisms (e.g. vancomycin and ceftazidime).
- Discuss treatment with microbiologist.
- Bear in mind possibility of yeast infection if no clinical response within 48 h (send blood cultures direct to mycology laboratory; ophthalmic examination).
- Consider using antibiotic 'lock' once sensitivities known (fill the CVC with antibiotic at a concentration of 1–5 mg/mL, mixed with 50–100 U heparin or normal saline, and leave in place when CVC not being used for PN).
- Usually treat for 10–14 days.
- Remove CVC if overwhelming sepsis (unless little prospect of alternative venous access for giving essential drugs); yeast isolated; continuing positive blood cultures despite appropriate antibiotics; septic embolism.

Occlusion of the CVC is another common problem complicating long-term PN. For prevention and management of partial or complete CVC occlusion:

- Use a suitable infusion pump for PN, with appropriate alarm settings.
- For flow rates <20 mL/h, pressure should be set at 30–40 mm Hg greater than the resting pressure.
- For flow rate ≥20 mL/h, infusion pumps may be used with occlusion alarms at 100 mm Hg.
- The infusion pressure should be recorded 4 hourly.
- A trend of increasing pressure measurements indicates developing occlusion; early intervention at this point may prevent complete blockage.

If the pump alarms repeatedly:
- Are the clamps open?
- Are there kinks or twists in the tubing?
- Is the flow rate too high for the catheter being used?

If none of these apply:
- Flush the CVC with saline/heparln sodium (10 units/mL) using an aseptic technique
- If the CVC resists flushing, an unblocking agent is required (see below).

When attempting to unblock a CVC
- Use a small syringe (delivers greater pressure).
- Start with a 5 mL syringe, and work down to 2 mL, then 1 mL.
- NB: Excessive force may rupture the CVC.
- Repeated gentle 'pull and push' on the syringe may clear the obstruction.
- If required, use the treatments below in turn until occlusion is cleared (the CVC lumen is filled with the solution and aspiration/flushing attempted after a short period of time).

Urokinase lock
- Add 1 mL of water for injection (WFI) to a vial of 25 000 units of urokinase:
  - child <1 yr, take 0.1 mL (2500 units) and make up to 1 mL with WFI; instil 1 mL into CVC
  - child >1 yr, take 0.2 mL (5000 units) and make up to 2 mL with WFI; instil 2 mL into CVC.
- Leave for 2 h, then aspirate and flush with 0.9% sodium chloride.

Alcohol lock
- Use absolute alcohol injection:
  - child <1 year, instil 1 mL into CVC
  - child >1 year, instil 2 mL into CVC
- Leave for 2 hours, then aspirate and flush with 0.9% sodium chloride.
- If the CVC is beginning to clear, repeat urokinase/alcohol before moving on to:

Hydrochloric acid lock
- Use 1 M hydrochloric acid:
  - child <1 yr, instil 1 mL into CVC
  - child >1 yr, instil 2 mL into CVC
- Leave for 20 min, then aspirate and flush with 0.9% sodium chloride.

Urokinase infusion
- Use only for patients with normal coagulation and platelets.
- Not suitable for a CVC that is completely blocked to manual flush.
- Make a 200 units/mL solution of urokinase in dextrose 5%.
- Infuse at 1 mL/kg/h for 6 h.

An important metabolic complication of prolonged PN is cholestasis, or intestinal failure associated liver disease (IFALD). In some cases this may progress to cirrhosis and liver failure, and is one of the main indications for liver and small-bowel transplantation. Important risk factors include:
- Premature delivery (immature hepatic function and reduced circulating bile salt pool)
- Recurrent sepsis
- Inability to tolerate enteral feed (very short bowel; severe dysmotility).

Management of **IFALD**
- Maximize enteral nutrient intake (e.g. overnight tube feed)
- Minimize risks of CRBSI through scrupulous aseptic technique
- Cyclical PN
- Ursodeoxycholic acid 10 mg/kg t.d.s. (given enterally)

- Trial of reduced intravenous fat intake (restrict to 1 g/kg/day)
- Empirical change to different lipid emulsion
- Consider trial of ceruletide (cholecystokin analogue)
- Treatment of small-bowel overgrowth.

References and resources

British National Formulary for Children: http://bnfc.org/bnfc/bnfc/current/129132.htm

Koletzko B; Goulet O; Hunt J et al. Guidelines on paediatric parenteral nutrition of the European Society of Paediatric Gastroenterology, Hepatology and Nutrition (ESPGHAN) and the European Society for Clinical Nutrition and Metabolism (ESPEN), supported by the European Society of Paediatric Research (ESPR). *J Pediatr Gastroenterol Nutr* 2005;**41** Suppl 2:S1–S4. www.jpgn.org. Select 'archive', and then November, Volume 41, Supplement 2.

Intestinal failure

The term intestinal failure (IF) refers to a functionally impaired gastrointestinal tract unable to maintain biochemical homeostasis and support normal growth. Short-bowel syndrome (SBS) is a common cause of IF and usually defined as a severe reduction in functional gut mass below the minimal amount necessary for digestion and absorption adequate to satisfy the nutrient and fluid requirements for growth. Other causes of IF include mucosal abnormalities giving rise to protracted diarrhoea, and neuromuscular disorders resulting in chronic idiopathic intestinal pseudo-obstruction syndrome (CIIPS). See Table 13.1.

Short-bowel syndrome

This refers to the physiological consequences of having insufficient small intestine to allow adequate absorption of fluids, electrolytes, and nutrients. Patients fall into two main groups: those with congenital bowel anomalies and those with an anatomically normal bowel who come to require resection of diseased gut.

Causes
These include:
- Congenital atresia of small bowel
- Gastroschisis with associated atresia, or bowel infarction (typically territory of superior mesenteric artery: from proximal small bowel to splenic flexure in colon)
- Malrotation with volvulus (may present with yellow or green vomit in the newborn period; symptoms may be intermittent)
- Necrotizing enterocolitis (usually in the preterm infant)
- Crohn's disease with resection.

The small bowel measures ~250 cm at birth and by adulthood has increased to 3–8 m. Nutritional consequences are likely to follow loss of >50% of small bowel. After massive gut resection there is a process of adaptation, ultimately resulting in an increased absorptive capacity, such that many children are dependent on parenteral nutrition (PN) for a time (sometimes years) but eventually manage to make the transition to full enteral feeding. Favourable factors for intestinal adaptation include >15 cm residual small bowel, presence of the ileocaecal valve, and preservation of the colon.

Adaptation involves mucosal hyperplasia, increasing surface area fourfold. Enteral nutrition is essential for this process, and should be given to the maximum tolerated without provoking severe diarrhoea. Intraluminal nutrition stimulates hyperplasia through contact of epithelial cells with nutrients, stimulation of secretion of trophic gastrointestinal hormones and upper gastrointestinal secretions. The process of adaptation can go on over a number of years. Failure to achieve full enteral feeding after 5 years of PN suggests there will be lifelong dependency on PN (but this is not invariable).

Management aims

These include:

- Maintenance of normal growth
- Use of oral/enteral nutrition rather than PN when gastrointestinal function allows
- Minimizing risk of complications of gut failure and nutritional support
- Optimizing quality of life.

Management should be by a multidisciplinary nutritional care team in a unit experienced in caring for such patients, and

- Is a multi-stage process, beginning with PN
- Starts with correction of fluid and electrolyte abnormalities
- Followed with cautious enteral feeding (1 mL/kg/h in newborn) with breast milk if available, or with hydrolysed protein/lactose-free feed
- Followed by slow increase in volume of continuous enteral feeding unless unacceptably high stool losses (i.e. >20 mL/kg/day from stoma)
- Moves towards cyclical PN, initially by having 1 h/day off PN and slowly increasing time as tolerated to 12 h on/12 h off (monitor for hypoglycaemia as time off PN is extended)
- May involve consideration of home PN in those patients in whom dependency is anticipated for >4 months (e.g. <30 cm small bowel in newborn).

Excessive diarrhoea

- More likely in children with jejunostomy; ingestion of water and hypotonic fluids dilutes luminal contents and exacerbates fluid losses because jejunal sodium concentration needs to be kept ~90 mmol/L; if this is diluted, sodium will diffuse into the lumen taking water with it.
- Gastric acid hypersecretion may occur for 3–6 months after resection due to lack of inhibitory hormones from intestine; high-dose H_2 receptor antagonist or proton pump inhibitors may be needed.
- Antimotility agents such as loperamide (up to 0.2 mg/kg q.d.s.) or codeine (1 mg/kg q.d.s.) may be helpful.
- Consider other causes (sepsis, partial/intermittent bowel obstruction, enteritis, residual bowel disease, drugs, bacterial overgrowth).

Colon present

- Ability to absorb fluid, making salt, water, and magnesium deficit less likely.
- Presence of ileocaecal valve slows small-bowel transit time and decreases risk of small-bowel bacterial overgrowth.
- Renal oxalate stones potential problem, since calcium in gut binds to unabsorbed fat rather than dietary oxalate as normal, allowing unbound oxalate to be absorbed, and excreted in urine; advise low-oxalate diet (i.e. avoid tea, rhubarb, spinach, beetroot, peanuts).

Other complications

- Intestinal failure associated liver disease (IFALD)
- PN-related (e.g. catheter-related bloodstream infection)
- Gallstones (disordered enterohepatic bile salt circulation)
- Vitamin B_{12} deficiency (loss of terminal ileum; may take years to develop)
- Fat-soluble vitamin deficiencies
- Thiamine deficiency (Wernicke/Korsikoff psychosis)
- D(-) lactic acidosis (from bacterial fermentation of dietary carbohydrate, causing confusion, ataxia, dysarthria, etc.).

Surgical interventions

- Aim to maximize mucosal contact with enteral nutrients without disturbing motility or reducing total absorptive surface area.
- Strictures should be removed and where possible, stomas closed.
- Intestinal tapering or plication are sometimes used to improve motility and in turn, absorption; bowel lengthening procedures are also used; these including the Bianchi procedure (longitudinal division of the bowel along its mesenteric and anti-mesenteric border), and more recently the serial transverse enteroplasty procedure (STEP).
- The precise indications and potential benefits of tapering, plication, and lengthening remain poorly defined.

Motility disorders

Chronic idiopathic intestinal pseudo-obstruction (CIIPS) is a heterogenous group of rare disorders, presenting with signs and symptoms of intestinal obstruction in the absence of an identifiable mechanical obstruction.

- Most cases present in infancy.
- There may be abnormalities in the enteric nervous system or gut musculature ('neuropathic' or 'myopathic').
- Sometimes other hollow viscera such as the bladder are involved.
- Hirschprung's disease and fabricated illness should always be considered as possible diagnoses.
- Manometric studies and full-thickness bowel biopsy may be necessary to fully clarify the diagnosis.
- Death or dependence on PN is more likely when the small bowel is short, and when there is malrotation, urinary tract involvement, or myopathic histology.

Mucosal disorders

These present in early life with severe diarrhoea (see Chapter 32) and include microvillus inclusion disease, tufting enteropathy, and glycosylation disorders. Most of these children require long term parenteral nutrition and ultimately need small-bowel transplantation.

Small-bowel transplantation

Indications are essentially life-threatening complications of PN, including:
- Liver failure from IFALD (small bowel and liver transplantation, or isolated liver)
- Venous thrombosis/occlusion jeopardizing continued venous access
- Recurrent overwhelming catheter-related bloodstream infection.

Relative contraindications include:
- Severe congenital or acquired immunological deficiencies
- Multisystem autoimmune disease
- Insufficient vascular patency to guarantee vascular access for up to 6 months after transplant
- Chronic lung disease of prematurity.

References and resources

Goulet O, Ruemmele F, Lacaille GF, Colomb V. Irreversible intestinal failure. *J Pediatr Gastroent Nutr* 2004;**38**:250–269

Gupte GL, Beath SV, Kelly DA, Millar AJW, Booth IW. Current issues in the management of intestinal failure. *Arch Dis Child* 2006;**91**: 259–264

Heneyke S, Smith VV, Spitz L, Milla PJ. Chronic intestinal pseudo-obstruction: treatment and long term follow up of 44 patients. *Arch Dis Child* 1999;**81**:21–27

Nightingale J, Woodward JM, on behalf of the Small Bowel and Nutrition Committee of the British Society of Gastroenterology. Guidelines for management of patients with short bowel. *Gut* 2006;**55** Suppl IV;iv1–iv12

Table 13.1 Causes of intestinal failure

Category	Disorder
Short-bowel syndrome	**Neonatal period**
	Gastroschisis
	Necrotizing enterocolitis
	Small bowel atresia
	Malrotation with volvulus
	Total aganglionosis
	Older children
	Crohn's disease
	Mesenteric infarction
	Radiation enteritis
	Tumours
	Trauma
Motility disorders	Hollow visceral myopathy
	Neuronal intestinal dysplasia
	Megacystis-microcolon-hypoperistalsis syndrome
	Abnormalities of interstitial cells of Cajal
Mucosal disorders	**Primary epithelial abnormalities**
	Microvillus inclusion disease
	Tufting enteropathy
	Congenital disorders of glycosylation
	Immune mediated
	Underlying immune deficiency states (e.g. severe combined immunodeficiency, pan-hypogammaglobulinaemia)
	Autoimmune enteropathy Syndromic intractable diarrhoea

Home nutritional support

Home enteral tube feeding (HETF)

Equipment supply is usually arranged through a home care company. Good communication between patient, family, and healthcare professionals is a prerequisite for effective discharge planning. The needs of the child and family must be clearly identified in order to prepare transfer from hospital to home. It is also essential that continuing care arrangements are in place with coordinated action from all involved (family, healthcare professionals, social services, education, voluntary bodies, etc.).

The aims of home nutritional support are to:
- Facilitate effective nutritional support.
- Facilitate patient and family autonomy, taking into account (for enteral feeding) their preference for route of feeding and care plan.
- Ensure safe and trouble free maintenance of nutritional support.
- Maximize potential for improved lifestyle as well as optimizing disease management.

Teaching in preparation for HETF

The following topics should be covered
- Information about the reasons for HETF and likely duration
- Safety aspects of care
- Checking tube placement
- Infection control issues
- Hand-washing techniques
- Feed preparation (use ready-made feeds whenever possible)
- Familiarity with feeding equipment
- Advice regarding social and practical implications for child and family
- Problem-solving advice and what to do in an emergency
- The importance to feeding of oral stimulation
- Telephone contacts of hospital and community staff
- Detailed information about how to obtain equipment and supplies.

Choice of feeding pump

Attributes
- Easy to operate
- Durable
- Small/lightweight/portable
- Accurate
- Option bolus feeding available
- Easy to clean
- Easy to set up
- Tamper proof
- Low noise level
- Alarm: occlusion/empty and low battery
- Excellent reliability

Teaching material
- Step-by-step guide to setting up
- Written instruction on side of pump and in pamphlet form
- Training video

Purchasing
- Identify servicing arrangements
- Information available from Medical Devices Agency
- Competitive cost.

Home parenteral nutrition (HPN)

HPN is usually considered when it can be anticipated that full enteral feeding is not likely to be established for at least 4 months. Clinical stability and severity of the underlying illness must be taken into account. When possible, PN is infused for 12 h overnight and the central venous catheter (CVC) 'locked' with heparin saline in the day. Cyclical PN may be helpful in preventing liver complications as well as freeing the child from the infusion pump in the day. Parents or carers need to be highly motivated and well trained, and to have adequate housing. Periodic re-admission to hospital with fever, CVC sepsis, or blocked catheter is common.

Teaching in preparation for HPN

The following topics should be covered:
- The child's underlying diagnosis and prognosis
- Placement and function of CVC
- Potential complications (e.g. infection, embolism, cholestasis)
- General overview of nutrients
- How to set up PN infusions
- How to adjust flow rates
- Maintenance and problem solving re infusion pumps
- Aseptic technique
- Emergency management of CVC: air, blockage, infection, rupture
- Management of hypoglycaemia
- Monitoring urine and blood glucose
- Understanding social implications of therapy
- Emergency contact numbers
- Support group contacts.

Parent-held records

Parents/carers should have an up-to-date set of health records for any health professionals they might encounter at different times who are unfamiliar with their child's care. These should include:
- Medical summary of condition
- CVC history
- CVC care protocols
- Feed prescription information
- Techniques for heparinizing CVC
- Unblocking a CVC
- Treatment of suspected sepsis
- How to respond to emergency situations
- List of hospital and community contacts
- Growth charts
- Record of biochemical monitoring.

References and resources

Holden C, Johnson T, Caney D. Nutritional support for children in the community. In: Holden C, MacDonald A (eds). *Nutrition and child health*, Baillière Tindall, Edinburgh, 2000, pp. 177–222

Mahgoub LEO, Puntis JWL. Longterm parenteral nutrition. *Curr Paediatr* 2006;**16**:298–304

Eating disorders

Eating disorders are defined as persistent disturbance of eating (± behaviour) that impairs physical health or psychosocial functioning or both and that is not secondary to any other medical or psychiatric disorder.

Anorexia nervosa

Anorexia nervosa is a complex disorder described in a number of different ways and recognized for >100 years. It involves voluntary self-starvation, with weight loss, or avoidance of weight gain during adolescence. Peak age of onset is in mid-teens, with a female to male ratio of 10:1, and a prevalence of around 1%. Genetic factors are important, with 55% of monozygotic twins being concordant for anorexia. Sociocultural factors are highly relevant, with the illness occurring predominantly in Western societies where thinness has become increasingly valued as an element of the feminine ideal. Reported mortality rates vary from 0 to 22%.

Diagnosis is based on the following features:
- Low weight; <85% expected weight for height (or BMI <17.5 kg/m^2), due to weight loss or failure to gain weight during the adolescent period.
- Due to deliberate dietary restriction, sometimes associated with use of appetite suppressants, self-induced vomiting, laxative abuse, excessive exercise.
- Associated with intense fear of fatness, and feeling fat even when underweight.
- Resulting in amenorrhoea in females past menarche, pubertal delay in early-onset cases, and loss of sexual interest in males.

Additional features
- Amenorrhoea (with long term risk of severe osteoporosis if >6 months)
- Hyperactivity
- Feeling asexual
- Binge eating
- Preoccupation with appearance and body
- Distorted body image
- Low self-esteem
- Denial of illness
- Misjudgement of food requirements
- Obsessional behaviour
- Rigid thought patterns
- Perfectionist
- Eating rituals
- Hypotension
- Bradycardia
- Cyanosis of extremities
- Increased growth of fine hair (lanugo).

Biochemical features

- Deficiency of Gonadotrophin Releasing Hormone (GnRH), low luteinizing hormone (LH) and follicle-stimulating hormone (FSH), normal prolactin, low oestrogen in females and testosterone in males
- Elevated plasma cortisol
- Low normal thyroxine, reduced T_3, and normal thyroid-stimulating hormone (TSH)
- Elevated resting plasma growth hormone (GH)
- Hypokalaemia, hyponatraemia, low magnesium, phosphorus, zinc, and copper are common.

Management

- Severe weight loss (<80% weight for height), severe depression, circulatory failure, dehydration, severe electrolyte disturbance warrant admission to hospital.
- Usually to psychiatric unit, but initially may be to paediatric ward under joint supervision of paediatrician and psychiatrist.
- Re-feeding programme involving correction of dehydration, electrolyte abnormality and nutritional deficiencies with gradual restoration of weight.
- Family therapy.
- Individual psychotherapy.

Occasionally severe weight loss gives rise to duodenal compression causing persistent vomiting: the superior mesenteric artery syndrome. Radiologically there is dilatation of the proximal duodenum and narrowing of the third part of the duodenum, apparently by the superior mesenteric artery. Weight gain may be followed by resolution of this problem; transpyloric tube feeding or even parenteral nutrition may be required.

Bulimia nervosa

Bulimia is an eating disorder characterized by binge eating followed by food elimination (purging) and an over-concern with weight and body shape. Large quantities (e.g. 10 000 kcal) of 'comfort' foods such as ice cream and cakes may be consumed in a few hours. During a binge, individuals feel unable to control their eating; they then focus on getting rid of the food eaten. This is usually by self induced vomiting, but may involve laxatives, diet pills, and vigorous exercise. The patients fear gaining weight and have often tried dieting with limited success. Most are of normal weight. The prevalence is estimated at around 1 in 10 000, but may rise to 1–2% among young females.

Clinical signs include hypertrophy of the salivary glands, skin changes on the dorsum of the hand used to stimulate the gag reflex, and erosion of teeth enamel. Sore throat, abdominal pain, oesophagitis, and electrolyte disturbance also sometimes occur.

Management

• Involves psychotherapy and occasionally hospitalization
• Roughly 1/3 to 1/2 of patients tend to recover or greatly improve within 1–3 years of seeking treatment.

Case study

A 16 year old girl was referred to the eating disorders clinic because of anorexia. She displayed many features of anorexia nervosa, but by hiding weights in her dressing gown at outpatient review managed to conceal the true extent of her condition. She was admitted to hospital after becoming drowsy and developing bilious vomiting; admission weight was only 22 kg (BMI 13). Radiological findings were consistent with a superior mesenteric artery syndrome (compression of the duodenum just to the right of the midline). Attempts at nasojejunal feeding were unsuccessful due to vomiting back of the tube. She was parenterally fed, initially to actual weight with a cautious increase in energy intake over a number of weeks and close monitoring of serum biochemistry (particularly potassium and phosphate). A multivitamin supplement including thiamine was given prior to nutritional intervention in case her altered conscious level was symptomatic of deficiency; she needed additional supplementation with sodium, potassium, phosphate, zinc, and magnesium. As her weight increased, vomiting ceased and from 40 kg, enteral tube feeding was re-established and PN discontinued. She required 24 h 'one to one' nursing to prevent removal of CVC and NG tube. While she was on the acute paediatric ward, medical and psychiatric teams liaised closely on a daily basis. Subsequently she was transferred to an inpatient psychiatric unit and made a full recovery, returning to school a year after admission.

References and resources

Wadge M, Hodgkinson P. Disordered eating behaviours and therapeutic interventions. In: Holden C, MacDonald A (eds). *Nutrition and child health*, Baillière Tindall, London, 2000, pp. 121–142

Difficult eating behaviour in the young child

Food refusal is common in early life. During the first year infants will try food because they are hungry, or because they are using their mouths to explore the environment. Later on, there has to be motivation to try new foods, and this usually comes from imitation of other people eating. In early childhood it is the presentation of safe and socially appropriate foods and their repeated ingestion that leads to them being liked.

Children may refuse food because of:
- Lack of appetite
- Lack of experience at certain developmental stages
- Poor oromotor skills
- Onset of the neophobic response in the second year (a 'biologically protective' dislike of new foods)
- Distaste or disgust at some foods
- Individual differences in food acceptance
- Parental anxiety and forced feeding.

Appetite

- From ~6 weeks of age infants regulate energy intake in accordance with energy needs
- Well toddlers will take the amount of energy they need for normal growth
- Children get hungry at the time they usually eat a meal, for the energy load they would usually eat
- From around 5 years, food intake is modified by social rules, e.g., 'clearing the plate', eating as a social or comfort activity.

Development

- At birth there is a preference for sweet-tasting food (sweet = biologically safe).
- At 3–5 months, ready acceptance of new tastes based on taste and smell; lack of experience at this stage may mean limited range of tastes accepted.
- At 6–12 months, start of self feeding with more solid foods; lack of experience at this stage may lead to poor acceptance of different textures.
- At 12–18 months, fear of new foods ('neophobia') develops; local features of food become important (e.g. biscuit must be whole, not broken).
- At 18 months–5 years, neophobic response strengthens, but overcome by imitation of adults and other children.

Modification of eating behaviour

- Move from mash to 'bite and dissolve' foods from 7 months.
- Encourage self-feeding as soon as possible, by the end of the first year.
- Allow the child to be messy at mealtimes and to enjoy eating.
- Putting a disliked food on a plate next to a liked food may lead to rejection of the liked food ('contamination').

- If one food is the reward for eating another, the food first offered is understood to be less nice.
- Repeated exposure to a food is the best way of it becoming accepted.
- Imitation (of adults or other children) also leads to an acceptance of new foods.
- If parents/carers do not eat particular foods, it is unlikely that the child will want to eat them.

The 'picky' child

Simple faddy eating is most likely to occur around 18 months.
- Take notice of satiety signals (e.g. closing mouth, turning away).
- Give frequent small meals.
- Take uneaten food away without comment.
- Give positive attention/encouragement when the child is eating.
- Don't force feed.
- Don't use one food as a reward for eating another.
- Don't give attention for not eating.
- Don't put liked and disliked food on the same plate.
- Don't expect all children to eat as well as each other.

(with grateful acknowledgement to Gill Harris)

Common feeding problems in 1–5 year olds

Problem	Solutions
Food refusal	Structured meal pattern; 3 meals and 2–3 small, nutritious snacks Offer variety of foods, with some favourites Small portions (second helpings if wanted) Do not 'force feed' Family mealtimes Happy, relaxed environment Do not offer sweets/other foods as reward
Excessive milk drinking	Limit milk intake to 500–600 mL/day Give milk after meals or at snack time Give water if thirsty between meals Use cup not bottle Offer milk in small cups
Excessive juice drinking	limit juice to no more than 1 cup/day Give drinks after meals Give plain water if thirsty Encourage milk; limit to 500–600 mL/day
Refuses to drink milk	Offer in small 'fun' cup through straw Add milk or cheese to foods e.g. mashed potato, scrambled egg Include other milk containing foods, e.g. yoghurt, custard, porridge Try flavoured milk or milk shakes
Refuses to eat fruits or vegetables	Try mixing vegetables into other foods such as soups or stews Add grated fruits and vegetables to other foods Include small amount of fruit and vegetable at each mealtime to allow opportunity to try Children learn by example; other family members to eat fruit and vegetables Some children prefer raw rather than cooked vegetables Try fruits cut into small pieces with yoghurt dips Make blended fruit drinks or milk shakes with added fruits

How to increase energy intake

Increasing the nutrient density of food can improve growth rate; some suggestions are listed below.

Weaning foods

- Add infant formula to dried baby foods or home-made puréed foods.
- Include puréed meats, add to vegetables.
- Spread butter or margarine on finger foods.

Normal table foods

- Add whole milk to mashed foods.
- Add extra dried milk powder to whole milk and milk puddings.
- Add oil or butter to mashed or puréed foods.
- Add cream to desserts and porridge.
- Add grated cheese or cream cheese to savoury foods such as mashed potato or scrambled egg.
- Encourage three meals a day and nutritious snacks between meals.

Case study

A 2 year old child was referred to the dietitian because of parental concern regarding eating. As a baby he had been reluctant to feed and had vomited with solids, taking only formula milk until 9 months of age. Subsequently, dry breakfast cereal, toast, crisps, chips, chocolate, orange juice, and certain biscuits were accepted. At mealtimes he would refuse to try any new foods and continued to request warmed milk from a bottle. He began to ask for help with feeding at mealtimes which had become increasingly stressful for the family. Height and weight had dropped from the 25th to the 10th centile, and a dietary assessment indicated that his intakes of energy and iron were sub-optimal. Iron was prescribed together with an energy-dense supplement drink; both were refused by the child. A video recording was made of a family mealtime, with analysis focusing on the interaction between child and carers. Guidance was then given to parents on behavioural modification; they were also encouraged to adopt a consistent approach to feeding and mealtimes.

References and resources

Green C. *New toddler taming*. Vermilion, London, 2006

Hutchinson H. Feeding problems in young children: report of three cases and review of the literature. *J Hum Nutr Diet* 1999;**12**:337–343

Mathisen B, Skuse D, Wolke D, Reilly S. Oral motor dysfunction and failure to thrive amongst inner-city children. *Dev Med Child Neurol* 1989;**31**:293–302

Skuse D. Identification and management of problem eaters. *Arch Dis Child* 1993;**69**:604–608

Food allergy

Food allergy most commonly affects preschool children and is being increasingly recognized. Careful history taking is central to making the diagnosis.

Definitions (World Allergy Organization)

- **Hypersensitivity:** objectively reproducible symptoms or signs initiated by exposure to a defined stimulus at a dose tolerated by normal persons.
- **Intolerance:** abnormal physiological response to an agent, which can be certain foods or additives; not immune mediated.
- **Atopy:** a characteristic that makes one susceptible to develop various allergies; it is defined as a personal and/or familial tendency, usually in childhood or adolescence, to become sensitized and produce IgE antibodies in response to ordinary exposures to allergens, usually proteins; as a consequence, these persons can develop typical symptoms of asthma, rhino-conjunctivitis, or eczema.
- **Allergen:** an antigen causing allergic disease.
- **Allergy:** a hypersensitivity reaction initiated by specific immunological mechanisms. When other mechanisms can be proved, the term **non-allergic hypersensitivity** should be used.

Food allergy is thus a term applied to a group of disorders characterized by an abnormal or exaggerated immunological response to specific food proteins that may be IgE or non-IgE mediated.

- **Psychologically-based food reaction (aversion)** is food avoidance for psychological reasons, or when there is an unpleasant bodily reaction caused by emotions associated with the food (rather than by the food itself); does not occur when the food is given in an unrecognizable form.
- Milk (2.5%), egg (1.3%), peanut (0.8%), tree nuts (0.2%), and fish (0.2%) are among the most prevalent causes of food allergy; soya and wheat allergy are also common.
- Food allergy resolves in most affected children, although peanut allergy may persist; 85% of children with cow's milk allergy in the first 2 years of life are tolerant by the age of 3, and 80% of children with egg allergy by 5 years.
- 20% of children under 2 years with peanut allergy are tolerant by school age; children with peanut specific IgE of 5 kU/L or less have around a 50% chance of losing their allergy.
- Risk of death from fatal allergic reactions to food is around 1 in 800 000 per year, with asthmatic children being at highest risk.

Types of allergic reaction

Reactions to allergens can be mild, moderate, or severe in nature. A mild reaction may involve itchy rash, watering eyes, and nasal congestion.

- Moderate reactions may spread to different parts of the body and include difficulty breathing.
- A severe reaction presents as anaphylaxis.
- IgE-mediated reactions cause symptoms almost immediately after food is ingested, with swelling of the lips and tongue sometimes together with vomiting, diarrhoea, asthma, and rarely anaphylaxis.
- Food dependent, exercise-induced anaphylaxis occurs typically in atopic young adults after vigorous exercise within several hours of eating an implicated food.
- Oral allergy syndrome involves itching, irritation, swelling, and urticaria in or around the mouth after ingestion of fresh fruit or vegetables.
- Non-IgE reactions (e.g. atopic dermatitis, eosinophilic gastroenteropathy, asthma) are mediated by allergen-specific lymphocytes and IgG antibodies.

Diagnosing and managing food allergy

In the history, enquire
- What foods are under suspicion?
- Time between ingestion and reaction?
- Amount of food needed to cause a reaction?
- Frequency and reproducibility of reactions?
- Signs and symptoms?
- Was food raw or cooked?
- Could there have been any cross contamination with other foods?

Skin prick testing with standardized allergen extracts can be positive in the absence of allergy, but are rarely negative in someone with true IgE-mediated allergic reactions. Quantitative measurements of food-specific IgE antibodies have a high predictive value for allergic reactions to certain foods.

Elimination diets and subsequent dietary challenges should be instituted with the help and supervision of a dietitian. Antihistamines and corticosteroids are useful for symptomatic relief of mild to moderate allergies. Adrenaline is used for severe reactions including anaphylaxis.

Cow's milk protein intolerance (CMPI)
- CMPI is the clinical syndrome(s) resulting from sensitization to one or more proteins in cow's milk.
- It frequently resolves spontaneously within the first 2 years of life, and almost always by 5 years of age.
- In most affected children, gastrointestinal symptoms (vomiting, diarrhoea, colic, constipation) develop in the first 6 months of life.

Other presentations include:
- Respiratory: wheeze, rhinitis, asthma
- Dermatological: atopic dermatitis, urticaria, laryngeal oedema
- Behavioural: irritability, crying, milk refusal.

Diagnosis is based mainly upon clinical history:
- Definite disappearance of symptoms after each of two dietary eliminations of cow's milk
- Recurrence of identical symptoms after one challenge
- Exclusion of lactose intolerance and coincidental infection.

Major foods to be excluded in a cow's milk protein free diet
- Cow's milk—all types, including modified (infant formula), skimmed, low fat, whole, dried, condensed and evaporated, buttermilk.
- Butter, ghee, some margarines, and low-fat spreads (check labels).
- Yoghurt, fromage frais, cream, ice cream.
- Cheese, cottage cheese, cream cheese, curds.
- Chocolate and other sweets containing milk solids.
- Check label of manufactured products and avoid 'non-fat milk solids', 'whey', 'casein', 'sodium caseinate', 'lactoglobulin', 'lactalbumin'.
- Goat's or sheep's milk should not be used as substitutes for infant formula as they are no less allergenic than cow's milk, contain a high solute load, and are deficient in vitamins.
- An extensively hydrolysed infant formula may be given as a milk substitute; cow's milk protein allergens are secreted in breast milk, and breast-feeding mothers may need to exclude cow's milk from their diet.
- Although more palatable than hydrolysed feeds, soya milk is not a suitable milk substitute since around 5–10% of infants who react to cow's milk will do so to soya; in addition, soya is not recommended for infants <6 months of age because of theoretical concerns regarding phytoestrogen content.

NB: For children on a cow's milk free diet, care must be taken to provide adequate calcium from other sources, such as cow's milk free formula, soya products fortified with calcium, or calcium supplements.

Food challenges
- Food challenges have a pivotal role in the diagnosis of food allergy.
- Unit protocols should be available for those foods commonly implicated.
- Challenges should be carried out in an appropriately staffed and equipped facility.

Challenges may be performed if:
- There is a history of recent uneventful dietary exposure.
- There is a negative skin prick/RAST test to antigen.
- There has been no severe reaction for at least 2 years (probably delay until teenage years if peanut allergy).
- Parents seek clarification (often pre-school entry) of need for antigen avoidance.
- Original diagnosis was based on dubious history/testing

Cow's milk challenge

This is an example of a protocol for non-blind food challenge of children who have had an allergic reaction to cow's milk in the past.

Proceed as follows at 20 min intervals, abandoning the test at any stage if a reaction is provoked:
- 1 drop of milk on skin
- 1 drop of milk on lips
- 1 drop of milk on tongue
- 5 mL of milk swallowed
- 15 mL of milk swallowed
- 30 mL of milk swallowed
- 45 mL of milk swallowed
- 60 mL of milk swallowed
- 90 mL of milk swallowed
- 120 mL of milk swallowed
- Resume normal diet.

NB: Adrenaline should be available in case of severe reaction.

Pseudo-intolerance/allergy

- Some parents become obsessed with the mistaken belief that their child has food allergy.
- Spurious pseudo-diagnostic techniques such as hair analysis and pulse testing may reinforce such beliefs.
- Unsupervised dietary restriction can lead to nutritional deficiency states and occasionally even to failure to thrive.
- In such cases, child protection issues arise and detailed multidisciplinary assessment is required.

Adrenaline injection

For patients who have had a life-threatening allergic reaction to food, emergency adrenaline treatment should be carried in the form of an EpiPen® or Anapen® Auto-injector 0.3 mg (>30 kg), or EpiPen® Junior/Anapen® Junior 0.15 mg (15–30 kg). Such a provision must, however, be part of an integrated management plan. These devices deliver 0.3 mL/0.3 mg or 0.15 mL/0.15 mg adrenaline intramuscularly. It is important for patients, carers, and doctors to be thoroughly familiar with their use.

In the event of anaphylaxis:

EpiPen®
- Remove the EpiPen® from its packaging.
- Remove the grey safety cap.
- Hold the EpiPen® with the black tip at right angle to the thigh and press hard until the auto-injector mechanism functions (there should be a click); hold in place for 10 seconds.
- Remove the EpiPen® and massage the area for 10 seconds.

Anapen®
- Remove the black needle cap.
- Remove the black safety cap from firing button.
- Hold Anapen® against outer thigh and press red firing button.
- Hold Anapen® in position for 10 seconds.

Note that:
- Pens need replacing periodically (check contents are clear and colourless; check expiry date).
- Demonstrate use with each new prescription (see above).
- Provide a written management protocol to family, carers, school.
- Keep spare pen at school.
- Always carry pen.

References and resources

Baral VR, Hourihane J O'B. Food allergy in children. *Postgrad Med J* 2005;**81**:693–701

Johansson SGO, Bieber T, Dahl R et al. Revised nomenclature for allergy for global use: report of the Nomenclature Review Committee of the World Allergy Organization 2003. *J Allergy Clin Immunol* 2004;**5**:832–6

Vandenplas Y, Brueton M, Dupont C et al. Guidelines for the diagnosis and management of cow's milk protein allergy in infants. *Arch Dis Child* 2007;**92**:902–908

Chapter 18

Carbohydrate intolerance

Carbohydrates in the diet

Carbohydrates make up at least half the energy intake in the diet. The principal carbohydrates are the storage polysaccharides (starch, glycogen and cellulose), the disaccharides lactose and sucrose, and the monosaccharides glucose and fructose.

- D-Glucose is the most important carbohydrate in the diet and in the intermediate metabolism of carbohydrate in humans.
- It is a hexose (a six-carbon sugar molecule), with both α- and β- stereoisomers.
- When one glucose molecule is joined to another to form a disaccharide or a polysaccharide the link may be between the C1 of the first molecule and C4 of the second molecule (1–4 linkage) or between C1 and 6 (1–6 linkage).
- This linkage is via an oxygen bridge with either an α- or a β-glycosidic bond, depending on the stereoisomer.

Starch is made up of amylase and amylopectin. Amylose is composed of a chain of glucose units linked via a 1–4α-glycosidic bond. Amylopectin is also made up of a chain of glucose units but, in addition to the 1–4α linkages, there are 1–6α linkages at a number of branching points, approximately every 25 glucose units, along the chain.

- Lactose is made up of a molecule each of galactose and glucose, linked by a β-glycosidic bond.
- Sucrose, maltose, and isomaltose are linked by an α-glycosidic bond.
- Maltose consists of two glucose molecules linked by a 1–4 bond, whereas isomaltose (also containing two glucose molecules) is linked via a 1–6 bond.
- Sucrose (cane or beet sugar) consists of a molecule of glucose linked to a molecule of fructose via an α-linkage on the glucose side coupled to a β-linkage on the fructose side (α-glucosido-β-fructose).

Carbohydrate digestion

Salivary and pancreatic α-amylases act on starch to yield maltose, maltotriose (three glucose units), and α-limit dextrins (branched oligosaccharides with 1–6 linkages at the branching points, but otherwise 1–4 linkages containing an average of eight glucose molecules).

- Disaccharide hydrolysis occurs within the brush border of the small intestinal enterocyte.
- There is a single brush border β-galactosidase (lactase)
- There are three brush border α-glucosidases—sucrase, isomaltase (or α-dextrinase), and glucoamylase.
- Sucrase not only hydrolyses maltose and maltotriose but also splits sucrose to glucose and fructose.
- Isomaltase cleaves 1–6α as well as 1–4α links in oligosaccharides.
- After hydrolysis, the liberated monosaccharides are absorbed by active transport mechanisms.
- Glucose and galactose share the sodium-glucose-linked transporter (SGLT-1), whereas fructose has a different mechanism.

Congenital and acquired defects of disaccharidase activity have been described in children as well as congenital mutations within SGLT-1. These disorders lead to malabsorption of various sugars. Symptoms include nausea, watery diarrhoea, wind, and abdominal cramps. There is clearly overlap with cow's milk protein intolerance in young children, and functional bowel disorders (e.g. irritable bowel syndrome, recurrent abdominal pain). In many patients who believe themselves to be lactose intolerant, objective testing suggests otherwise.

Hypolactasia/lactose intolerance

- Low activity of lactase in the small intestinal brush border membrane is the most common cause of carbohydrate intolerance; symptoms are provoked following ingestion of milk or lactose-containing products but the symptoms do not always occur together and the association with lactose absorption may not be obvious.
- In many populations lactase activity is normal in the first few years of life, but then declines in older children and adults; prevalence varies, being >80% in Semitics, Africans, Asians, Inuit, and American Indians, but only 10% of northern Europeans; inheritance is thought to be autosomal recessive.
- Congenital lactase deficiency is extremely rare, presenting with watery diarrhoea as soon as breast or formula feeds are introduced.
- Secondary hypolactasia commonly occurs after infective gastroenteritis but usually resolves spontaneously in a short period of time (days–2 weeks).
- Affected individuals vary in the amount of lactose they are able to tolerate so that strict exclusion of all milk products is rarely necessary (fermented dairy products such as cheese and yoghurt, for example, may not cause symptoms).
- Lactose and fructose intolerance may coexist.
- There is interest in whether lactose intolerance affects the link between dairy intake and other diseases, such as cancer, but little evidence as yet that this is the case.

Congenital sucrase–isomaltase deficiency

- Sucrase and isomaltase activity always go hand in hand (both enzymes are synthesized together, inserted into the brush border membrane as one long protein, and subsequently cleaved into two units, which remain closely associated).
- Much less common than lactase deficiency it occurs in about 0.2% of North Americans and 10% of Greenland Inuit; it is autosomal recessive in inheritance.
- Typical symptoms of carbohydrate malabsorption occur when sucrose is introduced into the diet (e.g. fruit).
- Diarrhoea may be associated with failure to thrive (NB: A change to a feed containing glucose polymer as treatment for suspected cow's milk protein or lactose intolerance will not resolve the problem.)
- Symptoms can be mild, and may appear clinically as 'toddler' diarrhoea.
- Mucosal biopsy analysis will show normal lactase activity and low sucrase–isomaltase.
- Dietary restriction of sucrose may help alleviate symptoms, but enzyme replacement therapy (Sucraid®, Orphan Medical Inc.) is also available.

Glucose–galactose malabsorption

- Glucose–galactose malabsorption is the only known primary monosaccharide intolerance, exceptionally rare, and autosomal recessive in inheritance.
- Infants do not tolerate feeds containing lactose (glucose–galactose) or sucrose (glucose–fructose) and have severe diarrhoea from first feeds; they can tolerate fructose.

Confirmation of diagnosis of carbohydrate malabsorption

- Samples of liquid stool will show undigested sugars on chromatography.
- In patients without watery diarrhoea, a sugar challenge may be given to see if symptoms are provoked and for breath hydrogen testing (if child old enough to cooperate): 2 g/kg of sugar being tested given by mouth, baseline and half hourly breath hydrogen analysis for 2 h; if sugar maldigested, colonic bacteria utilize, and produce hydrogen with >20 ppm in exhaled breath (positive test)
- Analysis of small-bowel mucosal disaccharidases in biopsy obtained endoscopically is the 'gold standard'
- Clinical response to treatment (dietary modification; sacrosidase).

Case study: sucrase–isomaltase deficiency

A male infant thrived on a standard cow's milk formula but developed diarrhoea when fruit juices were given for the first time at 4 weeks of age. He was treated with oral glucose and electrolyte solution for suspected gastroenteritis and diarrhoea stopped, only to recur when a soy-based formula containing glucose polymer was introduced. He continued to be fed with this formula and was referred to a tertiary gastroenterology unit at the age of 8 months because of continuing diarrhoea and poor weight gain. Use of a modular feed with glucose polymer also caused diarrhoea, but this stopped if fructose was substituted as the carbohydrate source. Endoscopic duodenal biopsy specimens were obtained, and enzyme analysis showed normal lactase with very low sucrase–isomaltase activity. He was given a standard lactose-based cow's milk formula and had prompt resolution of his symptoms. Subsequently he avoided sucrose in his diet and as symptoms were minimal did not require treatment with enzyme replacement (oral sacrosidase).

References and resources

Newton T, Murphy S, Booth IW. Glucose polymer as a cause of protracted diarrhoea in infants with unsuspected congenital sucrase-isomaltase deficiency. *J Pediatr* 1996;**128**:753–6

Treem WR, McAdams L, Stanford L; Kastoff G, Justinich C, Hyams, J. Sacrosidase therapy for congenital sucrase-isomaltase deficiency. *J Pediatr Gastroenterol Nutr* 1999;**28**:137–142

Nutritional problems in the child with neurological handicap

Neurological handicap is common, with around 15 000–20 000 children in the United Kingdom having cerebral palsy. Of these, 50% are reported to have feeding problems, rising to 85% in more severely affected children (e.g. those with spastic quadriplegia). In an Oxford-based community study of feeding and nutritional problems in children with neurological impairment:

- 89% needed help with feeding
- 56% experienced choking with food
- 38% of parents considered their child to be underweight
- 28% reported prolonged mealtimes
- 20% reported stressful mealtimes
- 64% reported that to their knowledge feeding and nutritional status had never been formally assessed.

Reduced energy intake as a consequence of feeding difficulties or vomiting (gastro-oesophageal reflux disease, GORD) may lead to poor growth, and micronutrient deficiencies including calcium, iron, zinc, and fat-soluble vitamins are commonly encountered. Feed intolerance may be associated not only with acid reflux, but also with delayed gastric emptying, diarrhoea, or constipation. Changing from bolus to continuous feeds; decreasing the rate of infusion; concentrating the feed to decrease the volume; selecting an alternative feed; and treating GORD, delayed gastric emptying (prokinetics), and constipation may all help.

Achieving and maintaining optimal nutritional status in children with disabilities helps them maximize their potential in life and is as important as it is in healthy children. Undernutrition adversely affects cognitive function and makes children apathetic and miserable. Underweight children with severe motor impairment are more likely to develop pressure sores. Overweight/obesity in the child with walking difficulties may further compromise mobility.

Assessment

In taking a feeding history it is important to enquire about the following:
- How long do meal times take?
- Are they enjoyable?
- What type and quantity of food is consumed?
- Is there coughing, choking or vomiting?
- Is there a history of chest infection (?aspiration)?
- Is there a history of constipation? (delays stomach emptying, exacerbates GOR, reduces appetite).

Nutritional status and determinants
- Nutritional status using standard anthropometry
- 'Height/stature' can be estimated by measuring upper arm length, lower leg length, or knee height as follows:
  - $21.8 + (4.35 \times \text{upper-arm length})$
  - $30.8 + (3.26 \times \text{lower leg length})$
  - $24.2 + (2.69 \times \text{knee height})$.
- Oromotor skills and safety of swallow best assessed by experienced speech and language therapist (may advise videofluoroscopy of swallowed liquid and solids)
- Occupational therapist to assess seating for mealtime, and appropriate eating aids
- Dietitian for assessment of energy needs and developmental age appropriate food; recommended daily amount (RDA) may overestimate energy needs when there is severe growth delay; energy requirements also influenced by variation in muscle tone and levels of physical activity.

Suggestions for optimizing oral intake

- Change of posture, special adaptive seating, soft cervical collar, use of wide-bore straw
- Treatment of oral hypersensitivity (speech and language therapist)
- Thickening of foods
- Use of energy supplements
- Treatment of: GOR, oesophagitis, slow gastric emptying, constipation.

Tube feeding

Indications
- Severely compromised swallowing
- Repeated aspiration pneumonia
- Malnutrition despite 'optimizing' oral intake
- Administration of medication.

Potential benefits
- Improved nutritional status
- Improvement in general well being
- Less time spent on feeding, more on other forms of interaction
- Oral feeding for pleasure still possible
- Easier to give medication
- Easier to keep well hydrated.

Long-term (>6 weeks) tube feeding is usually by percutaneous endoscopic gastrostomy (PEG). Gastrostomy requires careful discussion with family. It is not without risks and may be seen as evidence of 'failure' by some parents. The purpose is to improve quality of life for families and children; long-term follow-up is important. If energy intake exceeds energy expenditure, excessive weight gain will result. Children with impaired mobility or severe cognitive dysfunction may have a relatively low energy expenditure. Resting energy expenditure is also low in children with reduced lean body mass. In severe spastic quadriplegia, around 2/3 of recommended energy intake may be adequate for growth.

Gastro-oesophageal reflux disease (GORD)

Common (15–75%) in children with neurological impairments; may relate to:
- Persistent activation of vomiting reflex
- Generalized gastrointestinal dysmotility
- Hiatus hernia
- Prolonged supine position
- Increased intra-abdominal pressure secondary to spasticity, scoliosis, or seizures.

Although PEG may sometimes exacerbate or initiate significant GORD there is no need for 'prophylactic' fundoplication. An initial period of nasogastric tube feeding may be useful for assessing potential need for fundoplication (i.e. provocation of significant vomiting). 24 h pH monitoring pre-PEG is not generally predictive of who will need fundoplication.

Alternatives to anti-reflux surgery include:
- Jejunal feeding (e.g. PEG-J tube; surgical jejunostomy)
- Oesophago-gastric dissociation surgery (rarely needed).

Gastrostomy placement and subsequent care

An agreed pathway for children who need gastrostomy facilitates the process for children and their families; an example is given in Fig. 19.1.

Leaking, overgranulation and infection of the gastrostomy site are common problems; a high standard of general care is required together with periodic tube replacement. Some practical guidance for care and maintenance of gastrostomy tubes are given in Fig. 19.2.

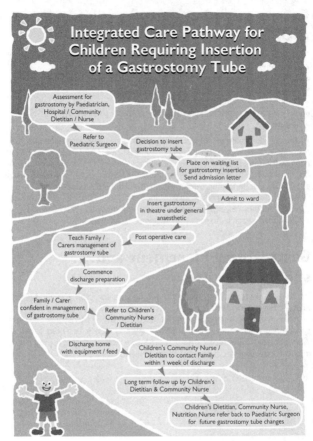

Fig. 19.1 Integrated care pathway for children requiring insertion of a gastrostomy tube (with grateful acknowledgement to Gill Lazonby and Cheryl Thomas, Children's Nutrition Nurse Specialists, Leeds General Infirmary).

CLEANING GASTROSTOMY STOMA SITE

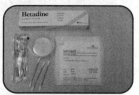

Collect equipment and wash hands thoroughly
Do not undo the fixation triangle for the first 4 days
following placement

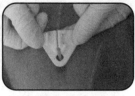

Ease the triangle up gently and clean with
soft guaze or cotton buds

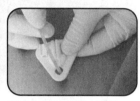

Lift tube out of fixation device and slide it down
the tube

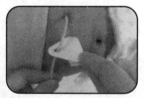

Check external length of tube

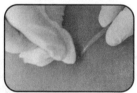

Clean around the tube with soft gauze or a
cotton bud. Use a clean piece each time, wiping
away from the gastrostomy stoma. Allow to dry
At least 4 days after placement and at
least once a week, open fixation device

Fig. 19.2 (a) Cleaning gastrostomy stoma site; (b) daily care of gastrostomy tube site; (c) management of overgranulation tissue; (d) persistent overgranulation tissue (e) management of a leaking gastrostomy stoma; (f) changing a balloon gastrostomy tube; (g) changing a button gastrostomy.

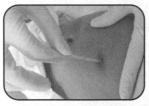

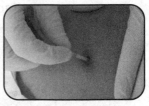

Gently push tube 1-3cm into stomach and turn the tube in a complete circle at least weekly and no more than once a day. This prevents the internal disc sticking to the stomach wall

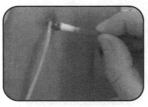

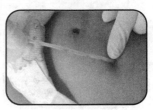

Apply antiseptic ointment (eg Betadine ointment) for the first 1-2 weeks following placement or if the gastrostomy site appears red. This reduces the risk of infection.

To check the external length of the tube, gently pull back until you feel the internal disc against the stomach wall.

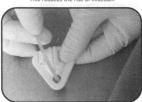

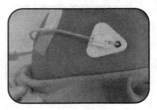

Slide the fixation device along the tube until it is close to the skin. Place your finger underneath the triangle and then press the yellow fixing clamp closed

Secure in position with a loop of tape, to prevent the tube pulling and stretching the gastrostomy stoma

Fig. 19.2 (a) *(Cont.)*

DAILY CARE OF GASTROSTOMY TUBE SITE

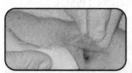

Clean around the tube with soft gauze or a cotton bud. Use a clean piece each time, wiping away from the gastrostomy site. Then clean the fixation disc

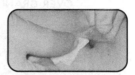

Dry around the skin and fixation disc thoroughly

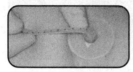

Turn the tube in a complete circle at least weekly and no more than once a day. This prevents the internal balloon sticking to the stomach wall. Gently pull back the tube and check the external length of the G tube is correct

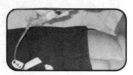

Flush the tube with cooled boiled water before and after feeds and medication and at least once a day if G tube not being used

Gastrostomy tube has migrated into stomach

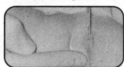

The tube appears shorter, the balloon may have migrated through the pylorus
Deflate the balloon and with drawn the tube to 6cm and then re-inflate the balloon. Gently pull back the tube until you can feel the balloon against the stomach wall and the slide the disc to skin level

If tube continues to slip through fixation device, wrap tape around the tube above fixation device.

Aspirate tube and test for gastric acid, pH1-5, to ensure gastric placement.

Fig. 19.2 (b)

MANAGEMENT OF
OVER-GRANULATION TISSUE

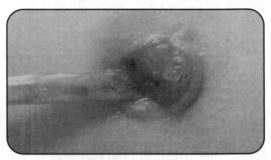

Over-granulation tissue

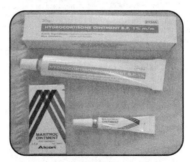

Use 1% Hydrocortisone, if no improvement
after 1-2 weeks change to Maxitrol ointment

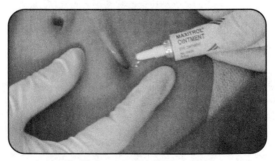

Applying Hydrocortisone or Maxitrol ointment.
Use twice a day for 10-14 days

Fig. 19.2 (c)

PERSISTENT OVER-GRANULATION TISSUE
(not responding to topical steroids/antibiotics)

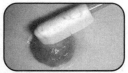

Persistent over-granulation tissue

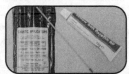

Use 75% Silver nitrate applicator
and yellow soft paraffin

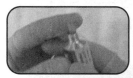 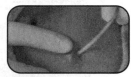

Apply soft paraffin to surrounding skin to prevent staining and damaging surrounding skin

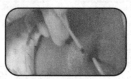

Apply silver nitrate to over-granulation
tissue, avoid touch gastrostomy tube as
this may damage the tube

Fig. 19.2 (d)

MANAGEMENT OF A LEAKING GASTROSTOMY STOMA

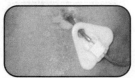

Tissue damage caused by gastric acid leakage.
Usually due to stoma being stretched by pulling or
excessive coughing/straining or a hole in the tube

Test leakage with pH paper to identify possible cause of leakage

pH1-5 indicates gastric
acid leakage.

pH 7-8 leakage is more likely
to be serous fluid /pus or
peritoneal fluid. This may
indicate infected gastrostomy
stoma site or misplaced tube.

If gastric leakage is confirmed,
clean skin with cooled boiled water
or saline and allow to dry

Use a skin barrier product such as Cavilon spray or sponge
wipe to protect surrounding skin

Fig. 19.2 (e)

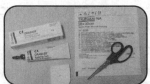

Use Orabase paste and a key hole foam dressing to reduce leakage and promote healing

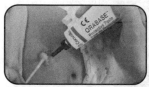

Apply Orabase paste generously around the tube. This creates a seal which will reduce leakage and protects surrounding skin

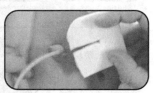

Apply key-hole foam dressing

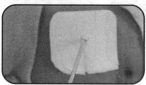

Hold in position with tape and gently pull tube back until you can feel the internal disc against the stomach wall

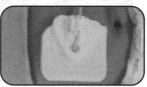

Close fixation device. Tape tube to skin to prevent the gastrostomy stoma site being pulled or stretched

- This treatment needs to be performed at least once a day.

- More frequent applications will be required if leakage is excessive.

- **Remember** that it will take regular applications of this treatment over 1-2 weeks to promote healing of the stoma and gradually reduce the leakage

- **Do not** stop treatment until leakage has stopped completely for 3-5 days

Fig. 19.2 (e) *(Cont.)*

CHANGING A BALLOON GASTROSTOMY TUBE
(G- TUBE)

Instil 5ml of sterile water/saline in balloon of new G tube and check balloon is a uniform shape.

Deflate the balloon on G tube in situ, using a male luer slip syringe

Lubricate the tip of the new G tube with gel. Insert G tube into stoma.

Deflate balloon and remove G tube.

Inflate the balloon with 5ml of sterile water/saline using a male luer slip syringe

Gently pull back the tube until you feel the internal balloon against the stomach wall

Attach extension set or attach catheter tip syringe directly onto the tube

Flush G tube with cooled boiled water

Test aspirate on pH paper, pH 1-5 indicates gastric placement

Check external fixation device is in correct position, use markings on the tube as a guide. The tube can be secured with tape to prevent it pulling on the stoma site. The tube can be secured with tape to prevent it pulling on the stoma site.

Fig. 19.2 (f)

CHANGING A BUTTON GASTROSTOMY
(low profile gastrostomy device LPGD)

Wash hands and collect equipment

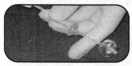

Check balloon on measuring device, if required

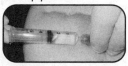

Deflate balloon on button/ g-tube insitu using a male luer slip syringe

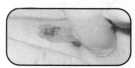

Remove button by placing fingers either side of the button. Ask patient to cough if possible.

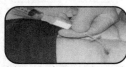

Lubricate tip of measuring device with gel, insert and inflate balloon with 5ml of water/saline

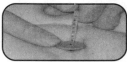

Note cm mark above the disc in both a sitting and lying position. Take an average of the two measurements to estimate shaft length

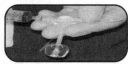

Select correct Fr size and cm length of button and check balloon for uniform shape

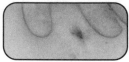

Remove measuring device

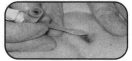

Lubricate tip with gel and insert the mini button

Fig. 19.2 (g)

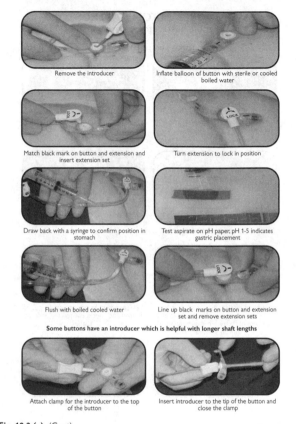

Remove the introducer

Inflate balloon of button with sterile or cooled boiled water

Match black mark on button and extension and insert extension set

Turn extension to lock in position

Draw back with a syringe to confirm position in stomach

Test aspirate on pH paper, pH 1-5 indicates gastric placement

Flush with boiled cooled water

Line up black marks on button and extension set and remove extension sets

Some buttons have an introducer which is helpful with longer shaft lengths

Attach clamp for the introducer to the top of the button

Insert introducer to the tip of the button and close the clamp

Fig. 19.2 (g) (Cont)

References and resources

Allott L. Feeding children with special needs. In: Holden C, MacDonald A (eds.) Nutrition and child health, Baillière Tindall, Edinburgh, 2000, pp. 143–160

Marchand V, Motil KJ and the NASPGHAN Committee on Nutrition. Nutrition support for neurologically impaired children: a clinical report of the North American Society of Pediatric Gastroenterology, Hepatology and Nutrition. J Pediatr Gastroenterol Nutr 2006;43:123–135 www.jpgn.org—go to 'archive')

Obesity

Weight gain in an individual is the result of an energy intake from food in excess of energy expenditure. Unhealthy diets and lack of physical activity are considered to be the leading causes of avoidable illness and premature death in Europe, and the rising prevalence of obesity is a major public health concern. There is a strong tendency for excess weight to continue to accumulate from childhood through to middle age. While 40–70% of the variation in fat mass between individuals may be genetically determined, environmental factors remain crucial. Important lifestyle choices predetermining health risks in adulthood are made during childhood and adolescence. Schools must come to play a key role in promoting healthy diets and enjoyment of physical activity.

Definitions

- Body mass index (BMI) = weight (kg)/height^2 (m)

BMI related to reference standards for age is the most practical measure of overweight/obesity. It is objective and provides a degree of consistency with adult practice. Current British Childhood BMI charts show the 91st, 98th and 99.6th centile lines, with a shaded area indicating healthy BMI range. The charts are also marked with the recommended International Obesity Task Force (IOTF) cut-offs for obesity and overweight in children; these equate with WHO adult definitions of obesity and overweight at 18 years—BMI 30 = obese, BMI 25 = overweight. There is still no universally agreed definition of obesity in childhood; a BMI >85% is regarded as overweight and BMI >95% severe overweight.

Because a high BMI by itself may not be a guarantor of obesity/overweight, a high waist centile will provide further evidence of fatness.

Epidemiology

In the European Union:
- Obesity levels have risen by between 10–40% over the past decade.
- Almost 1 in 4 children are overweight, with England and Poland showing the steepest upward trend.
- Obesity is an important risk factor for ischaemic heart disease (quadrupled risk in adulthood if BMI >29), hypertension, stroke, type 2 diabetes, cancers (breast, ovary, endometrium, prostate, bowel), depression, and social discrimination.
- Obesity across all ages accounts for up to 7% of healthcare costs.

Evaluation

When taking a history and conducting a clinical examination, assess the following:

- Family history of obesity and obesity related illness (e.g. diabetes, cardiovascular disease)
- Family structure
- Physical activity, diet, and eating patterns
- Psychological effects (e.g. low self-esteem, bullying, depression)
- School attendance and attainment
- Related morbidities (e.g. sleep apnoea, orthopaedic problems)
- Physical examination; height and weight, BMI, plotted on standard charts
- Features of rare causes of obesity (see below), particularly short stature
- Pubertal development; blood pressure
- Acanthosis nigricans—a dark, velvety appearance at the neck and axillae, a sign of insulin resistance.

Consider unusual causes of obesity:
- Endocrine
  - hypothyroidism, e.g. in Down syndrome
  - Cushing's syndrome (truncal obesity, hypertension, hirsutism, striae)
  - growth hormone deficiency (may have delayed puberty)
- Chromosomal abnormalities e.g. Prader–Willi (poor linear growth, developmental delay, small genitalia, dysmorphic)
- Drug related e.g. steroid treatment.

Predisposing factors
- Spina bifida
- Muscular dystrophy
- Other causes of immobility
- Polycystic ovary syndrome.

Consider further investigation if:
- Associated morbidity (e.g. apnoea, diabetes, arthritis)
- Short stature
- Precocious (<8 year) puberty, or delayed puberty (no signs at 13 years in girls, 15 years in boys)
- Symptoms/signs of genetic or endocrine abnormality.

Treatment

Given the lack of studies there is inadequate evidence to support particular interventions aimed at preventing obesity. On an individual basis, children who are objectively obese according to BMI should be treated providing the child and family are willing to make the necessary lifestyle changes. The aims of treatment include resolution of co-morbidity and changes in behaviour.

Weight management

- Probably best managed through community-based multidisciplinary team including GP, health visitor, school nurse, and dietitian.
- Strict diet and rapid weight loss are not appropriate for growing children.
- Aim for steady weight as height increases, or 'weight gain' less than 'height gain'.
- Involve the family and tailor interventions to the individual.
- Always set realistic (i.e. achievable) goals.

Promotion of physical activity

- Any increase in energy expenditure will help redress the input–output imbalance.
- Walking, cycling, using stairs instead of lifts.
- Whole family to be involved in more active lifestyle.
- Gym, swimming and organized sports may be unrealistic goals.
- Decrease time spent at computer or watching television.

Dietary changes

- Balanced, varied diet for the whole family.
- Regular meals (avoid grazing/snacking), smaller portions; avoid frying.
- Fruit rather than crisps, cakes, biscuits, etc.
- Less energy-dense food, e.g. semi-skimmed milk, low-fat products.
- Low-calorie drinks, preferably water.

Complications

Metabolic syndrome

- A constellation of metabolic risk factors that appear to promote the development of atherosclerotic heart disease, including high plasma triglycerides and low HDL-cholesterol, hypertension, insulin resistance.
- Non-alcoholic fatty liver disease (NAFLD) is considered the hepatic manifestation of metabolic syndrome.

NAFLD

- Thought to result from fatty infiltration of the liver due to obesity and insulin resistance, followed by inflammatory insults, possibly related to oxidative stress
- 10% of obese adolescents in USA have elevated alanine aminotransaminase.
- The most common cause of liver disease in the pre-adolescent and adolescent age groups.
- Histological changes range from simple steatosis, to steatosis with inflammation and cellular injury and fibrosis.
- Liver biopsy gold standard for diagnosis (applicability limited by risk and cost).
- Diagnosis usually based on elevated amino-transferases and/or fatty liver on ultrasound; other causes of liver disease (hepatitis B and C, Wilson disease, α_1-antitrypsin deficiency, autoimmune hepatitis, drug-induced liver injury) should be excluded.
- Although hepatic fibrosis is common (53–100%) in children with NAFLD, the incidence of cirrhosis is unknown.
- Interventions aimed at weight reduction are currently the only therapeutic option.

Case study

Jodie was 10 years of age when referred to outpatients because of concerns about her being overweight and the possibility of a 'glandular' problem. According to her mother she was getting on well at school, but did not like taking part in physical activities. Her records show that she began to put on weight rapidly from the age of 3 years; she was tall for her age, with a BMI on the 98th centile.

The aspects of Jodie's lifestyle that predispose to obesity should be assessed, together with any emotional and behavioural difficulties. Enquiry should be made regarding what Jodie and her family eat on a normal day, and details of physical and sedentary activities. Snoring at night and lethargy in the day may suggest sleep apnoea; musculoskeletal problems are common. There may be difficulties at school, with obese children being bullied or themselves bullying; they may be depressed. Take a family history with regard to whether anyone else is overweight and whether there is a history of heart disease at a young age, or diabetes.

Nutritional obesity is very common in comparison with other causes; children with endocrine problems and overweight are usually short. Since clinical examination of Jodie was normal apart from her obesity; it was not appropriate to investigate for endocrine or genetic abnormalities. The family were given advice regarding diet options aimed at reducing energy intake, and increasing levels of exercise.

References and resources

Alberti KGMM, Zimmet PZ, Shaw JE. The metabolic syndrome—a new world-wide definition from the International Diabetes Federation Consensus. *Lancet* 2005;**366**:1059–1062

An approach to weight management in children and adolescents (2–18 years) in primary care. Produced for the Royal College of Paediatrics and Child Health and the National Obesity Forum by P Gibson, L Edmunds, DW Haslam, E Poskitt; 2002. www.rcpch.org

Commission of the European Communities. Green Paper. Promoting healthy diets and physical activity: a European dimensions for the prevention of overweight, obesity and chronic diseases. Brussels, 08.12.2005 COM(2005) 637 final

National Institute for Health and Clinical Excellence. Obesity: the prevention, identification, assessment and management of overweight and obesity in adults and children. 2006. www.nice.org.uk

Public health strategies for preventing and controlling overweight and obesity in school and worksite settings. Department of Health and Human Services, Centers for Disease Control and Prevention 2005; vol. 54

Cystic fibrosis

The incidence of cystic fibrosis (CF) is around 1 in 2500. Cases are diagnosed as a consequence of population screening or high-risk screening, or following presentation with clinical symptoms typical of the disorder. The basic defect is in the CFTR (cystic fibrosis transmembrane conductance regulator) protein which codes for a cyclic adenosine monophosphate-regulated chloride transporter in epithelial cells of exocrine organs. This is involved in salt and water balance across epithelial surfaces. The gene is on chromosome 7. There are multiple known mutations, the most common being ΔF508.

CF is a multisystem disorder and the primary pathology is within the respiratory system, but it can present with primary gastrointestinal manifestations such as meconium ileus or chronic diarrhoea. Poor weight gain is common at diagnosis. This chapter deals with the gastrointestinal manifestations relevant to the assessment of children with gut disease, and the nutritional management of CF. The reader is referred to the publications listed under References and resources for a fuller account of this condition.

Gastrointestinal manifestations

Pancreatic disease

The pathophysiology of pancreatic disease is a failure of exocrine pancreatic secretion. Thickened secretions (low bicarbonate concentration) block the pancreatic ductal system; autodigestion by pancreatic enzymes follows and leads to a reduction in functional capacity.

- Pancreatic exocrine insufficiency occurs in up to 90% (80% in the first year).
- There is marked impairment of secretion of water, bicarbonate, lipase, amylase, and proteases from the pancreas into the duodenum resulting in maldigestion.
- Presentation is with chronic diarrhoea (steatorrhoea), poor weight gain, and occasionally hypoproteinaemic oedema.
- Pancreatic enzyme replacement is required and should be supervised by an experienced paediatric dietician; the dose needs to be carefully tailored to match food intake, prevent steatorrhoea, and promote weight gain.
- Energy needs are high as a consequence of the maldigestion, increased metabolic demands (primarily respiratory), and the impact of chronic disease on other body systems.
- A high-calorie diet is required but may be difficult to achieve when the child is unwell; energy-dense foods, supplements, or tube feeding are sometimes necessary.
- Fat-soluble vitamin replacement is required.
- Abnormal glucose tolerance occurs in up to 10% by the second decade and may lead to diabetes mellitus.
- Both acute and chronic pancreatitis may be seen.

Intestinal disease

Defects in CFTR lead to reduced chloride secretion with water following into the gut. This may result in meconium ileus at birth and in distal intestinal obstruction syndrome (DIOS) later in life. The basic pathophysiology results in dehydration of intestinal contents with clinical presentations as a consequence; 15% of children have meconium ileus in the neonatal period.

- Presents with delayed passage of meconium, abdominal distension and bile-stained vomiting.
- Management is by bowel clearance via an enterotomy using acetyl cysteine or Gastrografin®.
- Up to 30% require bowel resection.
- After bowel resection infants will be at increased risk of bacterial overgrowth and short-bowel syndrome.
- Not all children with meconium ileus have CF but it should be excluded in any child who presents in this way.
- Intussusception occurs more commonly and at a later age than in the general population.
- Rectal prolapse occurs in up to 15%; risk factors include frequent large stools, poor nutritional status, and raised intrathoracic pressure from coughing. Most cases improve with treatment of CF (NB: most children with rectal prolapse do not have CF).
- Distal intestinal obstruction syndrome (meconium ileus equivalent) results from the accumulation of thick faecal material in the terminal ileum, caecum, and ascending colon and may cause bowel obstruction. Differential diagnosis includes appendicitis, intussusception, and volvulus. Management is with intravenous fluids and laxatives; oral Gastrografin® or intestinal lavage is helpful in difficult cases.
- Constipation is very common; risk factors include poor fluid intake, inadequately controlled steatorrhoea, viscid intestinal secretions, energy-dense diets, dysmotility, plus all the other risk factors in the childhood population.
- Colonic strictures have been reported and are thought to be secondary to high-dose pancreatic supplementation.

Management of gastrointestinal symptoms in children with CF

The differential diagnosis of gastrointestinal symptoms in children with CF includes:
- CF-related complications
- Non-CF-related bowel disease
- Functional.

It is important to remember that the child with abdominal pain may have a complication of CF such as pancreatitis, non-CF-related bowel disease such as gastro-oesophageal reflux, peptic ulceration, or functional abdominal pain (recurrent abdominal pain of childhood). Gastro-oesophageal reflux is more common in children with respiratory disease, and may be exacerbated by energy-dense diets. Functional symptoms are very common in children with chronic illness, and psychosocial factors important to take into account in the overall assessment. During adolescence issues relating to acceptance of the underlying disease, acceptance by peers, and the gradual progression from dependence to independence are the most prominent.

Nutrition in CF

There is evidence that promoting good nutritional status can slow the progression of pulmonary disease and improve long-term outcome. Currently children born with CF can be expected to survive into their fourth decade.

Risk factors for malnutrition in CF

Increased resting energy expenditure
- Chronic cough
- Chest infections
- Impaired lung function

Increased nutrient losses
- Pancreatic maldigestion
- Reduced bile salt pool
- Expectoration of copious mucus
- Diabetes
- Vomiting

Poor energy intake
- Anorexia and fatigue during pulmonary infection
- Depression
- Anxiety regarding weight (girls).

Nutritional management

- Early diagnosis by neonatal screening and early intervention assists maintenance of nutritional status.
- Breast-feeding on demand or 150–200 mL formula/kg/day will support normal growth.
- Bowel resection leading to short bowel adds to complexity of nutritional management in some children presenting with meconium ileus.
- Cow's milk protein intolerance or gastro-oesophageal reflux may require specific management.
- Weaning foods should be introduced at 4–6 months.
- Consider use of high-energy infant formula and/or energy supplements if weight gain is poor.
- Full fat cow's milk can be introduced by 1 year.
- Regular review by experienced dietitian.
- Monitoring of growth and nutritional status
- Annual 1 day record of dietary and enzyme intake.
- Encourage high-fat diet with appropriate pancreatic enzyme replacement therapy.
- Enzyme supplementation needs to be adjusted as fat intake increases or fat composition of food changes.
- Food refusal occurs in some children; effective behaviour management strategies may be needed.
- During adolescence the need to be independent sometimes results in deteriorating dietary, vitamin, and enzyme intake with resulting negative impact on nutritional status and pulmonary function.

Pancreatic enzyme replacement therapy

- Start if any clinical evidence of fat malabsorption.
- Dose needed is variable; enteric-coated acid-resistant preparations most effective.
- In infants, initial dose is 2500 IU lipase/feed; capsules are opened and microspheres mixed with milk or fruit purée and given by spoon at start of feed.
- For a newly diagnosed older patient give 1–2 capsules per meal and half to one capsule with fat-containing snacks.
- Enzyme preparations should not be crushed or chewed.
- Gradually increase dose according to clinical symptoms, appearance of stools, and weight gain.
- Enzymes are best taken at the beginning, middle, and end of the meal, especially if it takes longer than 30 minutes to eat.
- The UK Committee on Safety of Medicines has advised a maximum daily intake of 10 000 IU lipase/kg/day (higher doses have been linked to fibrosing colonopathy).
- If higher intakes appear necessary, enzyme efficacy may be improved by reducing the gastric acid secretion with H_2 receptor antagonists or proton pump inhibitors.
- Persistent problems require investigation for other disorders (e.g. coeliac disease, cow's milk protein intolerance).

Vitamins

- Malabsorption of fat soluble vitamins is common with pancreatic exocrine insufficiency.
- All such patients should receive daily supplementation (see below) and have their biochemical vitamin status checked annually.
- Dosages for children under and over 1 year respectively:
  - vitamin A 400 IU; 4000–10 000 IU
  - vitamin D 400 IU; 400–800 IU
  - vitamin E 10–50 IU; 50–100 IU.
- Routine supplementation of water-soluble vitamins is not required.

Clinical features of vitamin deficiency

- Vitamin A: night blindness; xerophthalmia
- Vitamin D: gross deficiency uncommon, but sub-clinical deficiency may contribute to chronic bone disease (osteoporosis)
- Vitamin E: haemolytic anaemia; spinocerebellar degeneration
- Vitamin K: prolonged clotting.

Enteral tube feeding

- Used to maintain or restore nutritional status when dietary advice, optimization of enzyme replacement therapy and oral supplementation have failed.
- About 10% of UK CF population receive tube feeding.
- Usually whole protein, polymeric feeds with high energy density, delivered overnight.
- Institution of tube feeding may sometimes precipitate hyperglycaemia requiring insulin therapy.

References and resources

Balfour-Lynn IM. Newborn screening for cystic fibrosis: evidence for benefit. *Arch Dis Child* 2008;**93**:7–10

Borowitz D, Baker RD, Stallings V. Consensus report on nutrition for pediatric patients with cystic fibrosis. *J Pediatr Gastroenterol Nutr* 2002;**35**:246–259

Peebles A, Connett G, Maddison J, Gavin J. *Cystic Fibrosis Care: A practical guide*. Elsevier Churchill Livingstone, Edinburgh, 2005

Cystic fibrosis-associated liver disease

Cystic fibrosis (CF) is an autosomal recessive disease resulting from mutations in the gene coding for the cystic fibrosis transmembrane conductance regulator (CFTR) (see Chapter 21). CFTR functions as a transmembrane chloride channel in the apical membrane of most secretory epithelia and the disease thus affects lungs, pancreas, exocrine glands, gut, and liver. In CF-associated liver disease the biliary tract is most commonly involved in a spectrum from asymptomatic to biliary cirrhosis. The liver disease runs from mild and subclinical to severe cirrhosis and portal hypertension. Clinical disease is seen in 4–6% of cases, but there are biochemical abnormalities in 20–50%. At autopsy, fibrosis is present in 20% and steatosis in 50%.

Pathophysiology

The cause of liver disease in CF is not well understood, and is multifactorial. Reduced chloride channel function appears to result in reduction in water and sodium movement into bile, and there are abnormalities in the composition, alkalinity, and flow of the bile. It is unclear why all CF patients have abnormal CFTR in the biliary tree, but not all develop biliary disease. In the liver parenchyma, the most common pathology is steatosis, which is present in 50%. There is no relationship between the CF genotype and the phenotype of the liver disease. Risk factors for significant liver disease include pancreatic insufficiency, possession of HLA DQ6, male sex, and presentation with meconium ileus.

Clinical features

Neonatal (uncommon)

- Conjugated jaundice
- Fat malabsorption and failure to thrive
- Inspissated bile syndrome.

The cholestatic jaundice resolves over time, though residual fibrosis may remain. There is not thought to be an increased risk of subsequent cirrhosis.

Older children

- Asymptomatic hepatomegaly and/or splenomegaly
- Hypersplenism
- Complications of portal hypertension e.g. variceal bleeding
- Elevated transaminases, alkaline phosphatase or gamma-glutamyl transferase
- Malnutrition
- Cholelithiasis
- Sclerosing cholangitis
- Rarely ascites, jaundice.

Diagnosis

This can be difficult as liver function tests do not always reflect the severity of the disease.

Liver function tests

- Bilirubin normal unless disease is advanced
- Prothrombin time prolonged in severe liver disease or vitamin K deficiency
- Gamma-glutamyl transferase raised in >30% and in severe disease
- Intermittent rises in transaminases in 30% of patients
- Alkaline phosphatase elevated in 50% but not specific for liver disease.

Ultrasound

- Size and consistency of liver and spleen
- Heterogeneous liver parenchyma in steatosis
- Portal vein flow and splenic varices
- Cholelithiasis.

Liver biopsy

- Extent and severity of liver disease
- Changes of giant cell hepatitis in neonates
- Inspissated bile
- Steatosis in older children
- Focal biliary fibrosis
- Cirrhosis.

Endoscopy

- Oesophageal and gastric varices
- Portal hypertensive gastropathy.

Magnetic resonance cholangiopancreatography (MRCP)

- Sclerosing cholangitis
- Common bile duct stricture.

Management

Management is mainly symptomatic, i.e. avoiding fat-soluble vitamin deficiency, choleretic agents to improve bile flow, endoscopic management of bleeding varices, aggressive nutritional support, and liver transplantation in small number of patients.

Ursodeoxycholic acid

Ursodeoxycholic acid is a naturally occurring bile acid with choleretic, cytoprotective, membrane-stabilizing, antioxidant, and immunomodulatory properties. Treatment with ursodeoxycholic acid has been shown to improve biochemical and morphological parameters.

Endoscopy

Regular banding or sclerotherapy can provide good control of oesophageal varices and reduce the risk of bleeding.

Nutritional support

A dietician should be involved in the care of the patient, to give a high energy diet with an increased proportion of fat, and protein supplements. Gastrostomy tube placement is not usually recommended in those with portal gastropathy and varices.

Liver transplantation

Most centres would consider the following complications as indications for liver transplantation in the absence of severe impairment of lung function where multiorgan transplantation should be considered.
• Deteriorating quality of life due to significant liver disease
• Progressive chronic liver disease with increasing coagulopathy and falling albumin
• Intractable ascites
• Recurrent variceal bleeding not controlled with endoscopic procedures
• Severe malnutrition with liver disease unresponsive to aggressive nutritional interventions.

Vomiting

Vomiting is a common symptom of gut disease but can also reflect disease outside the gastrointestinal tract. Vomiting refers to the forceful expulsion of gastric contents. It generally occurs as a consequence of activation of the emetic reflex.

There are three phases of vomiting:
- Nausea
- Retching
- Expulsion.

Nausea may manifest as irritability, pallor, excess salivation, sweating, and tachycardia. In infants the three phases are not as easy to distinguish as in adults.

Vomiting is controlled through the emetic reflex by the vomiting centre. The vomiting centre is a functional rather than anatomical entity which responds through afferent stimuli from the cerebral cortex, cerebellum, vestibular system, and gastrointestinal tract. The vomiting centre and area postrema (previously called the chemoreceptor trigger zone) in the floor of the fourth ventricle triggers the cascade of events that results in vomiting (motor and autonomic). Endogenous (e.g. sepsis) and exogenous (e.g. drugs) factors can impact directly at the area postrema.

The threshold for vomiting may be altered by factors such as gastro-eosophageal reflux, gastrointestinal dysmotility (constipation, delayed gastric emptying), lifestyle factors (e.g. high-fat diet), and gut disease.

Vomiting should be distinguished from **regurgitation**, the effortless expulsion of gastric contents which is common in healthy infants and older children who eat in excess. **Rumination** is the frequent regurgitation of ingested food and is generally thought to be largely behavioural.

Assessment

The assessment and management of vomiting requires a careful history and examination considering the wide differential diagnosis as below with investigation dependant on the clinical features.
- Vomiting can be acute or recurrent (chronic or cyclical).
- Acute vomiting is more likely to be infectious, surgical or neurological.
- The differential to consider in recurrent vomiting is much wider.
- Bilious (green/yellow/brown) vomit suggests intestinal obstruction.
- Haematemesis suggests upper gastrointestinal pathology, e.g. oesophagitis, Mallory–Weiss tear, oesophagitis.

Differential diagnosis

The differential diagnosis of vomiting is wide and almost any pathology can present with vomiting as a symptom.

- Infection, e.g. urinary tract infection, gastroenteritis
- Intestinal obstruction, e.g. achalasia, pyloric stenosis, intestinal atresia, malrotation, volvulus
- Gastroeosophageal reflux, oesophagitis and peptic ulcer disease, Mallory–Weiss tear
- Food allergy and intolerance, e.g. cow's milk allergy, soy allergy, coeliac disease
- Metabolic, e.g. diabetic ketoacidosis, inborn errors of metabolism, porphyria, chronic renal failure
- Renal, e.g. pelvi-ureteric junction obstruction, renal stone
- Neurological, e.g. CNS tumour, epilepsy
- Functional, e.g. functional dyspepsia/non-ulcer dyspepsia
- Psychological, e.g. food refusal, anxiety
- Drug induced
- Induced illness (e.g. poisoning).

Management

The treatment is directed at the individual cause.

Indications to consider antiemetic therapy

- Motion sickness
- Postoperative nausea and vomiting
- Cancer chemotherapy
- Cyclical vomiting syndrome
- Gastrointestinal motility disorders.

Acute gastroenteritis

Gastroenteritis is one of the commonest conditions seen in childhood. Presentation to medical practitioners occurs where there is concern over inadequate intake and dehydration, and persistence of diarrhoea and vomiting.

Assessment of dehydration and consideration of the wide differential diagnosis are important factors in planning management.

Pathogenesis

Viral infections affect enterocyte function within the villi of the small intestine. Different pathogens have distinct methods of causing enterocyte damage, from toxin production to direct invasion. The damage caused leads to loss of the normal regulation of salt and fluid absorption. Inflammation can lead to a high osmotic load within the gut lumen precipitating further loss of fluid. Bacterial pathogens invade the lining of the small and large bowel and trigger inflammation.

Aetiology

In up to 50% of cases of gastroenteritis the aetiological agent is not found even when extensive investigations are undertaken. In preschool children where an agent is looked for the commonest cause is a viral pathogen, particularly rotavirus (see Table 24.1). Rotavirus is estimated to be responsible for up to 25% of deaths due to diarrhoeal disease worldwide.

Table 24.1 Aetiology of gastroenteritis

Viruses	Bacteria	Parasites
Rotavirus[a]	Campylobacter	Giardia llambia
Norwalk-like	Salmonella	Entamoeba histolytica
Adenoviruses	Shigella	Cryptosporidium [c]
Small round virus	E. coli [b]	
Astroviruses	Clostridium difficile	

[a] Rotavirus (commonest), seasonal, peaks late winter. Different pathogenicity of different strains, peak age for infection 6/12–2 years.

[b] Enteropathogenic E. coli, enterotoxigenic E. coli 0157:H7 (associated with haemolytic uraemic syndrome).

[c] Particularly in the immunocompromised host.

Clinical features

The clinical features are diarrhoea, vomiting, fever, abdominal cramps, and lethargy. A viral cause is more likely if there is a short period between ingestion of the pathogen and the development of symptoms. A bacterial pathogen should be suspected in a child with abdominal pain whose stools contain blood or mucus (colitis). Fever is more common in bacterial infection. A history of recent antibiotic administration in a febrile, systemically unwell child raises the possibility of *Clostridium difficile* infection. Foreign travel or contact with people who have been abroad widens the range of potential aetiological agents. Clinicians should also be aware of recent outbreaks of particular pathogens. The immunocompromised or malnourished child is at risk of infection with more unusual organisms, and infections are likely to be more severe with systemic sequelae.

Differential diagnosis

The differential diagnosis is wide. The symptoms of acute gastroenteritis—diarrhoea and vomiting—can be due to enteric infection or a symptom of infection elsewhere (for example urinary tract infection). It may also be the symptomatology of non-infective pathology in the gut (e.g. food intolerance) or another body system (e.g. diabetes mellitus, inborn error of metabolism).

Key differentials to consider

- Other infections—otitis media, tonsillitis, pneumonia, septicaemia, urinary tract infection, meningitis
- Surgical causes such as pyloric stenosis, intestinal obstruction including malrotation), intussusception, appendicitis
- Gastro-oesophageal reflux
- Food intolerance
- Haemolytic uraemic syndrome
- Drugs—antibiotics, laxatives

Specific pathogens

Giardia llambia

- A protozoal parasite which is infective in the cyst form.
- It also exists in the trophozoite form.
- It is found in contaminated food and water.
- Clinical manifestations vary; can be asymptomatic, acute diarrhoeal disease, chronic diarrhoea. Partial villous atrophy is occasionally seen.
- Diagnosis is by stool examination for cysts or examination of the duodenal aspirate at small-bowel biopsy.
- Treatment is with metronidazole and is often given blind in suspicious cases.

Clostridium difficile

- A Gram-positive anaerobe.
- Risk factor is disruption of the normal intestinal flora by antibiotics.
- Clinical features vary from asymptomatic carriage to life-threatening pseudomembranous colitis.
- Pathogenesis is through toxin production.
- Treatment is with vancomycin (oral) or metronidazole (IV or oral). Probiotics may have a role. *Saccharomyces boulardii* and *Lactobacillus spp* have been used.
- Relapse rate is 15–20%.

Assessment

This is to establish the diagnosis and the degree of dehydration (Table 24.2). A careful history needs to be taken. The risk of dehydration increases proportionally to the number of episodes of loose stool and vomiting, and in inverse proportion to age, thus the frequency and duration of symptoms needs to be established. A child who is extremely thirsty is likely to be dehydrated. The best measure of dehydration is documented weight change before and during illness, although this is rarely available.

The examination should help to exclude the differentials listed on p. 172 and also to exclude symptoms from systemic illness secondary to other infection such as meningitis, pneumonia, etc. The clinical assessment of degree of dehydration is difficult. There is a continuum from a child who is not dehydrated to a child in shock. Shock is apparent in a child with prolonged capillary refill (>2 s centrally) and tachycardia. Signs of decompensated shock include altered level of consciousness and hypotension. Shock requires urgent treatment with IV or IO fluid administration according to resuscitation guidelines. Dehydration can be determined on the basis of multiple clinical parameters. The presence of a prolonged capillary refill, an abnormal skin turgor, absent tears, and abnormal respiratory pattern (deep, rapid breathing without other signs of respiratory distress suggests an acidosis) are the most reliable signs. An active, playful child with moist mucous membranes and non-sunken eyes is unlikely to be dehydrated. A normal capillary refill time (<2 s) makes severe dehydration very unlikely.

Risk factors for dehydration
- Age <12 months (increased surface area to volume ratio, osmotic load of an exclusive milk diet, tendency to more severe vomiting)
- Frequent stools (>8 day)
- Vomiting (>twice a day)
- Bottle- rather than breast-feeding
- Previous poor nutrition.

Hypernatraemic dehydration
- Previously common, but with more modern refined infant formulae it is fortunately now rare.
- Should be suspected in a child with a history and symptoms compatible with a considerable degree of dehydration but who has minimal clinical signs other than a doughy texture to their skin and irritability.

Table 24.2 Assessment of dehydration

% Dehydration	Severity	Clinical features
3%		Undetectable
3–5%	Mild	Slightly dry mucous membranes
5 %	Moderate	Decreased skin turgor, slightly sunken eyes, depressed fontanelle, circulation preserved.
10%	Severe	All above more marked, drowsiness, rapid weak pulse, cool extremities, capillary refill time >2 s
12–14%		Moribund

Management

The vast majority of children with gastroenteritis can be managed at home.

Indications to consider hospital admission
- Age <6 months
- Diagnosis is unclear/complications have arisen
- Home management fails/unable to tolerate oral fluids/vomiting
- Significant other medical condition, e.g. diabetes, immunocompromised, cyanotic congenital heart disease (risk of thrombosis with dehydration)
- Poor social circumstances
- Difficulty to assess
- Inability to re-assess.

Investigations
- Serum electrolytes are not helpful in establishing the degree of dehydration, but they should be performed before and during intravenous rehydration to ensure correct fluid administration. They are also useful to confirm a clinical suspicion of hypernatraemic dehydration.
- Stool samples are not routinely necessary, but they should be obtained where there is a history of prolonged or bloody diarrhoea or a history of recent foreign travel, and in apparent outbreaks of gastroenteritis. Stool should be cultured for bacteria and samples tested for viruses, particularly rotavirus. Basic microscopy should detect ova cysts and parasites in stool. Stool should be sent for *Clostridium difficile* toxin if infection is suspected.

Rehydration
- Enteral rehydration using oral rehydration therapy (ORT) is the recommended treatment for children with mild to moderate dehydration. This can be given by the nasogastric route if oral fluids are not tolerated. Intravenous fluids should be reserved for children who are unable to tolerate fluids by either the oral or nasogastric route.
- Children with shock should have their fluid volume restored with appropriate boluses of normal saline. Once adequate circulation is established, further rehydration should be commenced by the enteral route.
- Water alone is not suitable for rehydration following diarrhoea and vomiting as these losses will be rich in electrolytes which also need to be replaced.
- Oral rehydration solutions (ORS) contain various quantities of electrolytes, glucose, and base. In developed countries where non-cholera-type gastroenteritis is the norm, solutions containing sodium concentrations of ~60 mmol/L and carbohydrate (non-cereal) concentrations of ~90 mmol/L are recommended. These solutions are slightly hypotonic to the serum osmolality of ~290 mmol/L. This enables the rapid absorption of fluid. Isotonic sports drinks are not ideal for correcting dehydration secondary to gastroenteritis because the concentration of electrolytes is less than required and their major component is carbohydrate.

- In developing countries, where cholera is a major killer, the lower-osmolality solutions recommended above increase the risk of hyponatraemia. Thus enteral rehydration is performed using hypertonic oral rehydration solutions containing a sodium concentration of 90 mmol/L. There is also evidence that using a cereal-based carbohydrate also decreases the duration of diarrhoea in this population.
- Enteral rehydration is labour intensive but can be given by parents orally or by nursing staff via nasogastric tube. Oral fluid can be given by bottle or syringe, or from lollies made of frozen ORS. Most ORS needs to be consumed within 1 h of being made, unless it is stored immediately in a fridge where it can be kept for 24 h.
- Rapid enteral rehydration is preferred. The fluid deficit should be calculated and replaced over 4–6 h. Maintenance fluid requirements should be given during this time and continuing excessive losses also replaced. If there is suspicion of hypernatraemia the fluid deficit should be corrected more slowly, over at least 12 h, with repeated electrolyte monitoring.
- If there are continuing stool losses or vomiting these should be replaced with ORS 10 mL/kg per stool or vomit, particularly if losses are large.

Feeding and gastroenteritis

Breast-fed infants should continue breast-feeding even during rehydration with ORS. Formula-fed infants should restart undiluted formula after rehydration. In the older child an age-appropriate diet should also be restarted early after rehydration. These measures reduce risk of further dehydration and lead to smaller stool volumes and faster recovery.

- There is no role for prolonged starvation except in some children with secondary lactose intolerance in which case feeds can be regraded 1/4 to1/2 to full strength 12–24 hourly

Other treatments

- Antibiotics are of no proven benefit in cases of uncomplicated gastroenteritis, and may cause harm.
- In the case of *E. coli* 0157 antibiotics may precipitate haemolytic uraemic syndrome.
- Antibiotics in uncomplicated salmonella gastroenteritis may prolong salmonella excretion as well as promote resistance.
- Antibiotics are of benefit in bacterial gastroenteritis complicated by septicaemia or systemic infections. This should be done in consultation with the local microbiology/public health department.
- Antibiotics should be considered in both immunocompromised and malnourished patients. They may be used in cases of prolonged infection, e.g. giardiasis and amoebiasis.
- There is no role for antiemetics
- There is no role for drugs to alter intestinal motility such as loperamide and opiate derivatives which have the potential to mask fluid losses by delaying gut transit.
- The role of probiotics in gastroenteritis, and particular type of these, is yet to be established. Some evidence suggests that *Lactobacillus* may be of benefit in reducing duration of symptoms.

Prevention

- Most gastroenteritis is spread by faeco-oral transmission and some results from uncooked or contaminated foods. Proper sanitation and attention to food preparation and storage as well as rigorous hand hygiene can prevent infection or control spread of disease.
- All cases of confirmed bacterial gastroenteritis should be notified to the local public health department.
- Within hospital during an episode of gastroenteritis children should be isolated from the general ward and especially from immunocompromised patients.
- Immunity to rotavirus infection develops during the first 2–3 years of life and is thought to prevent severe infection. As a result there has been much interest in developing an effective vaccine. One vaccine was voluntarily withdrawn after an increased risk of intussusception was identified. Subsequent vaccines have demonstrated good safety records, good immunogenicity and reduced hospital admissions and need for IV rehydration. Whether these results are applicable to all populations, particularly malnourished individuals, remains to be seen, and they are yet to become part of any routine immunization schedule.

Complications

- Dehydration, metabolic acidosis, and electrolyte disturbance (especially hypokalaemia, hyponatraemia and hypernatraemia).
- Carbohydrate intolerance is relatively common after acute gastroenteritis (particularly rotavirus infection), manifested by explosive stools. This can cause significant and rapid dehydration as an osmotic effect. Most is self limiting and, particularly if secondary to rotavirus infection, may respond to a slow regrade back on to a normal feed (see earlier). Monosaccharide intolerance (glucose malabsorption) is occasionally seen and requires a period on IV fluids. Persistent loose, frequent stool which often leads to damage to the perianal skin is usually transient. Stool reducing substances will be positive (>0.5%) and stool acidic; can be tested if diagnosis is uncertain. If symptoms persist a 4–6 week trial of a lactose-free diet is advised. Topical barrier creams prevent perianal ulceration.
- Post enteritis syndrome with enteropathy may respond to cow's milk/soya protein exclusion. (see Chapter 32, Chronic diarrhoea.)
- Complications can arise from inappropriate prescription of intravenous fluids to correct rehydration.
- Rapid correction of hypernatraemia can lead to cerebral oedema; serum sodium should be measured regularly and a gradual reduction aimed for.
- Haemolytic uraemic syndrome occurs in 6–9% of *E. coli* 0157 infections. It is characterized by sudden onset of pallor, lethargy, and oliguria after gastroenteritis. Examination findings are of a dehydrated child, with pallor and petechiae. Anaemia and thrombocytopenia are present on the full blood count. Blood film will show fragmented red cells, burr and helmet cells. Urinalysis often reveals mild microscopic haematuria and proteinuria.

Chronic diarrhoea

If diarrhoea persists for more than 2 weeks it is said to be chronic. This can reflect:
- Continued infection with the first pathogen
- Infection with a second pathogen
- Post enteritis syndrome
- Unmasking of a non-infective cause of chronic diarrhoea such as inflammatory bowel disease, food intolerance, coeliac disease, immunodeficiency, constipation with overflow, pancreatic insufficiency.

References and resources

Elliot EJ. Acute Gastroenteritis in children. *BMJ* 2007;334:35–40

Murphy MS. Guidelines for managing acute gastroenteritis based on a systematic review of published research. *Arch Dis Child* 1998;**79**:279–284

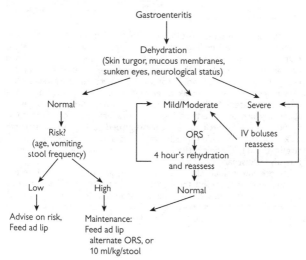

Fig. 24.1 Management of hydration in gastroenteritis. Reproduced with permission from Murphy (1998).

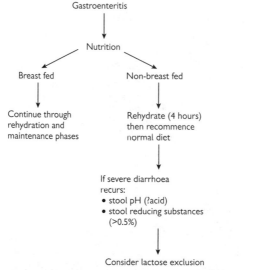

Fig. 24.2 Management of feeding in gastroenteritis. Reproduced with permission from Murphy (1998).

Case study

A previously well 6 month old infant (bottle fed) develops acute gastroenteritis manifest by frequent, watery explosive stools. She develops dehydration and requires admission to hospital. She is managed (as is conventional) by oral rehydration therapy for rehydration then a rapid return to normal diet. Stool is rotavirus positive. Her diarrhoea settles initially then recurs once milk is reintroduced. The stools are again frequent and watery. Stool is positive to reducing substances, suggesting secondary lactose intolerance. She requires a further period of oral rehydration therapy and is then gradually regarded back on to full strength milk (1/4 strength made up with oral rehydration solution, 1/2 then full strength) and her stools settle over the next few days by which time she is ready for discharge.

Lactose intolerance after rotavirus infection is common. If severe it can cause dehydration through the osmotic effect of malabsorbed carbohydrate (loose, watery, explosive stools). It is usually short-lived, responding either to a more gradual reintroduction of milk or to a period (4–6 weeks) on a lactose-free diet.

Gastro-oesophageal reflux

Introduction

Gastro-oesophageal reflux is very common. It refers to the passage of gastric contents into the lower oesophagus. It is a normal physiological phenomenon, particularly common in infancy. It is also seen in older children and adults, particularly after meals. It is secondary to transient relaxation of the lower oesophageal sphincter not associated with swallowing.

- **Physiological reflux** is normal in infancy, and is also normal in older children and adults who eat in excess.
- **Regurgitation** refers to the effortless return of gastric contents into the pharynx and mouth and is distinct from vomiting which is the forceful return of gastric contents into the pharynx and mouth.
- **Physiological reflux** is regurgitation without morbidity or clinical signs suggestive of gastro-oesophageal reflux disease. It is common and the natural history is resolution particularly as the child starts solids and becomes ambulant. More than 50% of normal infants regurgitate more than twice a day. A major factor is the high fluid volume per kilogram ingested at that age compared with older children/adults. In most infants the tendency to reflux resolves by age 12 months.
- **Adolescent rumination syndrome** is effortless regurgitation seen in older children and adolescents. The condition is benign providing complications such as weight loss do not occur.
- **Gastro-oesophageal reflux disease** (GORD) implies reflux with significant morbidity including failure to thrive, respiratory disease, and oesophagitis or complications of oesophagitis such as stricture.

The umbrella term gastro-oesophageal reflux therefore covers a considerable spectrum ranging in severity from an intermittent nuisance to life-threatening disease.

Reflux oesophagitis

Oesophagitis implies acid- or rarely alkali-induced damage to the lower oesophagus, which can be painful. Crying and irritability may be symptoms of oesophagitis in infants, similar to the adult complaint of heartburn and chest pain. Children with oesophagitis can develop a food aversion as a consequence of experiencing pain when they eat, and food refusal can be the presenting feature. This is likely to be a significant factor in the faltering growth seen in some children with reflux. This can be difficult to diagnose and requires treatment of the oesophagitis before a feeding program is instituted to deal with the food aversion.

Symptoms and signs of GORD

Typical
- Excessive regurgitation/vomiting
- Nausea
- Weight loss/faltering growth
- Irritability with feeds, arching, colic/food refusal
- Dysphagia
- Chest/epigastric discomfort
- Excessive hiccups
- Haematemesis/anaemia—iron deficient
- Aspiration pneumonia
- Oesophageal obstruction due to stricture.

Atypical
- Wheeze/intractable asthma
- Cough/stridor
- Cyanotic episodes
- Generalized irritability
- Sleep disturbance
- Neuro-behavioural symptoms—breath holding, Sandifer syndrome, seizure-like events, dystonia
- Worsening of pre-existing respiratory disease
- Apnoea/apparent life threatening events/sudden infant death syndrome

The association between gastro-oesophageal reflux and apparent life-threatening events is somewhat controversial and probably only relevant if the infant vomits, chokes, or goes blue during or immediately after feeds.

Investigation

- A full assessment of infants is essential including a careful feeding history. It is important to consider the differential diagnosis (see box on p. 185). Careful attention needs to be paid to symptom severity, impact on growth, and social factors that may be relevant, e.g. parental anxiety and stress.
- Mild or functional reflux is common. It rarely requires specific investigation and is a clinical diagnosis. However careful clinical assessment of cases and consideration of the differential diagnosis is necessary.
- More severe cases require further investigation/assessment. Investigation of reflux is often invasive and not necessarily precise, and needs careful planning. There are a number of different investigations. These must be done in conjunction with a careful history, including a feeding history and thorough examination.
- Difficult cases require specialist paediatric gastroenterological and/or paediatric surgical assessment.

Differential diagnosis of gastro-oesophageal reflux

- Infection, e.g. urinary tract infection, gastroenteritis
- Intestinal obstruction, e.g. pyloric stenosis, intestinal atresia, malrotation
- Food allergy and intolerance, e.g. cow's milk allergy, soy allergy, coeliac disease
- Metabolic disorders, e.g. diabetes, inborn errors of metabolism
- Psychological problems, e.g. anxiety
- Drug-induced vomiting, e.g. cytotoxic agents
- Primary respiratory disease, e.g. asthma, cystic fibrosis
- Rumination.

Gastro-oesophageal reflux and respiratory disease

- Obstructive apnoea with hypoxaemia and cyanosis can be the presenting feature in gastro-oesophageal reflux. There is some controversy about the causal relationship in that the obstructive apnoea may be the primary pathology with secondary gastro-oesophageal reflux. The mechanism probably relates to laryngospasm and can also manifest as intermittent stridor. Upper respiratory signs such as spasmodic croup, hoarseness or vocal cord nodules are seen in older children.
- There is a high incidence of gastro-oesophageal reflux in children with chronic respiratory disease, particularly asthma. This can be primary or secondary in that the respiratory disease may be secondary to reflux or the intrinsic lung disease (asthma, cystic fibrosis, immunodeficiency, tracheo-oesophageal fistula) may, through excessive coughing, result in reflux.

Indications for investigation of presumed gastro-oesophageal reflux

- Need to confirm the diagnosis
- Faltering growth
- Excessive vomiting
- Features suggestive of oesophagitis
- Abnormal electrolytes/acidosis
- Unexplained or difficult to control respiratory disease.

Barium radiology

- A barium swallow assesses the patient over only a short period. It will demonstrate reflux although is not particularly sensitive or specific. It can be diagnostic, but in less clear-cut cases may either miss pathological reflux or overdiagnose physiological reflux.
- It is, however, an essential investigation in the infant with severe symptoms suggestive of reflux when it will rule out large hiatus hernia, oesophageal stricture or web, atypical pyloric stenosis, gastric web, duodenal web, malrotation, volvulus, or other anatomical cause of recurrent vomiting.
- In older children it will exclude the above. It will also diagnose hiatus hernia, which functions as a reservoir for acid and increases the likelihood of reflux oesophagitis and so is relevant prognostically.

pH study

- This uses a probe to measure lower oesophageal pH and is considered by many to be the gold standard investigation.
- Its advantages are the ability to quantify reflux over a period of time (usually 24 h) and establish temporal relationships with atypical symptoms and events such as apnoea. It is particularly useful in children with respiratory or neuro-behavioural symptoms.
- Reproducibility is poor.
- The result is also affected by the clinical condition of the child on the day of the study which must, as far as possible, correlate with the normal state in terms of food intake and activity in particular.
- The recording should be interpreted as a whole in the clinical context. The time pH <4 (%) is quoted as the **reflux index**. In general 5–10% = mild reflux, 10–20% = moderate reflux which is usually controlled by medical therapy, 30% plus = severe and often requires surgical intervention.
- Children with physiological reflux do not require a pH study.

Specific indications for pH study

- Diagnostic uncertainty
- Poor response to medical treatment
- If surgery is being considered
- Children in whom doing the test will lead to a change in management.
- Symptoms suggesting occult reflux
- Unexplained or difficult to control respiratory disease.

The pH study may be falsely negative in the presence of alkaline reflux (reflux of alkaline stomach/duodenal contents). Either dual pH monitoring (electrode in stomach and oesophagus), oesophageal impedance or a radiolabelled milk scan is required to detect this. The radiolabelled milk scan will also give an estimate of gastric emptying.

Milk scan

- This uses continuous evaluation for up to an hour after a radio-labelled meal. It is independent of pH and so can detect alkaline reflux. It is after a physiological rather than an artificial meal. It is performed over a period of up to an hour with a delayed (24 h) film to look for aspiration. The technique is particularly useful in the diagnosis of non-acid reflux.
- It also gives an assessment of gastric emptying which is a useful indicator of overall gut motility. Markedly delayed gastric emptying is common in children with cerebral palsy in whom vomiting may reflect an overall gut dysmotility rather than GORD.
- The sensitivity for the detection of reflux is variable but can approach 95%.

Oesophagoscopy and oesophageal biopsy

- In children with suspected oesophagitis upper gastrointestinal endoscopy is a useful investigation and it should be considered in all children with severe symptomatic reflux.
- Biopsies need to be taken, as significant histological abnormality may not be obvious endoscopically.
- An eosinophilic infiltrate is characteristic of reflux oesophagitis.
- An excess of eosinophils suggests cow's milk allergic oesophagitis/eosinophilic oesophagitis.
- The distinction between reflux oesophagitis and eosinophilic oesophagitis is somewhat controversial.

Management

- Most patients with gastro-oesophageal reflux are managed in primary care by the health visitor and general practitioner.
- Simple measures are often effective including
  - explanation and reassurance about the natural history, parent education
  - review of feeding and feeding practice, e.g. check not being overfed, trial of smaller more frequent feeds, too small or too large a teat (both of which may cause air swallowing)
  - review of feeding posture
  - use of feed thickeners
  - use of anti-regurgitation milks.

Posture

Infants have significantly less reflux when placed in the prone position than in the supine position. However, prone positioning is associated with a higher rate of the sudden infant death syndrome (SIDS). In infants from birth to 12 months of age with reflux, the risk of SIDS generally outweighs the potential benefits of prone sleeping. In children >1 year it is likely that there is a benefit to right side positioning during sleep and elevation of the head of the bed.

Feed thickeners

Thickened feeds are helpful in reducing the symptoms of gastro-oesophageal reflux and this has been the subject of a recent Cochrane review. Feed thickeners and anti-reflux milks (which contain thickeners and thicken on contact with acid in the warm stomach environment) should be considered in children with persistent symptomatic reflux impacting on nutrient intake or through excessive vomiting on lifestyle, but are not indicated in healthy children who regurgitate. Feed thickeners include Carobel® (Cow & Gate) and Nestargel® (Nestlé). Some thickeners contain added energy and are unsuitable for infants. Anti-regurgitation milks e.g. Enfamil AR® (Mead Johnson) and SMA Staydown® are available over the counter. Both can be prescribed.

Milk exclusion

Children who have persistent symptomatic reflux, and evidence of atopy (positive family history, positive skin prick test) may warrant a trial of milk exclusion. The substitute milk should be with a protein hydrolysate (peptide or amino acid based, antigen free) feed. Examples include Nutramigen® (Mead Johnson), Neocate® (SHS). A 2 week trial is worthwhile. Solids need to be milk free. In some infants persistence to 6 weeks before making a decision about efficacy is sometimes necessary.

- Soya formulae should not be used. There is significant cross reactivity between cow's milk and soya protein and because of the presence of phytoestrogens in soya milks they are not recommended in infants <6 months.

Specific treatment

It is necessary to proceed to drug treatment in children with severe symptomatic reflux or symptoms and signs suggestive of GORD. The evidence base for drug treatment is well reviewed elsewhere.

Compound alginates

Compound alginates (e.g. Gaviscon®) are effective symptomatic treatment for gastro-oesophageal reflux. Gaviscon® works by reacting with gastric acid to form a viscous gel. Infant Gaviscon® comes in a dual sachet, 1 dose <4.5 kg, 2 doses > 4.5 kg, max 6 times a day. In infants Gaviscon® can be added to feeds, or for breast-fed infants dissolved in cooled boiled water and given by spoon after a feed.

Acid suppression

- H_2 blockers, e.g. ranitidine
- Proton pump inhibitors e.g. omeprazole.

Ranitidine is the most widely used. It is safe and well tolerated and can be considered before any further investigation in children who are thriving and in whom the diagnosis is robust. Dose is 2–4 mg/kg twice daily; the syrup can be used (75mg/5 mL).

Children with proven oesophagitis or severe symptomatic reflux proven on other tests are probably better treated with proton pump inhibitors; prescription is usually initiated by a paediatrician. Omeprazole is the most commonly used in children. It is available as a tablet or capsule. The tablet can be gently mixed or dispersed (not crushed) or the capsule broken for ease of administration in children. Dosage is 0.7–1.4 mg/kg per day although higher doses can be used. There are other proton pump inhibitors available including lansoprazole, which is available in a sachet that reconstitutes into a pink suspension with a strawberry flavour, although it has been used less in children.

Prokinetic drugs

These increase lower oesophageal sphincter pressure, improve oesophageal clearance and aid gastric emptying. Examples include metoclopramide, domperidone, and erythromycin. Metoclopramide is a dopamine antagonist. It is effective but because of concerns about the extrapyramidal effects is not widely used although a recent Cochrane review suggests it is probably underused and is effective. Domperidone, also a dopamine agonist has a much better side-effect profile although there is only limited efficacy data. Erythromycin has a role, although there is a significant gastrointestinal side-effect profile.

Role of surgery

Surgery is indicated when medical management of GORD has failed. Surgery is usually a fundoplication with a pyloroplasty if there is delayed gastric emptying. A gastrostomy for feeding is often done at the same time, particularly if there are feeding problems.

It is important to be aware of potential postsurgical problems which include recurrence of reflux (10%), retching, bloating, dumping, and intestinal obstruction which can be a late complication and in the absence of vomiting may not be diagnosed—with potentially disastrous consequences.

Patient groups at high risk of needing surgery
- Children with neurodisability
- Respiratory disease with intractable reflux (e.g. oesophageal atresia, bronchopulmonary dysplasia)
- Children with complications of oesophagitis such as stricture
- Barrett's oesophagus (rare in childhood)
- Tracheo-oesophageal fistula repair.

Barrett's oesophagus
- This refers to the presence of metaplastic columnar epithelium in the lower oesophagus. thought to be a consequence of long-standing gastro-oesophageal reflux.
- There is an increased risk of adenocarcinoma of the oesophagus.
- It is rare in childhood and requires aggressive medical treatment, of the gastro-oesophageal reflux and regular endoscopic surveillance.
- Surgery (fundoplication) is often considered.

Eosinophilic oesophagitis
- This condition, as part of the spectrum of eosinophilic gastroenteropathies/allergic disorders, is seen with increased frequency (see Chapter 45)
- There is a symptom overlap with gastro-oesophageal reflux.
- It is most common in older atopic boys.
- Dysphagia is a prominent symptom.
- Allergy testing is helpful. The pH study may be positive. There is an abundance of eosinophils on oesophageal biopsy.
- Treatments include those for gastro-oeosophageal reflux, trial of dietary elimination, steroids, anti-inflammatories, immunosuppression.
- There is a natural history of relapse, remission, and chronicity.
- Repeat biopsies are occasionally needed.

Feeding problems in cerebral palsy
Children with cerebral palsy commonly suffer from feeding difficulties of which gastro-oesophageal reflux is a component. Assessment of the contribution of gastro-oesophageal reflux requires considerable care. There are many potential causes of feeding difficulties:
- Bulbar weakness with oesophageal incoordination
- Primary or secondary aspiration
- Reflux oesophagitis
- Widespread gut dysmotility.
- Mobility and posture, degree of spasticity
- Poor nutritional state
- Constipation.

Children require careful multidisciplinary assessment by a feeding team including dietetics, speech and language therapy, occupational therapy and the neurodevelopmental paediatrician. A video barium assessment of the swallow is often indicated. GORD, if present, should be treated aggressively.

Attention to nutrition is of key importance and many children with feeding difficulties benefit from a feeding gastrostomy. A fundoplication is required if reflux is severe although in some cases improved nutritional status will result in improvement of the reflux.

Gut motility is a key factor in feed tolerance in children with cerebral palsy who may have delayed gastric emptying, which impacts significantly on the ability to feed particularly if nutrition is dependent on nasogastric or gastrostomy feeding. It is important to recognize this as a separate condition from reflux when the dysmotility is upper gastrointestinal only. Abdominal pain, bloating, and constipation are common feature of gut dysmotility. Therapeutic strategies include explanation and reassurance, prokinetic agent such as domperidone, laxatives, and occasionally (if there is a need for distal gut deflation) suppositories. It may be necessary to give feeds by continuous infusion. A milk-free diet for a trial period of 2–4 weeks can be helpful. Hydrolysed protein formula feed may be given as a milk substitute.

Differential diagnosis of reflux oesophagitis

Non-reflux causes of oesophagitis include:
- Cows' milk allergic oesophagitis (see above)
- Eosinophilic oesophagitis
- Candidal oesophagitis
- Chemical oesophagitis from caustic ingestion
- Achalasia
- Crohn's disease

References and resources

Fox M, Forgacs I. Gastro-oesophageal reflux disease. *BMJ* 2006;332:88–93

The reader is also referred to the comprehensive evidence-based guidelines produced by the North American Society of Pediatric Gastroenterology, Hepatology and Nutrition (NASPGHAN) and published on their website, www.naspghan.org

Rudolph CD, Mazur LJ, Liptak GS. Guidelines for evaluation and treatment of gastroesophageal reflux in infants and children: recommendations of the North American Society for Pediatric Gastroenterology and Nutrition. *J Paediatr Gastroenterol Nutr* 2001; **32**(S2): 1–31

Helicobacter pylori infection, peptic ulceration, and Meckel's diverticulum

Helicobacter pylori

- *H. pylori* is a Gram-negative organism. It is a very common infection worldwide. Infection is usually acquired in childhood, but prevalence rates are variable, being highest in developing countries. Most individuals infected with *H. pylori* do not experience symptoms or show signs.
- Persistent infection causes an antral gastritis, the most common manifestation in childhood, which may be asymptomatic.
- There is a strong relation between *H. pylori* infection and peptic ulceration in both adults and children.
- *H. pylori* is also a carcinogen (increased risk of gastric lymphoma, adenocarcinoma).
- There is no proven association between *H. pylori* infection and recurrent abdominal pain except in the rare cases where gastric or duodenal ulcer disease is present.
- Transmission is faeco-oral and familial clustering is common, with increased prevalence in institutions.

Investigation

- This should be considered in children with symptoms suggestive of peptic ulceration (epigastric pain, bloating, haematemesis, night pain) or proven peptic ulceration.
- The precise investigation (invasive or non-invasive) depends on the clinical picture, local prevalence and tests available.
- It is not indicated in children with recurrent abdominal pain or other chronic symptoms in the absence of features which suggests peptic ulcer disease.

Investigations available

- Urea breath testing (C-13 breath test, urea labelled with carbon-13): highly sensitive and specific for active (acute) infections. Need to stop antibiotics, proton pump inhibitors and H_2 antagonists before the test (local protocol), widely used to confirm eradication of *H. pylori* after treatment
- Stool antigen testing: under evaluation, highly sensitive and specific. Need to stop antibiotics, proton pump inhibitors and H_2 antagonists before the test (local protocol).
- Serology (IgG antibody): less specific, with high false-positive rate; positive serology persists for 6–12 months after infection, negative test excludes *H. pylori* infection
- Endoscopy allows the detection of peptic ulcer disease, gastritis, and oesophagitis with direct visualization of the mucosa and biopsy. Lymphoid nodular hyperplasia in the gastric antrum is commonly seen. Biopsies can be sent for culture (low yield) and PCR. Rapid urease testing can be done (e.g. CLO test) on biopsies at the time of endoscopy.

Treatment

- Treatment is indicated for *H. pylori* infection in the presence of peptic ulceration and, although controversial, antral gastritis if *H. pylori* positive.
- Treatment of children diagnosed through non-invasive testing is dependent on the clinical situation and factors such as the prevalence of *H. pylori* infection in the local population and family history need to be taken into account when the decision is made.
- There are various regimens. Drug resistance is common. Treatment is for 1 or 2 weeks; 2 week therapy offers the possibility of higher eradication rates although adverse effects and compliance are a major problem. The most commonly used regimens include omeprazole, amoxicillin, and metronidazole or clarithromycin. Local protocols should determine which combinations are first and second line. There is no need to continue with long-term proton-pump inhibitor therapy unless there is frank ulceration complicated by perforation or haemorrhage. The reader is referred to the current version of the British National Formulary (BNF) for Children for up-to-date treatment guidelines.
- Outcome after treatment is variable. Treatment failure usually indicates antibacterial resistance, re-infection within families or institutions, or poor compliance.

Other causes of antral gastritis and peptic (gastric and duodenal) ulceration

- Severe systemic illness—traumatic brain injury (Cushing ulcer), extensive burns (Curling ulcer)
- Non-steroidal anti-inflammatory drugs
- Corticosteroids
- Inflammatory bowel disease
- Eosinophilic gastritis
- Autoimmune gastritis (adults)
- Zollinger–Ellison syndrome
- Coeliac disease.

Risk factors for peptic ulceration

- Genotype
- Stress
- Alcohol
- Corticosteroids
- Smoking.

Zollinger–Ellison syndrome

This results from a gastrin-producing tumour of the endocrine pancreas, presenting with gastric acid hypersecretion and resulting in fulminant, intractable peptic ulcer disease.

Meckel's diverticulum

- Remnant of the vitellointestinal duct.
- Present in 2% of individuals.
- 50% contain ectopic gastric, pancreatic, or colonic tissue.
- Present in the distal ileum on the anti-mesenteric border within 100 cm of the ileocaecal valve and is around 5–6 cm long.
- Presents with intermittent, painless blood per rectum; bleeding can be quite severe and may require a blood transfusion; other presentations include intussusception (commoner in older males), perforation, and peritonitis.
- A technetium scan is used to look for ectopic gastric mucosa although it can be negative even in the presence of bleeding.
- Treatment is by resection of the diverticulum.

References and resources

Gold BD, Colletti RB, Abbott M. Helicobacter infection in children: recommendations for diagnosis and treatment. *J Paediatr Gastroenterol Nutr* 2000;**31**:490–537. Available from www.naspghan.org.

Cyclical vomiting syndrome

Cyclical vomiting was first described by Samuel Gee in 1882. It refers to intense periods of vomiting with symptom-free intervals. The incidence is unknown. It occurs principally in pre-school or early school age children. Epilepsy is a risk factor. Other risk factors include a history of recurrent headache, migraine (50%), travel sickness, and irritable bowel syndrome (50%) in children and their families.

Clinical features

More than 50% of sufferers have a predictable cyclicity with a consistent pattern of attack. Symptom onset is usually during the night or first thing in the morning. Episodes last several hours to days, although rarely >72 h. Episodes can end abruptly (suddenly better), end after sleep, or progress to severe dehydration.

There are three classical behaviours:
- Subdued but responsive
- Writhing and moaning
- 'Conscious coma'.

Nausea is characteristic with pallor, increased salivation, and lethargy. Epigastric discomfort occurs secondary to vomiting. Haematemesis/Mallory–Weiss tear can occur if vomiting is extreme. Autonomic features include hypertension, tachycardia, flushing. Neutrophilia and SIADH can occur. Behaviours include 'spit out' (won't swallow saliva), guzzling fluid followed by vomiting, intense thirst, irritability, inability to communicate (social withdrawal), and panic. Headache (25%), abdominal pain, fever, and loose stools are common.

Diagnostic criteria

- Recurrent severe, discrete episodes of vomiting
- Varying intervals of normal health in between
- Duration of vomiting from days to hours
- Other causes of the vomiting excluded
- Supportive criteria include—self-limiting, episodes stereotypical (true to form).

Triggers

Anxiety is a major factor. Emotional stress, life events (stressful and non-stressful, e.g. birthday), travel sickness, infections, and fatigue can trigger episodes. Often the precise trigger is unknown.

Cyclical vomiting syndrome plus refers to a subgroup of children with cyclical vomiting syndrome who develop early ketosis and have some additional neurodevelopmental problems such as neurodevelopmental delay, seizures, hypotonia, or attention deficit hyperactivity disorder. Can occur with mitochondrial disorders.

Investigation

It is important to take a full history and conduct a careful examination. Clinical examination is usually normal (apart from dehydration). Coexistent neurodevelopmental problems need to be excluded. Further investigation should be dependent on the clinical situation with a low threshold to investigate for other potential causes of vomiting, particularly if the presentation is atypical, with metabolic and neurological investigation if there are any risk factors. Causes of intermittent vomiting with symptom-free periods include metabolic disorders (e.g. urea cycle disorders), disturbances in gut motility, congenital abnormalities of the gastrointestinal tract (e.g. malrotation, duplication cyst), renal disorders, endocrine problems (e.g. adrenal insufficiency), pancreatitis, diabetes, and CNS lesions. It is also important to consider food intolerance, gastro-oesophageal reflux, peptic ulceration, constipation, and coeliac disease, all of which can present with significant vomiting.

Management

- There are no evidence-based recommendations.
- Chronic sufferers benefit from a named paediatrician and personalized management plan.

There are three phases:
- Prodrome
- Episode
- Recovery.

Prodrome
- This is the period between onset of symptoms and vomiting.
- Try ondansetron for nausea.
- Try lorazepam for anxiety.
- Simple analgesia for abdominal pain.

Episode
- This is characterized by intense nausea and vomiting; potential problems include dehydration (including hypovolaemic shock in extreme cases), electrolyte disturbance, haematemesis.
- Treatment needs to be initiated promptly particularly if there is a risk of dehydration.
- IV hydration with saline bolus and then maintenance fluids.
- IV ondansetron.
- Consider IV lorazepam, chlorpromazine.
- Consider other potential causes of vomiting.

Recovery
- Tend to recover rapidly, although can be prolonged.
- Consider prophylaxis and treatment plan for further episodes.

Prophylaxis

- Reduce triggers, e.g. anxiety, stress, food intolerance, prolonged fast.
- Anti-migraine prophylactic agents including pizotifen, amitriptyline, and propranolol have been tried.
- The long-term outcome is generally good

References and Resources

Useful treatment guidelines: www.cvsa.org.uk/treatmentframe.html

Pyloric stenosis

Infantile hypertrophic pyloric stenosis is a common cause of vomiting in infancy with an incidence of 2 to 3 per 1000 live births. Males are more commonly affected than females and there is a genetic predisposition. First-born males are more commonly affected.

- It results from hypertrophy of the pyloric muscle.
- Presentation is with vomiting.
- Vomiting is non-billions, effortless, and projectile.
- Onset usually between 3 and 8 weeks.
- Infant has a 'worried' look.
- Infant is generally active and alert and presents hungry after vomiting and with weight loss.
- Dehydration is common.
- Pylorus may be palpable (olive size) and visible gastric peristalsis present.
- Hypochloraemic, hypokalaemic metabolic alkalosis occurs as a consequence of vomiting gastric contents (rich in hydrogen and chloride), loss of potassium to preserve electrolyte equilibrium.
- Mild unconjugated hyperbilirubinaemia can be present.
- Ultrasound confirms the diagnosis demonstrating thickening of the pyloric wall. Barium radiology can be helpful in difficult cases and demonstrates the 'string' sign.
- Treatment is by pyloromyotomy (Ramstedt's procedure) after rehydration with correction of the electrolyte and acid–base disturbance.
- Preoperative fluids should be as 120–150 mL/kg of 0.45% saline 5% glucose with added potassium. Dehydration should be corrected if severe with a fluid bolus. Continuing losses should be replaced with 0.9% saline with added potassium. Electrolytes should be monitored and the replacement regimen altered accordingly.
- Most infants recover rapidly, feeding 6–12 hours postoperatively.
- Complications are rare.
- The differential diagnosis includes any other cause of vomiting presenting in early infancy. In particular urinary tract infection should be excluded. Gastro-oesophageal reflux should be considered. The differential diagnosis of pyloric outlet/duodenal obstruction includes duodenal web, duodenal stenosis, and malrotation.

Achalasia and malrotation

Achalasia

This is a motility disorder in which there is impaired peristalsis in the oesophagus and the lower oesophageal sphincter fails to relax with swallowing. This leads to food being held up in the oesophagus. Presentation tends to be in late childhood/adult life. Prevalence is around 1 in 10 000.

Clinical features include dysphagia, regurgitation, cough, chest discomfort, and weight loss. The differential diagnosis includes gastro-oesophageal reflux, hiatus hernia, eosinophilic oesophagitis, and functional causes (globus hystericus).

Investigation is by barium swallow with oesophagoscopy and biopsy if a mucosal lesion such as oesophagitis is suspected. Manometry, if available, is helpful. The appearance on barium swallow is characteristic with a fluid level and narrowing 'rat tail' appearance of the distal oesophagus. Secondary problems include reflux oesophagitis, aspiration, and poor weight gain. Achalasia can occur as a complication of anti-reflux surgery. Treatment options include balloon dilatation of the lower oesophageal sphincter, which will afford temporary relief, and Heller's myotomy. Botulinum toxin has been used in the elderly. There is an increased risk of oesophageal carcinoma in untreated achalasia.

Chagas disease

This is a parasitic infection seen in Central and South America that can mimic the changes of achalasia. Diagnosis is by serology.

Malrotation and volvulus

Malrotation of the small intestine is due to disordered movement of the intestine round the superior mesenteric artery during embryogenesis. The precise anatomy is determined by the stage of embryogenesis which was interrupted. In general the caecum (secured by Ladd's bands) remains in the right upper quadrant with the duodeno-jejunal junction in the right rather than left upper quadrant. There are serious potentially fatal sequelae.

There are two potential clinical syndromes:
- Duodenal obstruction from extrinsic compression from Ladd's bands
- Mid-gut volvulus (twisting) of the gut round a narrowed mesentery which can occur acutely causing complete obstruction or intermittently producing episodes of partial or complete obstruction. Symptoms of chronic 'intermittent' mid-gut volvulus include vomiting, abdominal pain, constipation, and diarrhoea (and malabsorption).

Malrotation is associated with duodenal atresia (1/3 of cases) and stenosis, exomphalos, gastroschisis, diaphragmatic hernia.
- Malrotation can be asymptomatic and an incidental finding on barium radiology.
- Most but not all of the cases that present clinically do so in infancy, mostly in the first few weeks.
- Malrotation with duodenal obstruction is part of the differential diagnosis of recurrent vomiting, particularly if bile-stained vomiting is present.
- Malrotation with volvulus can cause severe obstruction with ischaemia, perforation, and peritonitis.
- Bile staining may be green/yellow or brown, and vomiting can be inter-mittent with twisting and untwisting of the bowel.

Diagnosis of malrotation is by barium meal to assess the position of the duodeno-jejunal junction. Normal rotation is present if the duodenal C loop crosses the midline and places the duodenojejunal junction to the left of the spine at a level above or equal to the pylorus. If the barium meal does not confirm the presence or absence of malrotation, contrast enema may be indicated to clarify the position of the caecum.

Malrotation with volvulus can present as an acute abdominal pain with bile stained vomiting. The patient can be very unwell. This requires a rapid diagnostic work up and investigative laparotomy.

Management is by surgical correction of the malrotation. If either acute duodenal obstruction or malrotation with volvulus is suspected then this is a surgical emergency.

Ladd's procedure refers to the reduction of volvulus (if present), division of mesenteric bands, placement of small bowel on the right and large bowel on the left of the abdomen, and appendectomy.

Differential diagnosis of duodenal obstruction
- Duodenal atresia
- Duodenal stenosis
- Duodenal web
- Malrotation
- Annular pancreas
- Superior mesenteric artery syndrome

Superior mesenteric artery syndrome
This refers to duodenal obstruction caused by compression of the third part of the duodenum against the aorta by the superior meseteric artery and is seen following acute weight loss, e.g. anorexia nervosa, severe sepsis, immobilization (e.g. after scolioisis repair). The radiological appearance is characteristic. The condition usually requires nutritional restitution rather than surgical intervention. Nasojejunal feeding can be helpful.

Gastrointestinal bleeding

Overt gastrointestinal bleeding may occur as part of an acute illness or as a feature of chronic disease. Covert or obscure gastrointestinal bleeding may be uncovered in the investigation of anaemia.

Bleeding is alarming for parents. Assessment requires a balance between urgency when necessary and reassurance when the probable cause is less serious.

The priorities in assessment are to determine the severity of bleeding, the degree of systemic upset, the site, and the cause.

- In children bright red rectal bleeding may originate from the upper or lower gastrointestinal tract.
- The commonest cause of rectal bleeding in childhood is from anal fissure secondary to constipation.

Definitions

- Upper gastrointestinal bleeding:
  - **Haematemesis**—vomiting frank blood or black material ('coffee grounds', 'soil particles'). This needs to be distinguished from haemoptysis (Table 30.1, p. 214).
- Rectal bleeding:
  - **Melaena**—offensive black, tarry stools
  - **Haematochezia**—bright red or dark red blood per rectum.
- **Obscure gastrointestinal bleeding** is bleeding is from a presumed GI source when initial investigations, such as oesophago-gastroduodenoscopy (OGD) and colonoscopy, are normal.

Initial assessment

Resuscitation if actively bleeding

- Assess airway
- Assess breathing
- Assess circulation—if signs of compromise
  - prompt IV access with large-bore cannula
  - group and save/cross-match blood.
- Fluid resuscitate with 20 mL/kg 0.9% saline
- Re-assess
- Further 20 mL/kg 0.9% saline if necessary
- Re-assess
- 20 mL/kg blood if necessary.

Relevant history

- Colour of blood loss.
- Amount of blood lost.
- Is it definitely blood?
- Exclude bleeding from non-gastrointestinal source: haemorrhagic tonsillitis, epistaxis, dental work, haemoptysis, if breast-fed blood loss from a cracked nipple.
- Consider a bleeding disorder, thrombocytopenia.

- Ask about the presence of other gastrointestinal symptoms including diarrhoea, epigastric pain, abdominal pain or cramps, constipation, vomiting, previous diagnosis of irritable bowel syndrome, weight loss, steatorrhoea.
- Consider non-gastrointestinal symptoms including syncope, shortness of breath, dizziness, lethargy, palpitations, fever, rash.
- Include history appropriate to age, e.g. breast or bottle-feeding, was infant given vitamin K?
- Ask about recent foreign travel or infectious contacts.
- Ask about history of trauma
- Ask about current medications, e.g. non-steroidal anti inflammatory drugs (NSAIDS), warfarin, potentially hepatotoxic drugs
- Consider pertinent past medical history including presence of liver disease, gastrointestinal disorders, bleeding disorders
- Review the family history, e.g. inflammatory bowel disease, polyposis syndromes, bleeding disorder

Physical examination should aid in the assessment of the clinical stability of the child and may give clues as to the aetiology of the bleeding.

- It is important to look for signs of acute anaemia: pallor, tachycardia, gallop rhythm, hyper/hypotension and chronic anaemia: pallor, poor growth, lethargy.
- Assess whether the child is hypovolaemic or has signs of cardiovascular decompensation.
- Look for signs of chronic liver disease or coagulopathy.

Substances that can give the stool a bloody appearance

- Antibiotics
- Iron
- Liquorice
- Chocolate

Examination

Skin

- Pallor
- Jaundice
- Bruises
- Rashes.

ENT

- Tonsilitis
- Signs of bleeding.

Cardiovascular

- Tachycardia
- Hypotension/postural
- Prolonged capillary refill time.

Abdomen

- Tenderness
- Hepatosplenomegaly.

Perianal

- Fissure
- Excoriation or soreness/ bad nappy rash
- External haemorrhoids
- Fistulae or previous abscess: consider Crohn's disease.

Investigation

History and physical examination should guide the appropriate investigations (Tables 30.2 and 30.3). In acute bleeding blood results should be interpreted with caution as hypovolaemia leads to haemoconcentration and haemoglobin values can be artificially high. If a child loses half their circulating volume the haemoglobin concentration of the remaining volume takes time to dilute down to give a true reflection of blood loss. A full blood count should be repeated after fluid resuscitation. A 'group and save', urea and electrolytes and liver function including coagulation screen should also be performed. Renal function is helpful to assess degree of dehydration. Urea may be elevated secondary to absorption of blood (high protein load) from the gut.

Imaging

- If the source of bleeding is likely to be from the nasopharynx or the sinuses, CT scan should be considered.
- It can be difficult to differentiate between haematemesis and haemoptysis; in these cases a plain chest radiography may be helpful.
- In those with swallowing difficulties or epigastric pain an upper GI contrast study might be helpful, e.g. in the diagnosis of oesophageal strictures

- Technetium 99-m pertechnetate scan (Meckel's scan) will detect functional gastric mucosa in an ectopic location, e.g. Meckel's diverticulum, duplication cyst. A negative Meckel's scan does not exclude a Meckel's diverticulum.
- In patients with hepatosplenomegaly or other signs of chronic liver disease, abdominal ultrasound should be performed to look for evidence of portal hypertension and varices.
- Abdominal ultrasound can also be useful to look for bowel wall thickening which is suggestive of underlying inflammation.
- MRI angiography/technetium 99-m labelled red cell scanning has a role if the cause of blood loss remains uncertain.

Endoscopy

- OGD is indicated in children with haematemesis or melaena to establish the diagnosis and bleeding site; it is rarely necessary to perform diagnostic endoscopy when the child first presents. The degree of urgency depends on the likely cause of the bleeding and need to start treatment. Urgent endoscopy allows for rapid diagnosis but carries a risk of decompensation and poor visualization of the mucosa. It is carried out only if patients cannot be stabilized, surgical colleagues should be involved.
- Colonoscopy and ileoscopy should be performed in children with per rectum blood loss who do not have evidence of infective colitis or constipation/anal fissure. It is crucial that patients have had adequate bowel preparation before colonoscopy; otherwise the information obtained is very limited.
- Push enteroscopy/laparoscopy/ laparotomy should be considered if the source of bleeding remains obscure.
- There is increasing use of wireless capsule endoscopy in obscure gastrointestinal bleeding, with good potential to visualize the small intestinal mucosa directly.

Table 30.1 Difference between haemoptysis and haematemesis

	Haemoptysis	**Haematemesis**
Colour	Bright red and frothy	Dark red or brown
pH	Alkaline	Acid
Consistency	Mixed with sputum	Mixed with food
Symptoms	Gurgling, coughing	Nausea, retching

Can measure the amylase in saliva (high) to clarify if saliva is mixed with blood.

Table 30.2 Upper GI bleeding: aetiology and appropriate investigation

Age	Common aetiology	Investigations that may be appropriate
Neonate/infant	Swallowed maternal blood	APT test for maternal haemoglobin
	Oesophagitis/gastritis	FBC, U&E, LFT, coagulation screen, gastroscopy
	Vitamin K deficiency	
	Maternal NSAIDS	
	Maternal idiopathic thrombocytopenic purpura	Maternal full blood count
	Pulmonary haemosiderosis	CXR
	Factitious	
Child	Mallory–Weiss tear	FBC, U&E, LFT, coagulation screen
	Haemorrhagic tonsilitis	
	Oesophagitis/gastritis/peptic ulcer disease	Gastroscopy
	Oesophageal varices/Gastric varices	Abdominal ultrasound/ gastroscopy
	Pulmonary haemosiderosis	CXR
	Factitious	
Adolescent	Mallory–Weiss tear	FBC, U&E, LFT, coagulation screen
	Haemorrhagic tonsilitis	
	Oesophagitis/gastritis/ peptic ulcer disease	Gastroscopy
	Oesophageal varices/Gastric varices	Abdominal ultrasound/gastroscopy
	Factitious	

Table 30.3 Lower GI bleeding: aetiology and appropriate investigation

Age	Common aetiology	Appropriate investigations
Neonate/ infant	Swallowed maternal blood	APT test for maternal haemoglobin
	Anal fissure/constipation	FBC, U&E, LFT, Coagulation screen
	Allergic colitis/ cow's milk protein intolerance	Skin prick testing, milk RAST
	Necrotizing enterocolitis	AXR, CRP
	Hirschsprung's disease	Rectal biopsy
	Infective colitis	Stool specimen MC&S, Clostridium difficile
	Intussusception	Abdominal ultrasound
	Maternal ITP	FBC
	Meckel's diverticulum	Meckel's scan
	Vascular malformation	Contrast CT/MRI
	Factitious	History/diagnosis of exclusion
Child/ adolescent	Anal fissure/constipation	As above
	Threadworms	Examination of perineum/ Sellotape slide test
	Infectious colitis	As above
	Polyps	Endoscopy
	Inflammatory bowel disease	Endoscopy
	Intussusception	As above
	Meckel's diverticulum	As above
	Haemolytic uraemic syndrome	Blood film, urine dipstick
	Henoch–Schoenlein purpura	
	Vascular malformation	
	Factitious	As above

Differential diagnosis

Upper GI bleeding (Table 30.2)

Neonate and infant

- Significant haematemesis or melaena is rare in infants.
- Neonates can swallow maternal blood at delivery or amniotic fluid containing blood; breast-fed babies can swallow blood from cracked, bleeding nipples.
- Critically ill neonates can develop stress ulcers in the first days of life; these can present with significant GI bleed secondary to erosive gastritis or gastric ulcers.
- Mucosal bleeding can be secondary to coagulopathy caused by: vitamin K deficiency, maternal ITP or use of NSAIDS, haemophilia, or Von Willebrand's disease. It is rare for vitamin K deficiency or platelet defects to present with GI haemorrhage but relatively common for Von Willebrand's disease to present with mucosal bleeding.
- Significant non-gastrointestinal haematemesis can occur from ENT causes. This is rare in isolation in this age group, but can occur associated with coagulopathy. Pulmonary haemosiderosis commonly presents with haemoptysis. It is caused by recurrent bleeding into alveolar spaces and interstitial lung tissue. Chest radiograph shows alveolar infiltrates, and siderophages are found on bronchoalveolar lavage.

Older child

- In the patient with preceding retching and vomiting who then develops haematemesis a Mallory–Weiss tear with bleeding from the gastro-oesophageal junction/proximal oesophagus is a common cause.
- Infective, haemorrhagic tonsillitis can present with small-volume haematemesis (vomiting swallowed blood).
- As in infants, primary peptic ulcers are very rare but can occur secondary to multisystem disease such as head trauma or septicaemia with shock or secondary to medications.
- Helicobacter pylori gastritis can cause acute haematemesis.
- Variceal bleeding is a rare but important cause of significant haematemesis at all ages, and signs of chronic liver impairment should be looked for.

Adolescent

- As above
- Mallory–Weiss tears can occur following vomiting caused by alcohol ingestion.
- Primary peptic ulcers more commonly present at this age.
- Higher use of NSAIDS in this age group leads to a higher presentation of gastritis as a complication.

For all age groups, factitious/induced bleeding needs to be considered.

Mallory Weiss syndrome refers to bleeding from tears (Mallory Weiss tears) in the mucosa at the junction of the stomach and oesophagus, usually caused by severe retching, coughing, and vomiting.

Lower GI bleeding (Table 30.3)

Neonate/infant

- Constipation causing anal fissuring and bright red blood per rectum is probably the commonest cause of lower GI bleeding. It is not always possible to see obvious fissuring but the history is usually highly suggestive and the bleeding stops with appropriate treatment of the underlying constipation.
- Eosinophillic proctitis caused by dietary sensitivities, e.g. to cow's milk protein, is a common cause of bleeding per rectum. Allergy testing and trial of appropriate exclusion diet is usually very successful in establishing a diagnosis and stopping bleeding.
- Necrotizing enterocolitis is an important cause of bloody stools in the neonate. Clinical features and the classical radiological appearances of intramural gas or perforation usually make the diagnosis. Other causes of neonatal intestinal obstruction (e.g. volvulus) can present with blood per rectum.
- Hirschsprung's disease can present with enterocolitis.
- Infectious colitis is rare in this age group but can be a cause of bloody diarrhoea.
- Intussusception often presents with intermittent irritability, pallor, shock and, as a late feature, 'redcurrant jelly'-like stools.
- Meckel's diverticulum is the embryological remnant of the vitellointestinal duct, and is said to be present in 2% of the population. A Meckel's diverticulum can present with large quantities of painless rectal bleeding.
- Polyposis should be considered. Diagnosis is by endoscopy. The most likely type is a juvenile polyp. Polyps tend to produce bright red blood.

Older child/adolescent

- Children can have lower GI bleeding from many of the same causes as infants.
- In the older child with intussusception a lead point should be looked for.
- Patients with polyposis syndromes such as familial adenomatous polyposis coli (FAP) typically present in the older child. Diagnosis is by endoscopy. Management is dependent on the underlying syndrome.
- Inflammatory bowel disease often presents with bloody diarrhoea, particularly if there is a colitis. Other causes of an inflammatory colitis should be considered.
- Infection should be considered, e.g. salmonella, *Shigella*, *Escherichia coli*, *Clostridium difficile*.
- Local trauma, e.g. fissuring, prolapse, haemorrhoids, solitary rectal ulcer syndrome, sexual abuse should be considered.
- For all age groups factitious/induced bleeding should be considered.

Treatment

The management of GI bleeding requires accurate, prompt diagnosis and treatment of the underlying condition.

Gastrointestinal polyposis

Polyps generally present with painless rectal bleeding or through genetic screening of affected families with polyposis syndromes. There are various types, as listed in Table 31.1. Juvenile polyps (hamartomas) are the most commonly seen and generally benign.

Investigation requires full upper and lower gastrointestinal endoscopy. Barium radiology or push enteroscopy is required if small-bowel polyps are suspected.

Table 31.1 Classification of polyps

Hamartomas	Juvenile polyps
	Juvenile polyposis (multiple)
	Peutz–Jeghers syndrome
	Cowden's syndrome
	Bannayan–Riley–Ruvalcaba syndrome
Adenomas	Familial adenomatous polyposis
	Gardener's syndrome
	Turcot syndrome
Hyperplastic	
Inflammatory	

Hamartomas

Juvenile polyps
- More than 90% of polyps seen in childhood are juvenile polyps. They are hamartomas and have a stalk. They are usually easily detected by colonoscopy, usually presenting between ages 2 and 6 years with painless blood per rectum.
- Most polyps are solitary and located within 30 cm of the anus.
- Can regress but are seen in adults.
- Not premalignant.

Juvenile polyposis
- Juvenile polyposis (rare) refers to multiple (> 6) juvenile polyps.
- Polyps may be present throughout the gastrointestinal tract. Can be familial.
- Familial type is associated with autosomal dominant inheritance with variable penetrance.
- Premalignant.
- Prophylactic colectomy should be considered.

Peutz–Jeghers syndrome
- Rare: 1 in 120 000. Autosomal dominant inheritance.
- Hamartomatous polyps throughout the gastrointestinal tract associated with freckling and hyperpigmentation of the buccal mucosa and lips.
- Polyps tend to be large and pedunculated.
- Small bowel poyps may present as intussusception.

- Premalignant.
- Long term follow up with regular endoscopic screening required. Increased risk of pancreatic, ovarian, breast, cervix and testicular tumours

Cowden's syndrome
- Multiple hamartoma syndrome with orocutaneous hamartomas, fibrocystic disease of the breast, increased risk of breast carcinoma, thyroid abnormalities and hamartomatous polyps throughout the intestine. PTEN gene abnormalities in >50% (the *PTEN* gene provides instructions for making a protein that is found in almost all tissues in the body and acts as a tumour suppressor).

Bannayan–Riley–Ruvalcaba syndrome
- Gastrointestinal hamartomas, macrocephaly, speckled penis, developmental delay. PTEN gene abnormalities in >50%.

Adenomas

Familial adenomatous polyposis coli
- Inherited as an autosomal dominant trait. 1 in 10,000. Multiple polyps (>100) develop usually in the second decade.
- Polyps are premalignant with a lifetime risk of colonic neoplasia of 100%.
- They are often asymptomatic and a proportion present with carcinoma.
- Genetic testing is available for family screening. The gene is on the long arm of chromosome 5.
- Endoscopic surveillance should begin at age 10–12 years. Confirmation is by biopsy. Once the diagnosis is established prophylactic colectomy is advised. This is usually performed in late adolescence.
- Gastric and duodenal polyps develop in up to 50% and regular surveillance is recommended. There is an increased risk of thyroid and liver tumours.

Gardener's syndrome
- A variant of familial adenomatous polyposis including osteomas, skin tumours, desmoid tumours, carcinoma of the periampullary region of the duodenum and thyroid.

Turcot's syndrome
- The association of colonic adenomas with tumours of the central nervous system.

Hyperplastic polyps

- Single polyps, usually in the antrum or duodenum. Can cause abdominal pain. Benign.

Inflammatory polyps

- Can be multiple, common in inflammatory bowel disease, can be seen following 'other' inflammatory insults, e.g. post-infective, ischaemic.

Differential diagnosis of painless rectal bleeding

- Infectious colitis
- Allergic colitis
- Meckel's diverticulum
- Vascular anomalies
- Inflammatory bowel disease
- Anal fissure.

Chronic diarrhoea

- Diarrhoea is the passage of excessively liquid or frequent stools with increased water content.
- Chronic diarrhoea refers to diarrhoea that has persisted for more than 2–3 weeks.
- Children with chronic diarrhoea and faltering growth need further assessment, as the underlying cause may be a malabsorption.
- Assessment requires a careful history, physical examination including an assessment of growth, and basic investigations.
- Examination of the stool is essential.

Differential diagnosis

Common causes include:
- Infections, including postenteritis syndrome
- Coeliac disease
- Food intolerance, e.g. cow's milk protein sensitive enteropathy, soy protein enteropathy, lactose intolerance, eosinophilic gastroenteritis
- Bacterial overgrowth
- Short-bowel syndrome
- Pancreatic insufficiency, e.g. cystic fibrosis
- Immunodeficiency
- Inflammatory bowel disease
- Drug induced, e.g. antibiotics, laxatives.

Rare causes include:
- Abetalipoproteinaemia
- Intestinal lymphangiectasia
- Congenital microvillous atrophy
- Tufting enteropathy
- Glucose–galactose malabsorption
- Congenital chloride diarrhoea
- Autoimmune enteropathy.

The reader is referred to the larger paediatric gastroenterology texts for a more comprehensive differential diagnosis (see References and resources).

In children with chronic diarrhoea who are thriving, alternative diagnosis such as constipation with overflow, carbohydrate intolerance, and toddler's diarrhoea (chronic non-specific diarrhoea of childhood) should be considered.

Chronic constipation is a common cause, presenting as apparent diarrhoea which is in fact overflow soiling (variable consistency, stale stool). This occurs as a consequence of faecal leakage in the presence of a megarectum/incomplete rectal evacuation.

Assessment

- Is the child thriving?
- Is it true diarrhoea?
- Is the diarrhoea functional, secondary to malabsorption, or inflammatory?

The child with chronic diarrhoea and faltering growth

The most important part of the assessment of a child with chronic diarrhoea is a careful history and clinical examination including careful assessment of weight gain and linear growth.

The history includes the characteristics of the stool (watery, greasy [steatorrhoea], blood, mucous, overflow), stool frequency (e.g. night stool), presence of associated symptoms (e.g. pain, urgency, blood, weight loss), careful dietary history, assessment of general health, review of risk factors (e.g. chronic disease, previous surgery, antibiotic use), family history (e.g. cystic fibrosis, coeliac disease) and social history. Height and weight (with previous measurements) need to be plotted on a growth chart and interpreted in the context of family growth data. Puberty should be assessed in older children. Most children with chronic diarrhoea and failure to gain weight secondary to gastrointestinal pathology will be underweight for height. Height should be interpreted in the context of previous heights, midparental height, and pubertal status. A head-to-toe physical should be carried out. In particular this should include assessment of nutritional status by assessment of subcutaneous fat mass and muscle bulk. The perianal area should be visualized to exclude factors such as perianal excoriation from acid stool, rectal prolapse, soiling, or perianal signs of Crohn's disease. Rectal examination should be considered.

- There is no precise definition of diarrhoea.
- Diarrhoea can be osmotic or secretory or (mostly) a combination of the two.
- Osmotic diarrhoea occurs secondary to non-absorption of ingested solute (e.g. lactose intolerance). It will therefore stop if the child is made nil by mouth.
- Secretory diarrhoea implies an excess of secretion over absorption (e.g. inflammatory colitis).
- In the child with chronic diarrhoea of unknown aetiology in whom basic investigations are normal, factitious diarrhoea (e.g. laxative abuse, addition of urine/water to the stool) needs to be considered as a potential cause.

Chronic diarrhoea: red flags

Red flags in the history and examination for further investigation include:
- Continuous diarrhoea
- Night stools
- Acid stools
- Blood and mucus in the stool
- Faltering growth
- Associated symptoms that suggest organic disease —fever, rash, arthritis.

Investigation

- The precise investigation of chronic diarrhoea is very much dependent on the clinical situation that presents.

Stool testing

- Stool should be routinely collected and visualized to enable the best assessment of frequency, consistency, presence of blood/pus/mucus/fat, etc.
- Stools should be sent for microscopy and culture, virology, ova cysts and parasites and clostridium difficile toxin if suspected.

Other potentially useful stool investigations include:
- Stool for white cells/occult blood.
- Microscopy for fats/faecal fat collection (the latter is not popular with laboratories!).
- Stool reducing substances by clintest testing (>0.25% is abnormal) plus chromatography, which will detect reducing and non-reducing sugars and define which sugars are present.
- Stool chemistry is occasionally indicated if high stool electrolyte loss is suspected/diarrhoea is manifest as excess stoma loss.
- Faecal calprotectin, which is a stable neutrophil protein present in stool which is a non-specific marker of bowel inflammation.
- Faecal elastase, which is a pancreas-specific enzyme which is stable in faeces and a reliable indirect marker of pancreatic function. Low values in short gut and bacterial overgrowth.
- Faecal α_1-antitrypsin, which is a serum protein, not present in the diet with the same molecular weight as albumin. Faecal levels reflect enteric protein loss (e.g. protein-losing enteropathy).

Stool osmotic gap

- Stool osmotic gap = Stool osmolality − 2(stool Na + K)
- A significant gap suggests an osmotic diarrhoea with the gap reflecting the ingested, non-absorbed agent.
- No gap implies impaired electrolyte transport (secretory diarrhoea).
- Low stool osmolality suggests contamination of the stool with water or urine or an excess of ingested hypotonic fluid.

Blood testing

- Routine blood testing should include full blood count (including blood film), basic biochemistry including inflammtory markers, iron status, folate, B_{12}, serum immunoglobulins and coeliac antibody screen.
- Fat-soluble vitamins should be checked if a fat malabsorption is suspected
- Chronic diarrhoea may be an important manifestation of an immune deficiency. These can range from simple, relatively benign disorders such as IgA deficiency to major life-threatening immunodeficiencies such as severe combined immune deficiency (SCID). A full immunological work-up is required if an immune deficit is suspected. The precise tests are determined by the condition suspected.

Other investigations

- If laxative abuse is suspected, a urine laxative screen should be sent.
- Sweat testing/cystic fibrosis genotype are indicated if cystic fibrosis is suspected. Stool faecal elastase is a useful screen for pancreatic insufficiency.
- Hydrogen breath testing can be used to test for carbohydrate malabsorption, although there are significant false positive and false negative rates. The potential offending carbohydrate is given and breath hydrogen monitored with a peak (from fermentation) suggesting malabsorption.
- Pancreatic function testing is generally by indirect testing with faecal elastase. Direct assessment of pancreatic function can be made by duodenal intubation, stimulation of pancreatic secretion and measurement of the secreted enzymes.

Endoscopy

Gastroscopy with multiple duodenal biopsies is indicated if an enteropathy (e.g. coeliac disease, cow' milk protein sensitive enteropathy, postenteritis syndrome) is suspected. Gastroscopy and colonoscopy (plus barium radiology) are indicated if inflammatory bowel disease/colitis is suspected.

Infants with chronic diarrhoea in whom the diagnosis is not easily apparent should be referred to a paediatric gastroenterology unit for assessment.

Causes

See also the sections on short-bowel syndrome (Chapter 13), coeliac disease (Chapter 33), inflammatory bowel disease (Chapter 41), eosinophilic disorders (Chapter 45), and cystic fibrosis (Chapter 21).

Chronic non-specific diarrhoea (toddler's diarrhoea)

This is common, particularly in the run-up to toilet training. Children tend to pass frequent loose, often explosive stools. It can cause significant anxiety. Undigested food is frequently seen in the stool and is indicative of rapid transit. There are no additional features such as pain, blood in the stool, or night stools. Incomplete rectal evacuation may be a factor. The children are generally thriving. There are various potential factors implicated in causation—gut immaturity, dysmotility, diet (excess juice, excess fibre), and emotional stress. Fructose containing juices (e.g. apple juice) and excess sorbitol are common causes of chronic non-specific diarrhoea.

Management is by reassurance and general advice regarding potential triggers including avoidance of excess fibre and juice (particularly excessive hyperosmolar juice).

Carbohydrate intolerance

Carbohydrate intolerance is usually lactose intolerance, and acquired. The deficient enzyme is the brush-border enzyme lactase which hydrolyses lactose into glucose and galactose. The intolerance will present with characteristic loose, explosive stools. The diagnosis is made by looking for reducing substance in the stool following carbohydrate ingestion. This can be performed using Clinitest® tablets (which detect reducing substances in the stool); the detection of >0.25% is significant. Formal confirmation of the offending carbohydrate is through stool chromatography. Hydrogen breath-testing can be used to confirm a peak after lactose ingestion. Treatment is with a lactose-free formula in infancy and a reduced lactose intake in later childhood.

Following gastroenteritis, carbohydrate intolerance can be either to disaccharides or monosaccharides. It is usually in children who have been infected with rotavirus. Both types of intolerance are usually transient and both respond to removal of the offending carbohydrate. Both mono- and disaccharide intolerance will result in positive stool reducing substances.

Sucrose–isomaltase deficiency

This is a defect in carbohydrate digestion, with the enzyme required for hydrolysis of sucrose and alpha-limit dextrins not present in the small intestine. Symptoms of watery diarrhoea and/or failure to thrive develop after the introduction of sucrose or complex carbohydrate into the diet.

• Symptoms can be very mild.
• Reducing substances in the stool are negative, as sucrose is a non-reducing sugar.
• Diagnosis is by stool chromatography.
• Management is by removal of sucrose and complex carbohydrate from the diet.

Postenteritis syndrome

Acute gastroenteritis usually resolves in 7–10 days. Postenteritis syndrome refers to diarrhoea lasting >3 weeks, particularly if associated with poor weight gain/weight loss. This is usually seen in infants.

The continuing diarrhoea may be secondary to continuing infection, a further infection, carbohydrate intolerance (e.g. after rotavirus infection), enteropathy presenting as a severe malabsorptive syndrome which may reflect the 'unmasking' of another pathology (e.g. coeliac disease, cows' milk protein intolerance, or cystic fibrosis) or secondary to the initial infection. Enteropathogenic *E. coli* (EPEC), for example, can cause a severe enteropathy.

Postenteritis syndrome can be severe and require a period of parenteral nutrition. In most cases, however, treatment of the underlying condition (if unmasked) and/or a period of dietary exclusion using a cow's milk free diet using a protein hydrolysate (lactose free) as a substitute will suffice.

Coeliac disease

See Chapter 33.

Cow's milk or soya protein sensitive enteropathy

This implies enteropathy secondary to cow's milk or soya protein and improves following withdrawal of cow's milk, with a longer-term history of resolution in most cases.

- Disease of infancy presents with chronic diarrhoea with vomiting and malabsorption, faltering growth.
- More common in infants with other atopic features.
- Can present as postenteritis syndrome.
- Wide differential diagnosis.
- Diagnosis is based on biopsy, elimination, and challenge.
- Biopsy shows a patchy partial villous atrophy—patchy villous shortening, crypt hypertrophy, increased intraepithelial lymphocytes, eosinophilic infiltrate.
- Secondary lactose intolerance is common.
- Treatment is dietary protein exclusion with substitute feed under dietetic supervision.
- Soya products should not be used <6 months.
- Usually resolves in 1–2 years.

Protein-losing enteropathy

This refers to the excess loss of protein from the gut and can reflect altered permeability or lymph stasis or a combination of the two. The condition should be suspected in any child with chronic diarrhoea and unexplained hypoproteinaemia (hypoalbuminaemia the most prominent). It can occur in many different pathologies in the gastrointestinal tract as one of the factors in the disease process, e.g. Crohn's disease, coeliac disease, allergic gastroenteropathy, postenteritis syndrome, protein–energy malnutrition. Investigation is primarily directed to the likely underlying cause based on history and examination. Stool α_1-antitrypsin is a marker of enteric protein loss.

Intestinal lymphangiectasia

This refers to a functional obstruction of flow of lymph through the thoracic duct and into the subclavian vein which leads to fat malabsorption and a protein-losing enteropathy. It can be primary (congenital disorder of the lymphatic system) or secondary to other conditions e.g. pancreatitis, cardiac disease (pericarditis, post Fontan procedure), malignancy. Presentation is with chronic diarrhoea (steattorrhoea) and oedema. Lymphopenia is common. Diagnosis is by small-bowel biopsy (multiple sites as the lesion may be patchy), which shows dilated lymphatics in the absence of other pathology. Treatment is with medium-chain triglycerides—absorbed directly into the portal vein.

Short-bowel syndrome

See Chapter 13.

Pancreatic insufficiency

Pancreatic insufficiency manifests as chronic diarrhoea. This is a steatorrhoea (i.e. fat-containing stool) secondary to fat malabsorption. Management of pancreatic insufficiency is by pancreatic enzyme replacement.

Causes include:
- Cystic fibrosis (see Chapter 21).
- **Schwachman–Diamond syndrome:** This a rare autosomal recessive condition. Incidence is 1:20–200 000. The main features are pancreatic insufficiency, neutropenia, and short stature. Other features include metaphyseal dysostosis, mild hepatic dysfunction, increased frequency of infections, additional haematological abnormalities (including thrombocytopenia, increased risk of leukaemia).

Abetalipoproteinaemia

Abetalipoproteinaemia presents in early infancy with failure to thrive, abdominal distension, and foul-smelling, bulky stools. Symptoms of vitamin E deficiency (ataxia, peripheral neuropathy, and retinitis pigmentosa) develop later. The pathogenesis of this autosomal recessive inherited condition is failure of chylomicron formation with impaired absorption of long-chain fats with fat retention in the enterocyte. Diagnosis is by low serum cholesterol, very low plasma triglyceride level, acanthocytes on examination of the peripheral blood film, absence of betalipoprotein in the plasma, low plasma vitamin E, and fat-filled enterocytes on duodenal biopsy. Treatment is by substituting medium-chain triglycerides for long-chain triglycerides in the diet. Medium-chain triglycerides are absorbed via the portal vein rather than the thoracic duct. In addition, high doses of the fat-soluble vitamins (A, D, E, and K) are required. Most of the neurological abnormalities are reversible if high doses of vitamin E are given early.

Protracted diarrhoea/intractable diarrhoea of infancy

This refers to persistent diarrhoea starting in infancy and is less common.

Microvillous inclusion disease (congenital microvillous atrophy)

This presents as intractable diarrhoea from birth. The diarrhoea is secretory (i.e. persists when nil by mouth). An additional osmotic diarrhoea occurs with enteral intake. Pathology is an ultrastructural abnormality at the microvillus surface. Light microscopy reveals a partial villous atrophy. Special (PAS) staining is required. Electron microscopy is diagnostic. Microvilli are depleted on the apical epithelial surface and intracellular inclusions show apparently well-formed villi. Intestinal failure is profound with dependence on total parenteral nutrition (TPN) and failure to tolerate even minimal enteral intake. Fluid requirements are high as a consequence of continuing diarrhoea. Long-term nutritional support with TPN is required. Liver disease is common. Long-term survival is rare. Intestinal transplantation offers a potential cure.

Tufting enteropathy

This is rare. Presentation is similar to microvillous inclusion disease. The pathology is a primary epithelial dysplasia with the presence of 'tufts' of extruding epithelial cells on small-bowel biopsy. There is a combination of secretory and osmotic diarrhoea. Dependence on parenteral nutrition is usual, although unlike microvillous inclusion disease some gut function is present with the potential to tolerate a proportion of energy needs by the enteral route, which reduces the likelihood of liver disease.

Glucose–galactose malabsorption

This is a rare autosomal recessively inherited condition, characterized by rapid-onset watery diarrhoea from birth. It responds to withholding glucose (stopping feeds) and relapses on reintroduction. The diagnosis is essentially a clinical one. Reducing substances in the stool will be positive and small-bowel biopsy and disaccharide estimation normal. Treatment is by using fructose as the main carbohydrate source. Fructose is absorbed by a different mechanism from glucose and galactose.

Congenital chloride diarrhoea

This rare autosomal recessive condition is characterized by severe watery diarrhoea (associated with hypovolaemia) starting at birth—there is often a past history of polyhydramnios. Diarrhoea results from a failure of chloride reabsorption (in exchange for bicarbonate) in the ileum. There is a metabolic alkalosis. Serum sodium and chloride are low with a high stool pH and stool chloride (>90 mmol/L). Treatment is with sodium and potassium chloride supplements. Prognosis is good if diagnosis is made early. The gene defect is known.

A similar phenotype can occur (less common) due to defective Na^+/H^+ coupled transport. Stool Na^+ is high but Cl^- lower than Na+ and pH alkaline.

Autoimmune enteropathy

This refers to protracted diarrhoea presenting in infancy associated with the presence of circulating autoantibodies against intestinal epithelial cells. There is a partial villous atrophy with an inflammatory infiltrate on small-bowel histology. It is associated with other autoimmune conditions including renal disease and polyendocrinopathy (IPEX syndrome—immune dysregulation, polyendocrinopathy, enteropathy, X-linked). Treatment is with nutritional support and immunosuppression.

References and resources

Thomas PD et al. Guidelines for the investigation of chronic diarrhoea, 2nd edition. *Gut* 2003;**52**(suppl V):v1–v15. available from www.bsg.org.uk

Walker-Smith JA, Murch SH. *Diseases of the small intestine in childhood*, 4th ed. ISIS Medical Media, Oxford, 1999

Wyllie R, Hyams JS, Kay M. *Pediatric gastrointestinal and liver disease*, 3rd ed. Saunders Elsevier, Philadelphia, 2006

Coeliac disease

Coeliac disease is an immune-mediated enteropathy caused by a permanent sensitivity to gluten which is present in wheat, barley, and rye. It occurs in genetically susceptible children and adults. The classical presentation is with chronic diarrhoea, abdominal distension, and failure to thrive. The widespread availability of antibody screening has considerably changed the clinical spectrum of cases seen. The testing of children with less classical symptoms and screening of children at high risk has brought increasing recognition of the varied presentation and increased prevalence of this now very common condition.

The prevalence of coeliac disease based on either cross-sectional or population-based studies in developed countries is of the order of 0.3–2%, with a higher prevalence in at-risk groups. The vast majority of cases, however, remain undetected with seropositivity in apparently healthy individuals when populations are screened (silent coeliac disease). This is commonly referred to as the 'coeliac iceberg'.

The diagnosis of coeliac disease is confirmed by duodenal biopsy with classical histological features and prompt response to gluten exclusion (usually <2 weeks) in symptomatic individuals.

Who to investigate

There are three settings in which the diagnosis of coeliac disease should be considered:
- Children with frank gut symptoms
- Children with non-gastrointestinal manifestations
- Asymptomatic individuals with conditions that are associated with coeliac disease.

Coeliac disease presents after 6 months, i.e. after gluten has been introduced into the diet. The classical presentation is with irritability, weight loss, pallor, and abdominal distension in infants. More often children present later with a wide range of gastrointestinal symptoms including anorexia, generalized irritability, diarrhoea, abdominal pain, vomiting, constipation, anaemia of unexplained origin, intermittent abdominal distension, and faltering growth Recurrent abdominal pain/irritable bowel syndrome is a common presentation and coeliac antibody testing should be a routine part of the work-up of these common conditions. It is unclear what proportion of children with any combination of these symptoms will subsequently be diagnosed with coeliac disease. However, if symptoms are significant and clinical suspicion exists then coeliac serology is indicated and it is appropriate to test all children with chronic gut symptoms. Coeliac serology should also be considered in children with non-gastrointestinal manifestations of coeliac disease (see below). Short stature is an important specific indication with a high diagnostic yield and good catch-up growth once the condition is diagnosed. Screening should be considered in children at high risk. There is considerable controversy about whether coeliac screening should be extended to the general population.

Dietary compliance is difficult to establish in children who are picked up by either high-risk group or population-based screening, particularly if the child is, and perceives themselves as, asymptomatic as this will impact on acceptance of the diagnosis and compliance.

A **coeliac crisis** is a rare complication of coeliac disease seen at presentation characterized by explosive watery diarrhoea, dehydration (with hypovolaemia and hypoalbuminaemia), abdominal distension, and electrolyte disturbance. It responds to steroid treatment.

Non-gastrointestinal manifestations of coeliac disease

- Dermatitis herpetiformis (pruritic vesicular rash)
- Osteoporosis
- Dental enamel hypoplasia
- Short stature
- Delayed puberty
- Iron-deficiency anaemia not responsive to iron supplements
- Infertility

Conditions with an increased prevalence of coeliac disease

Children who are screened for any of these indications may have silent coeliac disease (abnormal small-bowel mucosa but no symptoms).

- Type I diabetes mellitus
- IgA deficiency*
- Down's syndrome
- Turner's syndrome
- Williams' syndrome
- First-degree relatives of those with coeliac disease (1 in 10)

* IgA deficient children are at increased risk of coeliac disease. Testing based on IgA antibodies will be negative (i.e. false negative). This is a potential diagnostic pitfall.

High-risk screening

It is important to remember that children in high-risk groups who are screened (see box, above) may have initially negative serology and develop positive serology later and repeat testing is indicated particularly if they develop suspicious symptoms. The North American Society of Pediatric Gastroenterology, Hepatology and Nutrition (NASPGHAN) guidelines recommend that screening should begin at 3 years in asymptomatic, high-risk children who have been on an adequate gluten-containing diet for at least 1 year prior to testing. Screening for first degree relatives in families with a child who has coeliac disease is also suggested by NASPGHAN. This should be done if other family members would like to have their serology tested or if they are symptomatic. Guidance from the National Institute of Clinical Excellence (UK) recommends screening of type I diabetics at diagnosis and then 3 yearly. The prevalence of coeliac disease in type I diabetes is probably 3–4%.

How to investigate

Measurement of IgA antibody to human recombinant tissue transglutaminase (TTG) and serum IgA is recommended for initial testing for coeliac disease. Sensitivity and specificity approach 100% although false positives are occasionally seen. IgA antibody to endomysium is observer-dependent and expensive. Antigliadin antibody tests are less accurate and not advised. It is important to exclude IgA deficiency as a cause of falsely negative serology. If coeliac disease is clinically suspected in children with IgA deficiency they should be referred for a small-bowel biopsy. IgG TTG serology may also be helpful as it is more likely to be positive in this group of patients than the general population.

It is crucial that children having coeliac testing are on a normal, gluten-containing diet prior to serological and histological diagnosis. Serology may be falsely negative if children are not on a normal gluten-containing diet. If children have already been started on a gluten-free diet or are eating insufficient amounts of gluten they should be referred to a paediatric dietitian and advised to recommence gluten in their diet for at least 3 months (preferably longer), with serial serological testing if there is a high clinical suspicion of coeliac disease and small-bowel biopsy following positive serology. After a period of gluten exclusion it may take many months for serology to turn positive once a normal diet is re-started.

Who should have a small-bowel biopsy

All children with positive serology should have an endoscopy with multiple duodenal biopsies before starting a gluten-free diet. The treatment of coeliac disease is for life and requires 100% confidence in the diagnosis before embarking upon it. Children for whom there is a high clinical suspicion, e.g. faltering growth or chronic diarrhoea, should be referred for consideration of a biopsy even if their serology is negative as other enteropathies may be found (see box, p. 237). Children who initially have positive serology with normal biopsies may subsequently develop mucosal abnormalities. This is referred to as **latent coeliac disease**. In such children a second biopsy (after an interval) is indicated for persistent positive serology.

Differential diagnosis of partial villous atrophy

- Coeliac disease
- Cows' milk-sensitive enteropathy
- Soy-protein-sensitive enteropathy
- Eosinophlic gastroenteritis
- Gastroenteritis and post-enteritis syndrome
- Giardiasis
- Small-bowel bacterial overgrowth
- Inflammatory bowel disease
- Immunodeficiency
- Intractable diarrhoea syndromes, e.g. autoimmune enteropathy
- Drugs, e.g. cytotoxics
- Radiotherapy

IgA deficiency

IgA makes up 15% of circulating immunoglobulin. In its secretory form it is the predominant immunoglobulin at respiratory and gastrointestinal surfaces. Selective IgA deficiency is a common disorder, with an incidence of 1 in 600. It is associated with an increased incidence of infection, atopic disease, rheumatic disorders, and coeliac disease. Immunoglobulin therapy is not worthwhile if isolated IgA deficiency is present. This is because there is only a small amount of IgA in immunoglobulin preparations and sensitization is therefore likely. If there is coexistent IgG deficiency or IgG subclass deficiency then immunoglobulin therapy may be appropriate.

Diagnosis

- Positive serology
- Biopsy with characteristic histology
- Response to treatment usually within 2 weeks.

Diagnosis is based on a small-bowel biopsy showing characteristic histological findings of partial or complete villous atrophy, crypt hyperplasia, and increased intraepithelial lymphocytes and a lamina propria plasma cell infiltrate in the presence of positive serology. Biopsies are usually taken endoscopically. Multiple biopsies should be taken, as the lesion can be patchy. Confirmation of diagnosis requires a response to treatment.

HLA typing can be considered in children for whom the diagnosis is uncertain. Coeliac disease is unlikely in those who are not HLA DQ2 or DQ8 positive.

A formal gluten challenge is rarely indicated particularly if serology is informative, the biopsy characteristic, and there is a good response to treatment. It should be considered in difficult cases particularly if there is diagnostic uncertainty (e.g. lack of clarity about the initial diagnosis, no serology at diagnosis, gluten exclusion with no biopsy) or the diagnosis is made in a child aged <2 years. The challenge should be supervised by a paediatric dietitian as it is crucial that during the challenge gluten intake is adequate (four medium slices of white bread). Gluten powder can be used as an alternative to normal diet if the families are concerned that a period back on a normal diet may result in problems with compliance subsequently if the diagnosis is confirmed. Serology should be monitored serially with biopsy once serology turns positive. There is no 'right period' on gluten. Relapse can occur rapidly or many months after challenge.

- **It is important to discourage gluten exclusion before diagnostic testing.**

The diagnosis is confirmed by complete symptom resolution on a strict gluten-free diet. Positive serology should revert to negative over time on a strict gluten-free diet. If there is no decline in anti-TTG after 6 months on a gluten-free diet, adherence with gluten exclusion should be reviewed. This may be as a consequence of inadvertent ingestion or non-compliance. A dietetic review is essential in such cases.

It is important to remember that there are other potential causes of a small-bowel enteropathy with partial villous atrophy, including cows' milk protein sensitive enteropathy, soy-protein-sensitive enteropathy, gastroenteritis and post enteritis syndrome, giardiasis, and autoimmune enteropathy (see box on p. 237).

Pitfalls in the diagnosis of coeliac disease

- IgA deficiency resulting in false negative serological testing
- Period of gluten exclusion prior to biopsy
- Inadequate gluten intake at the time of biopsy
- Poor-quality biopsy specimen.

Treatment

Gluten-free diet for life is the only effective treatment for coeliac disease (see Chapter 34). Children should all be seen regularly by a paediatric dietitian to help with compliance and assess the nutritional adequacy, considering the intake both of energy and of micronutrients. There are increased risks of morbidity and mortality in those with untreated coeliac disease. Good evidence exists that adherence to a strict gluten-free diet improves growth, normalizes haematological and biochemical markers, and reduces morbidity and mortality. A gluten-free diet is nutritionally complete and there are no known complications of the gluten-free diet itself.

A small proportion of individuals who are markedly symptomatic at presentation (usually with watery diarrhoea suggestive of lactose intolerance) and who fail to settle on gluten exclusion benefit from a 6–12 week period on a lactose-free diet, although this is rarely required long term.

There is very little data on the outcome of coeliac disease in children who are asymptomatic at presentation and picked up through screening, although a pragmatic presumption that the same long-term health benefits occur as in children symptomatic at diagnosis and therefore the recommendation is that all biopsy-positive children should be treated.

Iron status should be assessed and supplements given if necessary. Calcium and multivitamin supplements may be required in some children if intake is inadequate. DEXA scanning may be useful in children with inadequate calcium intake.

Although it has been shown that children with coeliac disease can tolerate oats, this is not recommended because oats are commonly cross-contaminated with other grains during processing.

Risks of non adherence to a gluten-free diet

- Persistent gastrointestinal symptoms
- Impaired nutrition
- Osteoporosis
- Impaired growth and pubertal development
- Reduced bone mineralization leading to osteoporosis
- Infertility/low birth weight infants
- Increased risk of gastrointestinal malignancy

Case studies

Child with positive coeliac serology, normal duodenal biopsy—what do you do?

This child is at risk (long term) of coeliac disease. The negative biopsy means that they don't fulfil the diagnostic criteria at the point it was taken. The biopsy should be reviewed by a paediatric/experienced gastrointestinal histopathologist. The child should continue on a normal diet. If positive serology persists, repeat biopsy is indicated. The interval before the next biopsy depends on the clinical situation but is usually not less than 1 year.

Child on gluten-free diet for 3 months (gut symptoms, positive family history, no diagnostic testing)—what do you do?

This is a common situation in the clinic. The child has been started on a gluten-free diet without diagnostic testing. There may have been gut symptoms and a positive family history of coeliac disease which have prompted the carers to make this decision. In this instance the family should be encouraged to put the child back on gluten for diagnostic confirmation (gluten challenge). This doesn't need to be done urgently. The timing will depend on the clinical situation, e.g. if the child is completely well on a gluten-free diet the challenge can be deferred.

Child undergoing a gluten challenge—how long should this be for?

Gluten challenge requires the reintroduction of gluten into the diet as a powder added to foods or normal foods. This needs to be under dietetic supervision to ensure adequate amounts of gluten are ingested. The onset of symptoms after challenge is usually within 3 months but can be prolonged (months to years) and late relapse following gluten challenge is well recognized. Children should be followed with serial serology then biopsy once serology turns positive.

Case of coeliac disease on gluten-free diet with persistent positive serology—does this matter?

The IgA-dependent coeliac serology (tissue transglutaminase or endomysial antibody level) should return to negative 3–6 months after starting a gluten-free diet. The failure of this to occur suggests poor compliance with gluten exclusion. In this instance clinical and dietetic review is indicated.

Coeliac disease (index case)—what about the family members?

Family members have a lifetime increased risk of coeliac disease and family members with gut symptoms should have coeliac disease excluded. Screening of first-degree relatives should be offered but has not been universally adopted. It is important to remember that a negative screen does not exclude the possibility of coeliac disease occurring later.

Follow-up and support

Follow-up should be with a paediatrician with an interest in gastroenterology. Monitoring includes general health, growth, compliance to and adequacy of diet, haemoglobin, iron status, albumin, and calcium. Serology should become negative and can be monitored as a marker of compliance if this is in doubt. Dietetic input is crucial and the paediatric dietitian involved should liaise with the child's school. Children should be seen 3 monthly until stable, then annually or biannually if very well. Any child for whom there is a difficulty in diagnosis, investigation, or management should be referred to a paediatric gastroenterology centre.

Families should be encouraged to join a parent support group such as Coeliac UK (see References and resources).

References and resources

The reader is referred to the comprehensive evidence-based guidelines produced by the North American Society of Pediatric Gastroenterology and Nutrition (NASPGHAN) and published on their website. www.naspghan.org

Hill ID, Dirks MH, Liptak GS, Colletti RB, Fasano A, Guandalini S, Hoffenberg EJ, Horvath K, Murray JA, Pivor M, Seidman EG. North American Society for Pediatric Gastroenterology, Hepatology and Nutrition. Guideline for the diagnosis and treatment of celiac disease in children: recommendations of the North American Society for Pediatric Gastroenterology, Hepatology and Nutrition. *J Pediatr Gastroenterol Nutr.* 2005 Jan;40(1): 1–19.

There is also guidance published on the British Society of Gastroenterology (BSG) and the British Society of Paediatric Gastroenterology, Hepatology and Nutrition (BSPGHAN) websites. www.bspghan.org.uk; www.bsg.org.uk

Patient information

Coeliac UK
PO Box 220
High Wycombe
Bucks HP11 2HS
Tel No 01494 437278
Helpline 0870 4448804
www.coeliac.co.uk

Nutritional management of coeliac disease

A gluten-free diet is the primary treatment for coeliac disease. This involves the complete exclusion of wheat, rye, oats, and barley, although the toxicity of oats is still in question. If properly treated, patients should be able to lead a normal, active life.

Patients and parents can be daunted by the prospect of avoiding these grains, which make up a large proportion of the Western diet. Avoiding many everyday foods impacts on the whole family's lifestyle as well as school and social activities. It is therefore strongly advisable that families receive advice and support from a paediatric-trained dietitian at the earliest opportunity after confirmation of diagnosis on a biopsy, and ongoing support as needed particularly in the months after diagnosis but also at regular scheduled reviews.

Gluten challenge

If a patient has been excluding gluten before diagnosis they will need a gluten challenge (period back on gluten). This must include 10 g of gluten daily (~4 medium slices bread) for at least 6–12 weeks (can be longer) to result in a conclusive diagnosis from a biopsy. 2 g gluten exchanges can be used (see box below). This quantity can be given as gluten powder disguised in food if gluten-containing foods are not acceptable, or there is anxiety that the switch to a normal diet will make subsequent acceptance of gluten exclusion difficult if the diagnosis is confirmed.

Food portions containing 2 g gluten

- 1 medium slice of bread
- 2 rusks
- 1 Weetabix or Shredded Wheat
- 3 chipolata sausages/ 2 large sausages
- 3 fish fingers
- 3 rich tea/digestive biscuits
- 1 slice of cake (~30 g)
- 30 g flour
- 4 tablespoons cooked or tinned spaghetti

Advice from the dietitian

Gluten-free diet

- All sources of wheat, barley, oats, and rye need to be excluded.
- There is no evidence that oats *per se* are harmful in the short term although there are too few studies showing the safety of long-term exposure. There is also the high risk of cross-contamination with gluten during processing and for this reason it is still currently recommended that children avoid oats.
- The exclusion of gluten is lifelong. Staple foods containing gluten such as bread, most breakfast cereals, pasta, biscuits, and cakes have to be avoided.
- The gluten-free diet should be based on naturally gluten-free staples such as rice, potatoes, and corn.
- Parents need dietetic support in providing suitable meals based around these that are acceptable to the child, and regular dietary review is required, keeping the diet as familiar as possible. This includes meals, snacks, treats, and meals taken outside the family home, e.g. at school and in restaurants.
- A small number of children who are particularly unwell at diagnosis, or in whom poor weight gain and diarrhoea persist on gluten exclusion despite adequate compliance, may benefit from a 6–12 week period of dairy exclusion.

Food labelling

- Wheat is widely used in processed foods as filler, binding agent, thickener, or flavour carrier.
- Patients, parents, and carers need to be taught to read and interpret food labels in order to identify gluten and associated derivatives.
- All pre-packaged food is covered by European Union food labelling legislation which now means that if any gluten-containing ingredient is included in the product, irrespective of quantity, it has to be included in the ingredients list. Manufacturers may state this as 'wheat', 'gluten', 'rye', or 'barley'.
- It is, however, not compulsory to list allergy information, such as stating if the product is 'gluten free'.
- Patients/parents are advised to be wary of packaging changes or 'new, improved' products which also may include a change in the ingredients making them no longer suitable. If there is any doubt, they should refer to the *Food and Drink Directory* produced by Coeliac UK, or manufacturers' information. If information is unobtainable patients are encouraged to be cautious and avoid the product.

Coeliac UK

- Coeliac UK is an independent charity for adults and children with coeliac disease. Parents and patients should be strongly advised to join for support and lifestyle information. They produce an annual directory of gluten-free food and drink which contains lists of gluten-free manufactured foods and is regularly updated in line with manufacturers altering their products. They have an excellent website (www.coeliac. co.uk), and publish a regular magazine for members and a range of leaflets covering many aspects of coeliac disease. Patients/parents should be made aware of the their helpline (see p.248).

- The dietitian should be able to supply application forms for membership of Coeliac UK and offer to help with completion and postage if necessary.

Gluten-free products

- An increasing number of proprietary gluten-free foods which mimic normal gluten-containing items are available for purchase or on pre-scription, e.g. bread, pasta, pizza bases, biscuits, and baking mixes. These are specially manufactured foods that comply with the International Gluten Free Standard. Codex wheat starch should contain less than 200 ppm gluten whereas naturally gluten-free foods should contain less than 20 ppm.
- Large supermarkets now stock a wide selection of these foods as well as ranges of their own label gluten-free foods. The dietitian should make families aware of these foods in order to improve variety in the diet and to supplement their prescription entitlement.
- Luxury gluten-free food items can be ordered and purchased through pharmacies. The use of gluten-free alternatives to previously eaten foods can help improve compliance.

Prescribable foods

- Basic gluten-free staple food items are available on prescription in the UK, and their use aids compliance.
- The dietitian should guide parents/carers about appropriate items and quantities then request the initial prescription from the patient's GP according to Prescribing Guidelines (see References and resources). Thereafter families can liaise with their GP to alter the prescription as they become more familiar with available products.

Monitoring

Children with coeliac disease should be seen by a dietitian at diagnosis and followed up at regular intervals in order that the following can be addressed:

- High rate of non-compliance.
- Height and weight recorded and plotted on growth charts.
- Faltering growth/poor nutritional status can be addressed.
- Compliance with the gluten-free diet reviewed either by 24 h recall or food diary.
- Recent history of bowel habits and gastrointestinal symptoms.
- Tissue transglutaminase antibody results are reviewed to monitor compliance with persistent tissue transglutaminase positivity despite gluten exclusion (>6 months) being a marker of poor compliance.
- Dietary calcium intake (meeting a minimum of the Reference Nutrient Intake 1992 recommendation). Supplements such as Calcichew® or Calcium Sandoz® syrup may be required if intake is not optimal, particularly in young children who are dairy restricted (Table 34.1).
- Dietary iron intake assessed particularly if low on blood testing.

If all aspects of the diet are assessed to be strictly gluten-free, consider other possible sources of ingestion:

- Any medications/supplements: advise patients/parents to seek advice from their pharmacist.
- Inhalation of wheat flour from cooking.
- Contamination during food preparation, e.g. from utensils, toasters, surfaces, communal use of butter/margarine/jam.
- Children playing with modelling dough (alternatives can be made with a gluten-free flour).

These reviews should be at least once a year but ideally 6 monthly. It is beneficial to offer an initial dietetic review at 3 months after diagnosis to check symptomatic improvement and that the gluten-free diet has been fully implemented. Additional telephone advice and support may be required.

Compliance

If there are problems with adherence to the gluten-free diet, patients must be seen by the dietitian and assessed at more regular intervals (3 monthly) until compliance is re-established.

Risks of non-compliance with gluten-free diet

- Persistent gastrointestinal symptoms, impaired nutrition
- Impaired growth and pubertal development
- Reduced bone mineralization leading to osteoporosis
- Infertility/ low birthweight infants
- Increased risk of gastrointestinal malignancy.

If appropriate, consider support from psychology/mental health team/ counsellor/education and social services.

Table 34.1 Reference nutrient intake (RNI) values for calcium

Age	RNI mmol/day	RNI mg/day
0–12 months	13.1	525
1–3 years	8.8	350
4–6 years	11.3	450
7–10 years	13.8	550
11–18 years (male)	25.0	1000
11–18 years (female)	20.0	800
Adults	17.5	700

From Dietary reference values for food energy and nutrients for United Kingdom.
Department of Health, London 1991.

References and resources

Coeliac UK, PO Box 220 High Wycombe, Bucks HP11 2HY. Tel: 01494 437278, Helpline: 0870 444 8804, www.coeliac.co.uk

Gluten free foods: a prescribing guide produced by British Society of Paediatric Gastroenterology Hepatology and Nutrition (BSPGHAN) in conjunction with an expert panel. These guidelines have also been approved by the British Dietetic Association (BDA), the Primary Care Society for Gastroenterology (PCSG), and Coeliac UK and are available at www.bspghan.org.uk/document/gluten-free_foods.pdf or from Good Relations Healthcare, Suite 2, Cobb House, Oyster Lane, Byfleet, Surrey, KT14 7DU

Bacterial overgrowth

Bacterial overgrowth refers to the syndrome of stasis of the small-bowel contents leading to bacterial proliferation and excessive numbers of bacteria being present in the small bowel (normally most of the gut bacteria are in the colon). It is also known as 'blind loop syndrome' or 'stagnant loop syndrome'.

- Symptoms include abdominal pain, distension, diarrhoea (both steatorrhoea and carbohydrate malabsorption), weight loss, and anaemia.
- Repeated courses of antibiotics, gut dysmotility, and previous surgery are risk factors.
- Stasis causes bacterial proliferation. The bacteria compete for nutrients, and both the bacteria and the degradation products result in damage to the small-intestinal surface and hence absorption capacity. Carbohydrate malabsorption is common.
- Deconjugation of bile salts occurs, with fat malabsorption resulting in steatorrhoea. Fat-soluble vitamin deficiency occurs.
- B_{12} deficiency is common.
- Diagnosis is by a high index of suspicion—particularly in patients with risk factors, e.g. multiple courses of antibiotics, previous gastrointestinal surgery (particularly involving loss of the ileocaecal valve, which normally prevents the reflux of colonic contents into the small bowel), strictures, short-bowel syndrome, small-bowel dysmotility, pseudo-obstruction, use of proton pump inhibitors to block gastric acid secretion.
- Any condition that reduces small-bowel motility is a risk factor.
- Culture of duodenal juice is helpful to isolate specific pathogens and inform treatment regimens. There is the potential for the emergence of resistant strains. Duodenal juice can be taken at endoscopy if performed.
- Hydrogen breath testing may be useful with an early hydrogen peak 30 min after ingestion of a carbohydrate load secondary to hydrogen production from the small-bowel bacteria (NB: the hydrogen peak occurs when bacteria metabolize the ingested carbohydrate, usually in the colon at 2 h).
- ^{14}C glycocholic acid (bile acid) breath testing with the detection of $^{14}CO_2$, which is elevated in bacterial overgrowth.
- Barium radiology should be performed if obstruction is suspected.
- Treatment involves appropriate management of the underlying cause:
  - Correction of any nutritional deficit, with supplementation of nutrients and fat-soluble and B_{12} vitamins if indicated. Lactose exclusion may be beneficial in the short term.
  - Metronidazole, which is effective orally and intravenously, is the antibiotic of first choice to normalize the gut flora. It may require use in combination or cyclically, e.g. in children with short-bowel syndrome. Local microbiological advice should be sought in difficult cases.
  - Probiotics have been used.

Acute abdominal pain

Introduction

The commonest surgical diagnosis in children who present to hospital with acute abdominal pain is appendicitis. The differential diagnosis is wide, however (see box below), and in >50% of admissions no specific cause is found.

The approach to assessment is through a detailed history and careful physical examination considering the wide differential diagnosis. Further investigations should be dictated by the clinical presentation. Age is a factor in the differential diagnosis. Other important factors in the assessment of the pain include the site, type, duration, time of day, associations, and the presence of associated symptoms including nausea, vomiting, urinary tract symptoms, or changes in bowel habit. Physical signs to assess include fever, pallor, abdominal tenderness and rigidity, presence of bowel sounds, faecal loading, and organomegaly. In boys a testicular examination is mandatory.

The urgent priority is to establish whether there is a surgical cause that requires intervention or a medical cause that requires urgent treatment. Initial investigations to consider include a basic blood screen including full blood count, inflammatory markers, serum amylase, and urine microscopy and culture. Plain abdominal radiograph is indicated if bowel obstruction is suspected, chest radiograph if there are any chest signs; abdominal ultrasound should be considered.

Differential diagnosis of acute abdominal pain

This is very wide, with abdominal pain being a common presenting symptom of pathology both within and outside the gastrointestinal tract.
- Appendicitis
- Intussusception
- Urinary tract infection
- Mesenteric adenitis
- Constipation
- Peptic ulceration
- Meckel's diverticulitis
- Pancreatitis
- Gastroenteritis
- Ovarian pathology, e.g. torsion/cyst
- Primary peritonitis
- Henoch–Schönlein purpura
- Hernia
- Testicular torsion
- Cholecystitis
- Renal colic
- Metabolic, e.g. acute porphyria
- Trauma
- Inflammatory bowel disease
- Pelvic inflammatory disease
- Sickle cell crisis
- Non-abdominal causes, e.g. pneumonia.

Appendicitis

- Appendicitis can occur at any age. Presentation can be as acute appendicitis, perforated appendicitis, or an appendix mass.
- The classical symptomatology is initial colicky central abdominal pain progressing to persistent localized pain in the right lower quadrant. Fever, anorexia, nausea and vomiting are usual. Loose stool or urinary symptoms may be an associated feature. The abdomen will be tender and there may be guarding in the right lower quadrant—'Mc Burney's point' (two thirds of the way along a line from the umbilicus to the anterior superior iliac spine). A pelvic appendicitis may not manifest with the classical abdominal signs. Rectal examination should be performed if pelvic appendicitis is suspected.
- White cell count is generally raised. Other investigation (urine, amylase) are to exclude differential diagnosis. Ultrasound is increasingly used as an acute investigation which can be diagnostic although even in experienced hands there is a false negative rate particularly if the appendix cannot be seen or is retrocaecal. CT is occasionally required.
- Management is by appendectomy unless there is an appendix mass in which case a period on intravenous antibiotics with an interval elective appendectomy is preferred. Laparoscopic techniques are widely used.

Intussusception

- The peak incidence at age 6–9 months although it can present later, with a male to female ratio of 4:1.
- Presentation is with spasmodic pain, pallor, irritability, and inconsolable crying. Vomiting is an early feature and rapidly progresses to being bile stained. Passage of blood-stained ' redcurrant jelly' stools often occurs and a ' sausage shaped' mass is frequently palpable. The presentation is often atypical, however, and requires a high index of suspicion in children who present with acute abdominal pain.
- The intussusception is usually ileocaecal, the origin being either the ileocaecal valve or the terminal ileum.
- An identifiable cause is commoner in those who present later, par- ticularly children who present aged >2 years — Meckel's, small-bowel polyp, cystic fibrosis, duplication cyst, lymphosarcoma, and Henoch– Schönlein purpura being examples. Preceding viral infection is a common trigger.
- Diagnosis is usually on clinical grounds. Confirmation is by plain abdom- inal radiography, ultrasound, or air-enema examination.
- Resuscitation with saline is often required.
- Treatment is either with air-enema reduction (if the history is short, <24 h) or surgically at laparotomy.
- Contraindications to air enema include peritonitis and signs of perforation.
- Recurrent intussusception occurs in ~5%.

Miscellaneous conditions

Henoch–Shönlein purpura

This is a vasculitis that affects the skin, gut, joints, and kidneys. Gastrointestinal manifestations include abdominal pain, gastrointestinal bleeding, and intussusception. Pain can be severe and corticosteroids can be used. Abdominal pain occurs secondary to the vasculitis. If intussusception occurs it tends to be in the proximal small bowel and difficult to treat, with parenteral nutrition required for difficult cases. Ultrasound is the best initial investigation.

Acute porphyria

Porphyrias are rare inherited or acquired disorders of the enzymes of haem biosynthesis, and can manifest with skin (erythropoietic) or neurological (hepatic) problems or both. Acute porphyria primarily affects the nervous system resulting acute abdominal pain, vomiting, neuropathy, seizures, and mental disturbance. Abdominal pain can be severe and chronic. Constipation is common. Diagnosis is by estimation of urinary porphyrins which should be raised during an acute attack. Treatment is with a high carbohydrate load or dextrose infusion if severe.

Recurrent abdominal pain

Introduction

- Recurrent abdominal pain is common in school-aged children and is a frequent presenting complaint in general practice and general paediatric and paediatric gastroenterology clinics. Patients often have vague symptomatology and investigation usually results in a low yield of organic disease. Treatment strategies are varied and often subjective with very little evidence upon which to base them.

- Apley described the syndrome of recurrent abdominal pain in childhood as three episodes of abdominal pain occurring during a period of 3 months, which were severe enough to affect daily activities. Prevalence is between 10 and 30%.

- The symptom of abdominal pain in childhood is so common that it is unusual for a child to go through school years without experiencing it at some stage and up to half of all children with recurrent abdominal pain do not present to the doctor although their pain is often as severe as in those who do. Therefore, this symptom is often considered trivial by the patient or family, presumably because of mild severity or transient nature. Usually, it is only when the pain impacts on the functioning of the child or family that medical help is sought.

- The differential diagnosis is wide and one of the early priorities in the assessment of children with recurrent abdominal pain is the exclusion of serious underlying organic pathology. The various significant organic disorders are dealt with in the relevant chapters of this book. In most patients the aetiology is functional or unclear.

- Multiple factors have been implicated in the aetiology of childhood abdominal pain, including psychological stress, visceral hypersensitivity, previously undiagnosed organic disorders, infection with *Helicobacter pylori,* gastrointestinal motility disorders, abdominal migraine, food intolerances, and constipation.

- The psychological environment within the family may be relevant in the aetiology. The biophysical model proposes that recurrent abdominal pain is the child's response to biological factors, governed by an interaction between the child's temperament and the family and school environments.

- Acceptance by parents and child of a biopsychosocial model of illness is an important factor for the resolution of symptoms.

- Many cases of childhood recurrent abdominal pain respond to acknowledgement of the symptoms and reassurance regarding the lack of serious underlying organic disease

Classification

It is useful in the clinical assessment to classify cases by subtype (see Table 37.1):
- Functional abdominal pain
- Functional dyspepsia
- Irritable bowel syndrome
- Abdominal migraine.

Table 37.1 Classification of recurrent abdominal pain according to the ROME 111 criteria

Functional dyspepsia	*Criteria must be fulfilled for at least 2 months before diagnosis and must include all of the following:* Persistent or recurrent epigastric pain or discomfort not relieved by defecation or associated with change in bowel pattern (i.e. not IBS) No structural/metabolic abnormalities to explain symptoms
Irritable bowel syndrome	*Criteria must be fulfilled for at least 2 months before diagnosis and must include all of the following:* Abdominal discomfort or pain that has 2 out of 3 features: Relieved with defecation Onset associated with change in stool frequency Onset associated with change in form of stool No structural/metabolic abnormalities to explain symptoms.
Functional abdominal pain	*Criteria must be fulfilled for at least 2 months before diagnosis and must include all of the following:* Episodic or continuous abdominal pain in a school-aged child No relation of pain with physiological events (e.g. eating) Some loss of daily functioning The pain is not feigned Insufficient criteria for other functional gastrointestinal disorders that would explain the abdominal pain
Abdominal migraine	*Criteria fulfilled two or more times in the preceding 12 months and must include:* Paraxysmal episodes of intense, acute periumbilical pain that lasts >1 h Intervening periods of normal health Pain impacts on functioning Two of the following features: Anorexia Nausea Vomiting Headache Photophobia Pallor No structural/metabolic abnormalities to explain symptoms.

Modified from Rasquin A, Di Lorenzo C, Forbes D, et al. Childhood Functional Gastrointestinal Disorders. Child/Adolescent. *Gastroenterology* 2006;**130**:1527–37.

However, not all children can be easily classified into one group.

- Children with functional dyspepsia require consideration of organic disease such as gastro-oesophageal reflux, peptic ulceration, or *H. pylori* infection. Night pain should prompt referral for endoscopy. Constipation should be excluded, as severe constipation with loading can present as epigastric discomfort/bloating. Dyspeptic symptoms may follow a viral illness.
- It is estimated that 10–20% of adolescents have symptoms suggestive of irritable bowel syndrome. The diagnosis of irritable bowel syndrome is supported by abnormal stool frequency (frequent, infrequent), abnormal stool type (loose, hard, mixed), abnormal stool passage (pain, incomplete rectal evacuation), passage of mucus, and bloating/distension. There are many physical and psychosocial factors that can impact on symptoms, with functional and family factors being relevant.
- It is probably the case that abdominal migraine, cyclical vomiting syndrome, and migraine headache are different clinical presentations of the same disorder along a disease spectrum. The diagnosis of abdominal migraine is supported by a positive family history of migraine headache. Many patients have a history of travel sickness. Dietary triggers include caffeine and foods containing nitrites or amines.
- Children with functional abdominal pain are often the most difficult to manage.
- Stress is often a major factor. It is important, however, to remember that stress can be either physical or psychological or a combination of the two, and reflects the response to external factors of the inherent personality type.

Personality type and family factors

Children with functional symptoms tend to be rather timid, nervous, anxious characters. They are often perfectionists—overachievers with an increased number of stresses, who are more likely to internalize problems than other children. School absence is common. There may be a degree of school refusal or separation anxiety in the younger child. There may be specific issues of importance in the school environment.

There may be significant stresses within the family environment, such as marital discord, separation, divorce, excessive arguing, extreme parenting (over-submissive or excessive punishment). Factors such as a family history of alcoholism, antisocial, or conduct disorders or the presence of somatization disorders within the wider family setting may be relevant.

Children with recurrent abdominal pain that becomes chronic often come from families with a high frequency of medical complaints, particularly recurrent abdominal pain, nervous breakdown, migraine, or maternal depression.

Common stresses in children with recurrent abdominal pain

Physical stresses
- Recent physical illness
- Postviral infection which can present as a postviral gastroparesis.
- Food intolerance—poor diet, wheat, carbohydrate intolerance, excess sorbitol
- Different and/or multiple medications, e.g. NSAIDs, anti-spasmodics
- Constipation
- Lack of exercise
- Chronic illness.

Psychosocial stresses
- Death of a family member
- Separation of a family member—divorce, child going to college
- Illness in parents or sibling
- School problem
- Altered peer relationships
- Poverty
- Geographical move.

Therapeutic options

The evidence base for therapeutic interventions is poor, probably reflecting the wide spectrum of different aetiologies and considerable differences in clinical phenotypes and triggering factors. This means management that tends to be subjective and based largely on the experience of individuals working in the field

Standard medical care/reassurance

This is the cornerstone of effective medical management. Many cases will respond to acknowledgement of the symptoms and reassurance regarding the lack of serious underlying organic disease.

Psychological intervention

The aims of psychological therapy are to modify thoughts, beliefs, and behavioural responses to symptoms and the effects of illness. Therapeutic modalities include biofeedback, relaxation therapy, behavioural therapy, cognitive therapy, coping skills training, hypnosis or self-hypnosis, and family therapy.

Life style and dietary management

There is a lack of published evidence, but it seems sensible to recommend healthy eating including plenty of fruit and vegetables, regular sensible meals, and plenty of fluids. Food that can potentially aggravate symptoms (e.g. fatty food, spicy food, fizzy drinks) should be avoided. Dietary triggers should be avoided in abdominal migraine. Dietary strategies should go hand in hand with a daily routine which includes exercise and is not unduly sedentary. An extended part of this strategy is to promote school attendance if that is an issue.

Pharmacological therapy

Many pharmacological interventions have been tried in treatment of recurrent abdominal pain but few have been tested in clinical trials.

- Medication that can aggravate symptoms should be avoided, e.g. NSAIDs in functional dyspepsia.
- Commonly prescribed agents include simple analgesics and antispasmodics.
- Pizotifen is probably of use in abdominal migraine (see Table 37.1).
- There is a role for H_2 antagonists and probably proton pump inhibitors and prokinetics such as domperidone in children with functional dyspepsia. They should be given on a trial basis and continued only if effective.
- Peppermint oil is useful in children with irritable bowel syndrome.
- Laxatives are helpful when constipation or incomplete rectal evacuation is felt to contribute to recurrent abdominal pain. This can be a feature in children with functional dyspepsia secondary to faecal loading or irritable bowel syndrome.

Outcome

Recurrent abdominal pain may be the antecedent of irritable bowel syndrome in adults, but here have been few long-term studies. Retrospective data suggest an increased incidence of psychiatric disorders in adulthood, particularly anxiety disorders.

The acceptance of the biopsychosocial model by the patients and their families is an important factor in the response to therapy

Recommended clinical approach

1 Exclude organic disease

The history and examination should be carefully scrutinized for features suggestive of organic pathology, bearing in mind the wide-ranging differential diagnosis of organic disorders that may present with recurrent abdominal pain.

- It is important to recognize that diet, lifestyle, and constipation may be significant factors in the child with recurrent abdominal pain.
- In the absence of likely underlying organic disease, it is often useful to elicit clinical features known to be associated with recurrent abdominal pain, such as psychological stress and anxiety. Many of these will become apparent while taking a detailed social history. Typical adverse social factors leading to psychological stress include bereavement, altered peer relationships, school problems, and illness of a family member. High achievers are at risk, particularly those who have excessive out-of-school activities. It is important not just to ask about illnesses in the family but also to ask about how those illnesses impact on the family. In some families there is an 'illness model' and this puts the child at increased risk of functional symptoms. This part of the assessment may also reveal a family history of anxiety disorders, or an anxious temperament in the child.

2 Classify by symptomatology

The next logical step is to attempt to classify the abdominal pain according to symptom subtypes, as documented in the ROME criteria (see Table 37.1). Although these criteria are not strictly validated, they do allow the clinician to target further investigation and management.

Important organic causes
- Gastro-oesophageal reflux/oesophagitis
- Peptic ulcer disease
- *Helicobacter pylori* infection
- Food intolerance
- Coeliac disease
- Inflammatory bowel disease
- Constipation
- Urinary tract disorders
- Dysmenorrhoea
- Pancreatitis
- Hepato-biliary disease
- Anatomical abnormalities, e.g.:
  - Meckel's diverticulum
  - malrotation

Symptoms suggestive of organic disease
- Age <5 years
- Constitutional problems:
  - fever
  - weight loss
  - delayed growth
  - skin rashes
  - arthralgia.
- Vomiting—particularly if bilious
- Nocturnal pain that wakes the child
- Pain away from the umbilicus
- Urinary symptoms
- Family history:
  - inflammatory bowel disease
  - coeliac disease
  - peptic ulcer disease
- Perianal disease
- Bloody stool (gross or occult).

Suggested initial investigations
- FBC
- ESR/CRP
- Renal and liver function
- Coeliac antibody testing
- Urine microscopy and culture

3 Targeted investigations

The mainstay of management of these patients is reassurance. Nevertheless, the symptoms may impact on the child's and family's functioning enough to warrant further investigation. For such cases, suggested initial investigations are listed in the box on p. 262.

The role of initial investigations is to help identify organic disease. However, secondary investigations may be indicated if there are suggestive symptoms and signs, initial investigations are suggestive of organic disease symptoms or symptoms are atypical. It is logical to use a targeted approach to further investigation according to symptom subtype. If initial investigations are normal and based on the clinical assessment organic pathology unlikely it is important to avoid doing more tests and emphasize the normal results.

Second-line investigations that might be appropriate include ultrasound of the abdomen, renal tract and pelvis, barium radiology, and endoscopy

4 Treatment/therapeutic approach

- The mainstay of treatment is reassurance, and the emphasis being on rehabilitation. Therefore, the first step is to acknowledge to the family and child that the pain is a real symptom.
- It is then necessary to recognize and treat any underlying or contributing factors. This may include a tendency to constipation
- Avoid excessive medications such as NSAIDs.
- Promote a healthy diet and lifestyle. Assessment by a dietitian may be helpful. It is worthwhile identifying dietary triggers, and suggesting alternatives.
- If the patient has an anxious temperament or is missing an excessive amount of school, consider psychology/mental health assessment. Many families are looking for an explanation for the symptoms and need to have discussed with them the inseparability of physical and psychological causes of symptoms, e.g. stress following viral illness, 'sick with worry', anxiety (with 'butterflies') prior to exams.
- Graded rehabilitation with goal-based approach, setting simple targets such as optimizing school attendance, graded exercise programme, and reducing NSAIDs.
- Many children can be discharged once the diagnosis has been made. The more severe and long-standing cases in whom, for example, school attendance is poor may benefit from psychological support and require follow-up until symptoms resolve and to give an opportunity for any psychiatric co-morbidity to emerge.

References and resources

Berger YM, Gieteling MJ, Benninga MA. Chronic abdominal pain in children. *BMJ* 2007;**334**:997–1002

Plunkett A, Beattie RM. Recurrent abdominal pain in childhood. *J Roy Soc Med* 2005;**98**:101–106

Spiller R, Aziz Q, Creed F et al. Guidelines on the irritable bowel syndrome: mechanisms and practical management. *Gut* 2007; **56**:177–98. Available from www.bsg.org.uk

Chronic constipation

Chronic functional constipation is a common problem in childhood. Without early treatment the condition is likely to impact on all aspects of the child's life, including education and psychological well-being as well as physical growth and development.

The key to successful management is early diagnosis and prompt treatment with an emphasis on practical management strategies with multidisciplinary support where needed. Conventional treatment relies on patient education, behavioural modification, and drugs.

- Constipation is defined as a delay in the passage of stool leading to distress and may include other symptoms such as pain, discomfort, anorexia, soiling, or encopresis.
- Soiling refers to the leakage of stool in the context of a megarectum.
- Encopresis (inconsistently defined in the medical literature) refers to the passage of normal stool at an inappropriate time/in an inappropriate place in the absence of constipation.
- The recently published Paris Consensus on Childhood Constipation Terminology (PACCT) Group's recommended terminology is shown in Table 38.1.
- The mean stool frequency in the first week of life is around 4/day, although some breast-fed normal infants may not pass a stool for several days.
- In general, the trend throughout childhood is a decreasing stool frequency up to the age of 4 years, at which time stool frequency is the same as in adult life with most schoolchildren in the range between 3/day and 1 every 2 days.

The prevalence of constipation in childhood varies with age. The peak incidence of occurs around toilet training (age 2–4) although prevalence remains high throughout childhood and into adult life.

Pathogenesis

The physiology of normal defecation depends on the interplay of multiple factors:

- Stool is moved through the distal colon by peristaltic contractions of the bowel wall.
- This movement is influenced by colonic tone, which in turn is influenced by diurnal variation and the gastrocolonic reflex (altered colonic tone in response to a meal).
- Once the stool enters the rectosigmoid junction, distension of the rectal wall results in reflex rectal contraction with concomitant relaxation of the internal anal sphincter.
- Stool is therefore presented to the anal canal and enters the so-called 'firing position'.
- Stool is perceived in the anal canal, and a decision to expel or withhold the faeces is made.
- Interruptions at any stage during this process may lead to constipation.

The commonest interruption is a painful stimulus perceived during defaecation at around the time of toilet training (e.g. anal fissure secondary to the passage of hard stool). Once the painful stimulus has occurred, the child may learn that voluntary withholding of stool prevents recurrence of the stimulus. This may lead to a stool-withholding cycle, which may ultimately lead to faecal impaction and overflow faecal incontinence. Prolonged faecal impaction can lead to chronic rectal distension and eventual loss of normal rectal sensation. This can lead to further impaction of stool and megarectum. This is known as functional constipation—i.e. constipation in the absence of underlying organic disease. It is the cause of childhood constipation in ~95% of cases.

Chronic functional constipation may coexist with other functional disorders. One example of this is irritable bowel syndrome (IBS), which may exist as in a 'constipation-predominant' form. The symptom of incomplete rectal evacuation is likely to be a factor and although there is no good quality evidence that IBS may improve with laxatives in children, there is some evidence from adults.

Table 38.1 Paris Consensus on Childhood Constipation Terminology (PACCT) group's recommended terminology

Suggested terminology	PACCT group definition
Chronic constipation	The occurrence of two or more of the following characteristics, during the last 8 weeks: Frequency of bowel movements <3/week >1 episode of faecal incontinence per week Large stools in the rectum or palpable on abdominal examination Passing of stools so large that they may obstruct the toilet Display of retentive posturing and withholding behaviours Painful defecation
Faecal incontinence	Passage of stools in an inappropriate place.
Organic faecal incontinence	Faecal incontinence resulting from organic disease (e.g., neurological damage or sphincter abnormalities).
Functional faecal incontinence	Non-organic disease which can be subdivided into: Constipation-associated faecal incontinence. Non-retentive (non-constipation-associated) faecal incontinence.

Benninga M, Candy DC, Catto-Smith AG, et al. The Paris Consensus on Childhood Constipation Terminology (PACCT) Group. *J Pediatr Gastroenterol Nutr* 2005;40(3):273–275.

Differential diagnosis of chronic constipation

- Hirschsprung's disease
- Anorectal anomalies (e.g. anal stenosis)
- Neuronal intestinal dysplasia
- Spina bifida
- Neuromuscular disease
- Hypothyroidism
- Hypercalcaemia
- Coeliac disease
- Food allergy/intolerance
- Cystic fibrosis
- Perianal group A streptococcal infection
- Anal fissure
- Pelvic/spinal tumours
- Child sexual abuse
- Drugs

Clinical assessment

Key features in the history

- Delay in passage of meconium: the vast majority of infants will pass meconium within 48 h of birth; a delayed passage of meconium raises the possibility of Hirschsprung's disease.
- Age at onset of symptoms: typical age of onset for functional constipation is 2–4 years, around the age of toilet training.
- Consistency/nature of stool: infrequent, very large stool (large enough to block the toilet) is common in chronic functional constipation.
- Painful or bloody stools: the differential diagnosis should include anal fissure, perianal group A streptococcal infection or, rarely, sexual abuse.
- Abdominal pain: a very common symptom in childhood, and is a feature of many organic and functional disorders. Many constipated children have recurrent abdominal pain, which may be relieved by the periodic passage of large stool.
- Stool withholding behaviour: voluntary stool withholding may manifest as unusual behaviour, which may be mistaken for straining.
- Soiling: occurs as a result of involuntary passage of liquid stool around faecal impaction in the rectum. It is almost always associated with psychological distress in the child or family.
- Diet: children with chronic constipation may have a history of anorexia, poor energy intake, poor fluid intake. Low fibre intake is common. Cow's milk allergy may be a factor in some children, particularly if other atopic features are present.
- Urinary symptoms: urinary tract infections, urinary frequency and nocturnal enuresis are common in chronically constipated children.
- Family history of constipation/irritable bowel syndrome.

Key points in examination

- General health, nutritional status, and growth.
- Abdominal palpation: this will reveal a faecal mass in at least half of all chronically constipated children. The size of the mass reflects the extent of rectal/colonic involvement. Usually the mass is palpable in the suprapubic area, but in severe cases may extend above the umbilicus. If the child is obese or if the stool is soft (e.g. after laxatives have been introduced). palpation can be difficult.
- Perianal inspection: the perianal area should be carefully inspected for signs of soiling, inflammation (which may be due to streptococcal infection), anal fissure, or congenital abnormalities such as anterior anus. In rare cases there may be signs of sexual abuse.
- Rectal examination: if the clinical features are typical of functional chronic constipation, the digital rectal examination is unlikely to add further useful information. Furthermore, a rectal examination is invasive and may compound the underlying fear of anal pain and toileting. However, if there are clinical features suggestive of underlying organic pathology (e.g. Hirschsprung's disease, anal stenosis particularly in infancy) a single rectal examination be indicated to assess anal tone, calibre, position, and the presence of stool in the rectum.
- Neurological assessment including inspection of the lumbar-sacral spine and examination of the lower limbs is essential.

Investigation

If the history and examination are typical of chronic functional constipation, further investigations are not generally indicated. The following lists some of the investigations that can be considered but should not be routine.

- Abdominal radiograph: useful to demonstrate underlying spinal abnormalities and to delineate the extent of faecal loading. Only indicated in rare cases, where there is a strong suspicion of neural tube defect, or the abdominal examination is not conclusive. This should not be routine as there is a high radiation dose.
- Bowel transit studies: segmental colonic transit time may be assessed by measuring the position of swallowed radio-opaque markers on plain abdominal radiographs. This is a specialist investigation and its diagnostic use is questionable, since up to 50% of chronically constipated children may be shown to have normal colon transit time, although severely delayed transit is associated with a poor prognosis.
- Anorectal manometry: this is an invasive investigation not indicated as first line, the main purpose being to demonstrate the normal relaxation of the internal anal sphincter in response to rectal distension.
- Full thickness rectal biopsy: diagnostic of Hirschsprung's disease and indicated only if there is a strong clinical suspicion.
- Coeliac antibody screen: coeliac disease is common and constipation can be the presenting feature.
- Electrolytes, micronutrients, endocrine assessment: iron deficiency is common in childhood constipation. Electrolyte (e.g. hypercalcaemia) and endocrine abnormalities (e.g. hypothyroidism) should be considered if the history and examination are suggestive.
- Allergy: in children with atopic features (rhinitis, dermatitis, or bronchospasm) and evidence of proctitis or perianal erythema, investigation for cow's milk allergy/allergic colitis should be considered.

Practical management

The practical management of chronic constipation is not just about laxatives. Patients and their families need a full clinical assessment as outlined above, emphasizing in particular family and social factors that may impact on the condition and its management. If, for example, there is a coexistent behavioural or emotional problem then the management of that will be relevant to the management of the constipation. The successful management of the constipation, particularly when soiling is a major factor, may impact on the behavioural problem.

Emphasis on the many factors relevant in the aetiology of chronic constipation is fundamental from the outset.

There are seven general principles of management, of which drug therapy plays a major role. Unless the first six principles are considered, drug therapy is rarely effective.

1 Explanation of normal bowel function

Careful explanation of this process to the parents (and child if appropriate) helps the family understand the disorder and aids compliance with therapy. A basic understanding of the pathophysiology may also relieve tensions in the family associated with blame and guilt.

2 Diet/fluids and exercise

A high-fibre diet is recommended, along with adequate fluid. Dietary fibre/bulking agents help retain water in the gut lumen by osmosis, and stimulate peristalsis by adding bulk to the stool. Regular exercise promotes intestinal peristalsis and helps with bowel transit.

3 Behavioural advice

Gaining a child's trust is important. Time needs to be spent reassuring children about their condition and the treatment. The psychological principle of ignoring failure and rewarding success is important. Anything that helps relax the child will help with the defecation problem, whether it is fear of pain or persistent soiling. Conflict should be avoided. It is vital that the child wants to get better.

4 Toilet training advice

Regular toileting is a crucial part of the management. Children need to be encouraged to sit on the toilet on waking, after all meals, and before bed. It is important the child has a comfortable position, e.g. toilet seat with foot support. It must be stressed to the parents that this is the most important part of the child's management. It is important that the child sits on the toilet for long enough.

5 Simple reward schemes

Reward schemes can be highly effective in the behavioural management. The star chart can be used but any attractive variation of this can be used to appeal to each particular child (e.g. sticker charts, computer game time). Rewards can be given for compliance at first (e.g. sitting on toilet twice a day after breakfast and tea), and later rewards are given for success (e.g. bowels opened into the toilet).

6 Reassurance and encouragement

Parents ought to be reassured that constipation is common and that the prognosis is generally good.

Biofeedback training

Biofeedback training is a procedure that allows the muscle tone of the external anal sphincter to be displayed on a screen and has been used with constipated children to teach them how to tighten and relax their perianal muscles in order to pass bowel movements more efficiently.

Drug therapy

There is no right strategy for pharmacological intervention, and there is wide variation between different units in the regimens used. The evidence base is poor. There is no best fit for all patients and many cases require individual treatment plans. Open discussions are needed from the outset about compliance. Parents and the child need to be aware that any laxative regimen may in the short-term increase soiling particularly if the toileting regime is not being adhered to. Frequent support and follow up is required during the initial phases with encouragement not to give up as soon as the stools become loose. Many medications are available (see Table 38.2).

Disimpaction

The basic principle is to first disimpact if there is a megarectum in order to facilitate normal defecation dynamics and then give a sufficiently high laxative dose to ensure regular emptying.

Local therapy (manual evacuation, enemas, suppositories) can be used although can exacerbate the stool withholding and/or exacerbate toilet-phobic behaviour, which is usually present in children with chronic constipation, so oral therapy is often preferred. Options include senna, polyethylene glycol, sodium picosulfate elixir, bisacodyl, liquid paraffin, sodium docusate, Picolax,® or local therapy (e.g. Micralax® enema, phosphate enema) if the above fail.

It is essential that high doses are used and that mechanisms are put in place to monitor the child and ensure compliance. Increased soiling is often seen during the early phase of disimpaction.

Senna can be used as a sole agent given in the evening in stepwise increasing doses, increased by 5 mL (7.5 mg) at a time until at least daily evacuation is achieved. This can be usually done as an outpatient. Doses of 15–30 mL, as syrup or tablets, are generally required. It is important to make patients aware that senna takes 10–12 h to work and therefore an adequate evening dose should result in a bowel motion the next morning. It is important to stress that the child needs to sit on the toilet regularly for this to occur. The peak stimulant effect is in the morning and after breakfast there will be an enhanced gastrocolic reflex.

Polyethylene glycol can be used similarly as a sole agent in increasing doses until effective bowel emptying is achieved. It is best given in a twice-daily regimen.

In children in whom impaction is severe other agents may be needed including sodium picosulfate, as the elixir (5–10 mL) or Picolax® sachets (1/2–1) given daily or polyethylene glycol sachets at higher dose. All three are options and the regimen needs to be tailored to the needs of the individual child.

Regimens may take several days to take effect. Sodium picosulfate in particular has a significant osmotic effect and requires a high fluid intake.

Maintenance

Laxatives are often required for a prolonged period. The laxative regimen used needs to be consistent and given regularly, with weaning only after a sustained period of normal stooling with no soiling. The choice of laxative is probably less important than the compliance of the child and parent with the treatment regimen.

There is considerable debate about which laxative to use long term; long-term stimulant laxatives (other than as rescue) are not advocated in North America but they are widely used in the UK.

Senna given in the evening can be effective. Children with long-standing, severe constipation will often require high doses. The aim is to produce a formed or semi-formed stool regularly (hopefully daily), although some children on senna will always produce an unformed stool. It may take a few weeks to find the correct dose for an individual child; maintenance dose is usually 10–20 mL senna nocte. The maximum dose is usually not more than 30 mL.

Alternative laxatives can be used when senna fails. Many centres use polyethylene glycol as first line.

Weaning from high-dose laxatives

Treatment may be needed for many months, or even years in very severe cases. Eventually almost all children will require progressively less and wean off over time. The weaning regimen should be cautious, tailored to the individual child, and regularly reviewed. Early weaning will invariably result in relapse of the constipation.

Notes on commonly used laxatives

- **Lactulose** is a non-absorbable disaccharide of the sugars D-galactose and D-fructose. It is not absorbed from the small intestine because it is resistant to hydrolysis by digestive enzymes. It is fermented by colonic bacteria in the colon. The by-products of this process exert a local osmotic effect, resulting in an increased faecal bulk and stimulation of peristalsis. The side effects of treatment are predominantly secondary to intraluminal fermentation and gas production. This may lead to flatulence, bloating, and cramping abdominal pains. Lactulose may exacerbate soiling in the presence of faecal impaction. It is often the first line choice of drug prescribed for acute/ mild constipation in children.

- **Polyethylene glycol** has been used for some time in high dose for bowel lavage prior to gastrointestinal procedures. Recently, a lower-dose form (PEG 3350, Movicol,® Movicol Paediatric Plain®) has become available and been used successfully as an alternative treatment for acute and chronic constipation being effective in both the disimpaction and maintainance phases. Its large molecular size renders it unabsorbed in the intestinal tract. It therefore produces a local osmotic effect, preventing the absorption of water from the faeces. Unlike lactulose it does not result in the production of gas secondary to bacterial fermentation and consequently has fewer side effects (such as bloating and flatus).

- **Stimulant laxatives** include **senna, bisacodyl, sodium docusate** (also a softener), and **sodium picosulfate.** These agents work by increasing intestinal motility. A common side effect is, therefore, colicky abdominal pain particularly in the presence of retained stool. Stimulant laxatives are widely used in the management of chronic functional constipation—in both the disimpaction and the maintenance phase. They are both safe and effective. Despite the ubiquitous nature of the use of drugs such as senna, docusate and sodium picosulfate, there is very little empirical data to support their use. A recent Cochrane review of the use of stimulant laxatives for the treatment of constipation and soiling in children found no randomized controlled trials that met the selection criteria for analysis. The authors concluded that there is insufficient evidence to guide the use of stimulant laxatives and more research is needed. Nevertheless, in the UK, senna in particular is commonly used in the maintenance phase of treatment. Its longer mode of action compared with other agents such as lactulose make it more applicable to the school-aged child, where an evening dose may precipitate a bowel motion the following morning.

- **Liquid paraffin (or mineral oil)** is a petroleum derivative. Historically it has been a popular choice of drug for the treatment of constipation and faecal impaction. Its main effect is thought to be as a stool lubricant (although the conversion of the oil to fatty acids also exerts an osmotic effect). Although widely used in North America, it is not commonly used in the UK.

- **Enema therapy** is occasionally required in acute faecal impaction or oral medication fails. Children find this treatment unpleasant and it can exacerbate stool-withholding behaviour. There have been numerous reports about toxicity of phosphate enemas secondary to absorption, leading to profound metabolic changes.

> **Key points in management**
> - Chronic functional constipation is a common problem in childhood with soiling a significant issue. The morbidity is high and treatment complex.
> - There is a very poor evidence base for the drug treatments used and considerable differences in practice in different units.
> - The key to successful management is early diagnosis and prompt treatment with multidisciplinary support where needed.

Table 38.2 Pharmaceutical agents used in the treatment of constipation: mode of action

Class of drug:	Mode of action/ properties	Example drugs
Osmotic agents	Increase quantity of water in large bowel by osmosis	Lactulose Macrogols, e.g. polyethylene glycol Magnesium sulfate Phosphate enema
Stimulant laxatives	Increase intestinal motility	Anthraquinones, e.g. senna Bisacodyl Docusate Picosulfate
Lubricants/softeners	Lubricate/soften impacted stool	Mineral oil, e.g. arachis oil, liquid paraffin Docusate
Bulking agent	Increase faecal mass and therefore stimulate peristalsis	Fibre Bran Isphagula Methylcellulose Erythromycin
Other agents	Prokinetics	

Plunkett A, Phillips CP, Beattie RM. Management of chronic constipation in childhood. Pediatr Drugs 2007;9(1):33–45

Outcome

Children with chronic constipation require follow up until full recovery and then benefit from a consolidation period. There is a high frequency of relapse. It is usual practice therefore to offer long-term follow-up. The length of follow-up depends on time to full recovery and the likelihood of relapse.

Indications to refer for specialist advice

- Children in whom aggressive bowel clearance, e.g. picosulfate, needs to be considered
- Children in whom significant behaviour/psychosocial problems are impacting on the management of their constipation.
- Failure to respond to high doses of laxatives.
- Persistent soiling despite laxatives.
- Structural/physical cause cannot be excluded.
- Concern re nutrition/poor growth.
- Anal fissure or rectal prolapse if there is failure to be cured by a reasonable course (three months) of laxatives.

References and resources

Education and Resources for Improving Childhood Continence, www.eric.org.uk

Tough Going, www.nhslothian.scot.nhs.uk/quicklinks/RHSC_CONSTIPATION2.PDF

Case study 1

A 3 year old boy (previously toilet trained) presents with constipation. He has just recovered from an acute gastrointestinal illness. He is off his food, irritable, and stooling only once every 3 days passing hard stools with pain and fresh blood per rectum. He is rather pale. Growth is normal. He has palpable stools and perianal soreness. Basic investigations are normal including urine culture, perianal skin swab, and coeliac antibody screen. He is in a stool-withholding cycle whereby it is painful to pass stool so he doesn't, but resisting the urge to pass stool compounds the problem. This is managed with laxatives (at reasonable doses), regular toileting, and explanation and reassurance.

Case study 2

A 10 year old boy presents with soiling. He is a rather picky eater and doesn't eat breakfast. His fluid intake is poor. He has had recurrent urinary tract infections and wets at night. He has behavioural problems although is in mainstream education. He is constantly teased. He was born preterm. His brother has attention deficit disorder. Clinical examination is unremarkable apart from palpable faecal loading and old stool around the anal margin. Basic investigations are unremarkable. His faecal loading suggests that the soiling is secondary to overflow. The normal defecation dynamics have been lost as a consequence of his permanently distended rectum. Management is with high-dose laxatives (disimpaction then maintenance) with attention to diet, fluids, and regular toileting particularly after meals. He is clean within a few days, but laxative dependent for several months. He continues with his early morning routine of breakfast (with a drink), then toileting. He gradually becomes dry at night. His confidence and behaviour improve.

Hirschsprung's disease

Hirschprung's disease

Hirschsprung's disease is the absence of ganglion cells in the myenteric plexus of the most distal bowel. Presentation is with constipation. Incidence is 1 in 5000. Long-segment Hirschsprung's disease is familial, with equal sex incidence. The gene is on chromosome 10. It is associated with Down's syndrome and there is a high frequency of other congenital abnormalities.

- Usually presents in infancy in the first months of life with failure to pass meconium and abdominal distension.
- Can present acutely with an enterocolitis.
- Patients can be very unwell at diagnosis.
- One of the common differentials of intestinal obstruction in the neonatal period.
- Presentation in the older child is rare, the most common cause of chronic constipation in this age group being functional.
- Most children with Hirschsprung's will have never had a normal bowel habit and have failed to respond to reasonable doses of laxatives given regularly.
- The definitive test is a full-thickness rectal biopsy to confirm the absence of ganglion cells in the submucosal plexus; histochemistry will demonstrate excessive acetylcholinesterase activity and the absence of ganglion cells.
- Surgery is excision, usually with temporary colostomy followed by pull-through anastamosis at a later stage.
- Hirschsprung's enterocolitis (which is poorly understood) can occur before or after surgery. Treatment is with fluid resuscitation, bowel rest, and intravenous antibiotics.
- 90% of cases the aganglionosis affects <40 cm of colon
- Prognosis for long-term continence is reasonable, although up to 10% have long-term problems with constipation, night soiling, and night stools in particular.
- Children with Down's syndrome and other learning disability rarely achieve continence and may be better left with a stoma.
- Long-segment Hirschsprung's disease (rare) may extend into the small bowel. This can result in such severe bowel dysfunction that the infant is parenteral nutrition dependant. Bowel adaptation is poor. The prognosis in this instance is poor particularly if the child is dependent on TPN, with TPN-induced cholestasis.
- Ultra-short-segment Hirschsprung's disease (<2 cm) is very rare and can present significant diagnostic difficulty for the histopathologist as the very distal rectum is usually hypo- or aganglionic. Rectal manometry can be helpful.

Neuronal intestinal dysplasia

This is a controversial condition in which there is hyperplasia of the myenteric plexus with increased numbers and size of ganglion cells. The presentation can be with symptoms similar to Hirschprung's disease. The histopathological entity can exist in children with only minimal symptoms.

Intestinal pseudo-obstruction

This is the term used to describe patients with symptoms and signs of intestinal obstruction in whom there is no mechanical obstruction. This can be acute, e.g. associated with chronic disease/medication.

Primary chronic intestinal pseudo-obstruction is rare. This is a heterogenous group of conditions. The underlying cause can be neurological (visceral neuropathy) or muscular (visceral myopathy). There are no definitive diagnostic tests. Management is complex and requires strategies to enable feeding. In the most severe cases long-term parental nutrition may be required.

Perianal disorders

The perianal examination is an important part of the examination of the gastrointestinal tract. This is best done by inspection with the patient lying in the left lateral position. The perianal region can be inspected by gently parting the buttocks.

Perianal redness is most commonly seen.

Differential diagnosis of perianal redness

- Poor perineal hygiene
- Soiling/encopresis
- Perianal streptococcal infection
- Threadworm infestation
- Lactose intolerance (acidic stool)
- Anal fissure
- Inflammatory bowel disease
- Cow's milk protein allergy
- Sexual abuse (rare).

Anal fissure

- Commonly seen, often caused by the passage of a hard stool and results in 'stool withholding' cycle exacerbating constipation if present.
- Presents with pain and bright red blood either on the surface of the stool or post defecation.
- Usually anterior or posterior and if lateral more suggestive of inflammatory pathology.
- May be a skin tag at the site of a healed fissure.
- Treat underlying cause (e.g. constipation).
- Local treatment rarely indicated.
- Most settle conservatively.
- Inflammatory bowel disease should be considered if fissures are atypical/resistant to medical treatment.
- Child sexual abuse should be considered if fissures are atypical/resistant to treatment.

Perianal streptococcal infection, 'soggy bottom'

- Common cause of perianal redness.
- Can present as constipation or perianal pain or both.
- Characterized by erythematous, well demarcated, tender perianal margin.
- Secondary to group A β-haemolytic streptococcus infection.
- Perianal skin swab should be sent for diagnostic confirmation.
- Treatment is with penicillin for 7–10 days.
- There may be a need for a period on laxative therapy as there is a risk even after treatment of the child developing stool-withholding behaviour secondary to perianal discomfort.
- Infection can recur and require a more prolonged course of antibiotics. Choice of antibiotics should where possible be determined by sensitivities.

Threadworm infestation

- This is very common secondary to *Enterobius vermicularis* (pinworm).
- Common cause of perianal redness and itch.
- Transmission is faeco-oral.
- The life cycle is 6 weeks.
- Eggs are layed on perianal skin.
- Commonest symptom is itch, results in scratching; eggs on fingers are then swallowed, which perpetuates the infective cycle.
- Diagnosis is mostly clinical based on the presenting symptoms and signs.
- Can do a Sellotape slide test whereby the tape is placed at on the skin around the perianal margin and then taped onto a slide and sent for microscopy to look for eggs.
- Treat with mebendazole (single dose) or piperazine (two doses, 2 weeks apart). Re-infection is common. The whole family needs to be treated and bedding changed to try to reduce this.

Rectal prolapse

- This is the abnormal protrusion of the rectal mucosa through the anal margin.
- Usually spontaneously reduces.
- Aetiology includes chronic straining, chronic diarrhoea, malnutrition, polyps, cystic fibrosis as a manifestation of chronic diarrhoea (15%).
- Surgical management (usually injection) is rarely indicated.

Solitary rectal ulcer syndrome

- This rare condition is poorly understood.
- Occurs usually in adults but can occur in children with chronic constipation (particularly those who strain) and may be due to injury to the rectum.
- Usually manifests as a single ulcer (or occasionally multiple/polypoid mass) in the rectum.
- Symptoms include rectal bleeding, straining during bowel movements, constipation, soiling (particularly mucous), and a feeling of incomplete evacuation.
- Treatments include regular toileting, attention to diet and fluid intake, laxatives. In resistant cases biofeedback or surgical intervention can be considered as an option. If surgery is contemplated the advice of a colorectal surgeon should be sought.

Inflammatory bowel disease

- The presence of perianal abscess, persistent fissuring (usually lateral), skin tags, and fistula should raise the possibility of perianal Crohn's disease.

- Fissures are resistant to treatment and at atypical sites, e.g. lateral.
- Skin tags are generally large and 'fleshy'. Although minor skin tags are seen in up to 10% of the normal population, (particularly at the site of healed fissures), larger tags are strongly suggestive of inflammatory bowel disease. Need careful histological examination with multiple layers looking for granulomas if resected. Pathologist needs to be told that Crohn's disease is suspected.
- Fistula with discharge may be present.
- There is often surprisingly little discomfort in the presence of extensive perianal Crohn's disease (in the absence of perianal abscess formation).
- Management is complex, with anti-inflammatories and immunosupressive agents. MRI is useful. Surgery should be minimal (abscess drainage, seton placement, diversion).

Inflammatory bowel disease: introduction

- 25 % of inflammatory bowel disease (IBD) presents in childhood, usually as Crohn's disease or ulcerative colitis. The UK incidence is 5.2/100 000 children <16 years of age. Crohn's disease is the more common. Family history of Crohn's disease or ulcerative colitis is common. Both diseases can occur in the same family.
- **Crohn's disease** is a chronic inflammatory disease that can affect any part of the bowel, from mouth to anus. The most common sites are terminal ileum, ileocolon, and colon. The typical pathological features are transmural inflammation and granuloma formation, which may be patchy.
- **Ulcerative colitis** is an inflammatory disease limited to the colonic and rectal mucosa. The characteristic histology is mucosal and submucosal inflammation with goblet cell depletion, cryptitis, and crypt abscesses but no granulomas. The inflammatory change is usually diffuse rather than patchy.
- **Colitis** is inflammation of the colon. Characteristic features include abdominal pain, tenesmus, bloody diarrhoea, and blood and mucus per rectum. Children with inflammatory bowel disease who have colitis can have either ulcerative colitis or Crohn's disease.
- 10–15% of children with inflammatory bowel disease have colitis which is **indeterminate**, which means the histology is consistent with inflammatory bowel disease but not characteristic of Crohn's disease or ulcerative colitis.
- The precise aetiology of inflammatory bowel disease is unknown and reflects a complex interaction between genetic predisposition, immune dysfunction and environmental triggers. Smoking is a risk factor for Crohn's disease but protects against ulcerative colitis.
- The differential diagnosis of inflammatory bowel disease is wide and should be considered in the diagnostic work-up.
- Inflammatory bowel disease runs a chronic relapsing course, with a significant morbidity particularly during the adolescent growth spurt.
- Growth and nutrition are key issues in the management with the aim of treatment being to induce and then maintain disease remission with minimal side effects.
- Diagnosis is by upper and lower endoscopy and barium radiology or some other modality (e.g. ultrasound, MRI) to assess the small bowel.
- Management is by careful clinical assessment and multidisciplinary management as part of an inflammatory bowel disease service led by a physician with expertise in the condition

Differential diagnosis of inflammatory bowel disease

Infective

- *Salmonella*
- *Shigella*
- *Campylobacter pylori*
- *E. coli* 0157 (and other strains of *E. coli*)
- *Yersinia enterocolitica*
- *Ameobiasis*
- *Giardia llambia*
- Tuberculosis
- Cytomegalovirus
- *Entamoeba histolytica*
- Pseudomembraneous enterocolitis (*Clostridium difficile* infection).

Non-infective

- Eosinophilic gastrointestinal disorders including eosinophilic gastro-enteritis, eosinophilic colitis, eosinophilic proctitis
- Vasculitis and autoimmune conditions eg Henoch Schönlein purpura, haemolytic uraemic syndrome
- Polyposis syndromes
- Immunodeficiency states (e.g. chronic granulomatous disease)
- Coeliac disease
- Intestinal lymphoma
- Ischaemic colitis
- Hirschprung's enterocolitis
- Necrotizing enterocolitis (newborn)
- Behçet's disease
- Solitary rectal ulcer syndrome
- Carbohydrate intolerance
- Laxative abuse
- Non-steroidal anti-inflammatory drug-induced enterocolitis
- Lymphoid nodular hyperplasia.

Chronic granulomatous disease

- Can present with granulomatous inflammation in the gastrointestinal tract (Crohn's like).
- Mostly X linked.
- Defect of neutrophil killing.
- Presents with recurrent bacterial infections, abscesses, osteomyelitis usually in the first year of life.
- Diagnosis is by detection of the impaired neutrophil respiratory burst using the nitroblue tetrazolium test (NBT).
- Treatment is with prophylactic antibiotics, anti-inflammatories and corticosteroids if there is significant gut inflammation.
- Bone marrow transplant offers the potential for cure.

Behçet's syndrome

- Oro-genital ulceration with/without non-erosive arthritis, thrombophlebitis, vascular thromboses, or CNS abnormalities including meningoencephalitis.
- Treatment of orogenital ulceration is often unsatisfactory, however local/systemic steroids may be used acutely.
- Other drugs that have been used in prophylaxis include azathioprine and thalidomide.

Crohn's disease

Introduction

Crohn's disease is a chronic inflammatory disease that can affect any part of the bowel, from mouth to anus. Family history is common. 25% of patients present in childhood (age <18 years), most commonly during the adolescent growth spurt.

- The diagnosis should be considered in children who present with abdominal pain, diarrhoea, weight loss, unexplained growth failure, and pubertal delay.
- The clinical course is one of recurrent relapses.
- Particularly in adolescence, the disease impacts significantly on growth and development.
- Assessment includes upper and lower gastrointestinal endoscopy and barium radiology.
- Medical management is complex, requiring multidisciplinary input and a major emphasis on nutrition.
- Surgery is frequently required in resistant Crohn's disease but the relapse rate is high and continued medical therapy usually required.

Clinical features

The disease may be florid at presentation or insidious in onset. The diagnosis may therefore be delayed, sometimes for many months or even years. Most cases are underweight and up to 50% have significant growth failure, usually associated with delay in pubertal development. Growth failure can be the presenting feature

The commonest presenting symptoms are abdominal pain, diarrhoea, and weight loss. In the British Paediatric Surveillance Unit (BPSU) survey this triad was seen in only 25% of children. Abdominal pain was the commonest symptom occurring in 75%, nearly 60% had weight loss preceding diagnosis, 56% of children had diarrhoea while only 45% reported both diarrhoea and weight loss (Sawczenko A. Sandhu B. K. Logan R. F. et al Prospective survey of childhood inflammatory bowel disease in the British Isles. *Lancet* 2001; **357**:1093–4). Abdominal pain is, however, common in children. The presence of additional features such as vomiting, diarrhoea, blood per rectum, weight loss, joint pains, and/or systemic upset, particularly if growth failure is present, should always prompt consideration of Crohn's disease and further evaluation and/or investigations if appropriate.

- The perianal examination is crucial in the assessment of such children as perianal skin tags, fistulae, and resistant fissures make Crohn's disease likely.
- Large, fleshy skin tags are strongly suggestive of Crohn's disease.
- Perianal visualization is therefore an essential part of the assessment of a child with abdominal pain, particularly if chronic.

Nutritional status is frequently compromised at diagnosis. This is multifactorial.

- There is decreased food intake because of anorexia and abdominal pain following food which reduces the desire to eat.
- There may be reduced absorption in the presence of bowel mucosal inflammation.
- There is also an increase in energy requirements, chronic inflammation being associated with an increased metabolic rate.

Investigation

- Basic investigation includes a full blood count, basic biochemistry, liver function tests, and inflammatory markers,
- Most (not all) children with active Crohn's disease will have raised inflammatory markers at presentation,
- Inflammatory markers are less likely to be raised in ulcerative colitis, particularly if not florid.
- Infective colitis should be excluded by stool culture (including ova, cysts, and parasites), Stool should be sent for Clostridium difficile toxin.
- **Endoscopy is indicated in all cases in order to get a tissue diagnosis and assess disease extent.**
- Endoscopy should include upper gastrointestinal endoscopy and ileo-colonoscopy.
- A positive family history should lower the threshold for investigation.

Most children in the UK have endoscopy under general anaesthetic, although some centres will investigate children using controlled sedation. Adequate bowel preparation is essential, as a good mucosal view will only be obtained if the bowel is clear. Ileocolonoscopy and upper gastrointestinal endoscopy with biopsy provide information about disease severity and extent (in conjunction with barium radiology) as well as a tissue diagnosis in most cases. The disease extent will influence the choice of treatment and follow-up. It is essential to take biopsies as there may be no endoscopic abnormality but significant histological change.

- Small-bowel disease is best assessed by either barium meal and follow-through or small-bowel enema. Ultrasound will assess bowel wall thickening and is specific but less sensitive.
- White cell scanning can be used to assess colitis but is not a particularly sensitive investigation for small-bowel disease. It may, in selected cases, help with the ongoing assessment of colitis.
- MRI is useful in the assessment of difficult perianal disease.
- Histology is indeterminate in a significant number of children with colitis (indeterminate colitis) and in these cases serological markers may help in the assessment (pANCA positive in 70% of UC, pASCA positive in >50% of Crohn's disease).

Growth failure

Occurs as a consequence of:
- Nutritional impairment
- The systemic consequences of gut inflammation
- Disturbances of the growth hormone/insulin-like growth factor axis
- The side effects of corticosteroids when used.

Some extraintestinal manifestations of Crohn's disease

- Joint disease in 10%
- Skin rashes—erythema nodosum, erythema multiforme, pyoderma gangrenosum, cutaneous Crohn's disease
- Liver disease (rare in childhood)—sclerosing cholangitis, autoimmune liver disease
- Iritis/uveitis
- Osteoporosis.

Complications of Crohn's disease

- Growth failure with delayed puberty
- Emotional disturbance—difficulty with friendships, impact of a chronic disease with chronic symptoms, impact of pubertal delay
- Treatment toxicity, e.g. corticosteroids
- Osteoporosis
- Long-term cancer risk.

Diagnostic work-up in children with suspected inflammatory bowel disease

- Full blood work-up including inflammatory markers
- Stool culture
- Gastroscopy
- Ileocolonscopy
- Barium meal and follow-through.

Clinical course

Crohn's disease runs a chronic relapsing and remitting course. A single episode of active disease followed by a sustained clinical remission is rare. The chronic nature of the inflammatory process (and frequent need for steroids) leads to ongoing growth failure, usually with delayed onset of puberty. Many children will miss periods of schooling, and their illness may disrupt their social and psychological well-being. They often look younger than their peers and are treated accordingly. Children who are chronically ill and who lag behind physically, educationally, and socially may struggle during their adolescent years and into adulthood.

Management

A multidisciplinary approach is important. Key professionals include paediatric gastroenterologist, general paediatrician, paediatric surgeon, radiologist, histopathologist, paediatric dietician, nurse specialist, and psychologist. Close liaison with education is essential. Appropriate strategies need to be in place for transition to adult services.

- The aim is to induce remission and to normalize growth and development minimizing treatment impact and complications.
- The initial treatment will be determined by the clinical state of the child and the disease extent.
- Local therapy may be appropriate for local disease.
- In most children exclusive enteral nutrition is appropriate as first line treatment.
- Corticosteroids are indicated in severe colitis.
- Additional therapies are often required, however, because of the frequently relapsing nature of the disease and surgical input required in up to 50% of cases.
- Basic anthropometry, including height and weight together with pubertal status, is an essential part of the initial clinical and follow up assessment.
- Multidisciplinary care with attention to disease control and social, family, and educational issues is a fundamental part of management.

Exclusive enteral nutrition

The use of liquid dietary therapy as a substitute for normal diet for a period (6–8 weeks) will induce disease remission in 70–80% of children if cases are selected appropriately and compliance is good. Large volumes are required, with individualized volume and feed concentration to achieve weight gain and to prevent hunger. The volume of feed is increased over 5–7 days depending on tolerance. Often children require 120% or more of their predicted calorific requirements. Most children tolerate their feed orally, divided evenly through the day. The formula can be flavoured to improve compliance. Nasogastric feeding is an option, and is most useful in children who cannot tolerate a volume large enough to meet their calorific needs by mouth.

The formulation used most frequently in the UK is Modulen IBD® (Nestlé). This is a polymeric feed specifically designed for use in inflammatory bowel disease. EO28 (SHS), an elemental feed, is an effective alternative but less palatable. There have been no published controlled trials comparing the types of feed. Both induce improvement in symptoms. Often an improvement in well-being is felt in a matter of days. Weight gain is frequently established in the first week when the feed is well tolerated. Inflammatory markers almost universally improve within 2 weeks of treatment in children who are going to do well.

Motivation (patient, family, and healthcare professionals) is key and ongoing support is needed to maintain compliance. Food reintroduction after a period of enteral nutrition is staged and begins with low-residue foods, new food groups being added every few days over a period of 2–3 weeks. Enteral nutrition is weaned slowly during this period in order to ensure nutritional requirements are met during the weaning period.

Corticosteroids

Corticosteroids are considered in children with severe disease or isolated colitis, or in those who do not respond to enteral nutrition alone. They are an effective treatment for Crohn's disease with a similar efficacy to enteral nutrition although can impact on growth, at least in the short term.

Steroids are usually given as prednisolone 1–2 mg/kg (maximum dose 40–60 mg) by mouth although occasionally intravenous steroids are required. High-dose prednisolone is continued until remission is achieved, and then the dose is weaned by reducing the daily dose by 5 mg each week. Soluble rather than enteric-coated preparations should be used. Calcium and vitamin D supplements given as Calcichew D3 forte® should be given to children at risk of deficiency, particularly during the adolescent growth spurt. DEXA scanning of bone mineral density is useful although needs to be interpreted in the context of height, weight, and pubertal status. An antacid preparation may be required in children with gastritis.

Budesonide (which has a high first-pass metabolism and therefore less toxicity) has been used with good effect in ileocaecal (right-sided) disease.

Side effects of steroid therapy

- Immunosupression with increased susceptibility to infection
- Cushingoid facies (moon face)
- Inappropriate weight gain (central obesity) and fluid retention
- Acne, hisutism and striae
- Osteopenia/osteoporosis/aseptic necrosis
- Hypertension
- Glucose intolerance
- Pancreatitis
- Hyperlipidaemia
- Depressed mood
- Growth suppression, adrenal suppression, delayed puberty
- Cataract.

Maintaining remission
- 50–90% of people diagnosed with Crohn's disease will relapse within the first 12 months.
- Maintaining remission is therefore a major challenge.
- 5-ASA derivatives are widely used but of little proven benefit; however, they are useful to control continuing active disease or for the management of acute flare-ups. High doses are generally used. Sulfasalazine in syrup form is most appropriate for the younger children, with mesalazine given as either controlled or delayed release preparations in older children. Controlled release preparations (e.g. Pentasa)® work better proximally and delayed release preparations work better distally (e.g. Asacol®).
- Continued emphasis on good nutrition is essential with a number of children electing to remain, long term on nutritional supplements. Most children require higher than normal requirements, particularly when well. Children with long-term nutritional needs may benefit from gastrostomy placement for supplementary feeding.
- Repeated courses of exclusive enteral nutrition and/or steroids can be given.
- Corticosteroids are not effective as maintenance therapy.

Further management
- **Azathioprine** (or 6-mercaptopurine, a metabolite of azathioprine) is a steroid-sparing agent that is effective in 60–80% of cases inducing a sustained remission and growth spurt in many cases. Azathioprine is used more commonly in the UK. More than 50% of children with Crohn's disease are likely to need azathioprine. The usual indication is to give after 2–3 relapses, particularly if over a short period. Growth failure is a factor in the decision to treat, particularly if steroid requirements are high. Azathioprine is increasingly being used at diagnosis in severe cases. It can take 3–6 months to take effect. There is significant potential toxicity, with flu-like symptoms, gastrointestinal symptoms, leucopenia, hepatitis, pancreatitis, rash, and infection. The dose of azathioprine is 2–2.5 mg/kg per day and for 6-mercaptopurine 1–1.5 mg/kg per day, given as a single daily dose. Thiopurine methyl transferase (TPMT) is important in the metabolism of thiopurine derivatives. Genetic polymorphisms for this enzyme will increase the risk of toxicity and consideration should be given to checking this before starting. There is small increase in the risk of lymphoma with long-term use of thiopurine derivatives. Frequent blood monitoring is required. There are various suggested regimens. The BNF for children recommends a weekly full blood count for 4 weeks, then 3 monthly. Parents/children should be told to report any symptoms or signs of bone marrow suppression (bruising, bleeding, infection) acutely.
- **Methotrexate**, initially given parenterally, is used in children who are intolerant to or fail to respond to thiopurine derivatives.

Refractory disease

Refractory disease refers to disease that fails to respond to the standard therapies.

Infliximab

Tumour necrosis factor(TNF)-α is a proinflammatory cytokine produced in lymphocytes and macrophages that has been implicated in the pathogenesis of Crohn's disease. There are several therapeutic modalities that antagonize its effects. These include anti-TNFα antibodies including the mouse–human-derived infliximab. It is indicated for induction of remission in refractory paediatric Crohn's disease, including fistulating disease and in such children given every 8 weeks as maintenance therapy. Infliximab however is not without side effects, some of which can be significant. Reactivation of latent tuberculosis has been reported and an increased risk of lymphoma has been shown in patients receiving infliximab in combination with other immuno-suppressive agents, including hepatosplenic T cell lymphoma associated with infliximab use for Crohn's disease, mainly in adolescents. This type of lymphoma is rare (~100 published cases worldwide) but uniformly fatal and why there is an increased incidence in this group is unknown. This reported toxicity should not preclude its use in appropriate cases, but does necessitate a full risk benefit discussion with the patient and their family before starting it. The National Institute of Clinical Excellence (NICE) has provided specific guidance for the use of infliximab in adults which can reasonably be applied to children. There is the potential for infliximab dependency or loss of response, in which case other biologicals such as a Adalimumab can be tried.

Indications for infliximab use in adults (NICE)

- Active disease unresponsive to immunosuppressant therapy and not amenable to surgery (i.e. localized resection)
- Treatment-resistant fistulizing disease

Surgery

Surgery is indicated for acute complications such as perianal abscess or stricture. Emergency surgery may be needed in the child who presents with acute toxic colitis and colonic dilatation. Elective or semi-elective surgery is indicated in children with chronic disease resistant to the medical therapy, particularly if there is chronic symptomatology, chronic steroid use, and/or growth failure. Surgical options range from removal of isolated disease segments or strictures to extensive panproctocolectomy and the possibility of permanent stoma formation. Surgical resection of active disease can lead to rapid increases in growth and a prolonged period of disease remission therefore timing of surgery relative to the pubertal growth spurt is crucial.

Specific situations

Oesophagitis

Most children with oesophageal involvement present with disease elsewhere in the bowel. Treatment of symptomatic oesophagitis or gastritis with a proton pump inhibitor is helpful, particularly if corticosteroids are being given in addition.

Oral disease

Oral manifestations of Crohn's disease may occur as recurrent aphthous ulceration, as orofacial granulomatosis (swelling of the lips and cheeks), or as a manifestation of panenteric disease. Orofacial granulomatosis implies oral disease in isolation without disease elsewhere in the gastrointestinal tract. Management can be local or systemic. Oral disease may also respond to enteral nutrition. Benzoate- and azo-free diets have been used. Systemic antibiotics, corticosteroids, and thiopurines are required in difficult cases. Intralesional corticosteroids can reduce swelling and improve cosmesis.

Perianal Crohn's disease

Active perianal disease can occur in isolation, although it is often associated with active Crohn's disease in other locations. Treatment of the active disease will often result in improvement of perianal disease and/or closure of fistulae. Specific therapeutic strategies used include 5-ASA derivatives; local and systemic corticosteroids and other immunosuppression including azathioprine; and antibiotics, particularly metronidazole. Tacrolimus may be administered topically, although systemic treatment can be used if the conventional treatments fail. Infliximab has been used in difficult cases with reasonable efficacy. Surgical management is by abscess drainage, Seton placement to encourage fistula drainage, and diversion in the most resistant cases.

Case study

A 15 year old boy presents with a 6 month history of abdominal discomfort, loose stools and weight loss and has a reduced height velocity (<4cm/year) over the last 12 months. He has not yet entered puberty. He has missed more than 50% of school. He looks pale and unwell. Basic investigations show a mild normochromic anaemia, thrombocytosis, raised C reactive protein and a low serum albumin. Crohn's disease is suspected – further investigation including upper gastrointestinal endoscopy, ileo-colonoscopy and barium radiology confirm ileo-caecal Crohn's disease.

Management priorities include getting him well, establishing weight gain, promoting growth and the onset of puberty and getting him back into school.

He is treated with Enteral Nutrition given as sole therapy for 8 weeks, which induces a clinical remission. He is then well for more than 6 months with good weight gain. He does unfortunately relapse and requires a further course of enteral nutrition. Steroids are avoided because of the potential toxicity (on growth in particular) and Azathioprine introduced as steroid sparing therapy. He then has a more sustained remission with improved liner growth and the onset of puberty. His final adult height is normal.

Medical therapy will suffice in most cases of ileo-caecal Crohn's disease particularly with the early introduction of Azathioprine as steroid sparing medication. Newer agents eg infliximab can be used. If the disease proves resistant to medical management particularly if there are persistent symptoms or structuring disease and/or persistent growth failure then ileo-caecal resection is appropriate which will affect a remission, although recurrent disease is common.

References and resources

Beattie RM, Croft NM, Fell JM, Afzal NA, Heuschkel RB. Inflammatory bowel disease. Arch Dis Child 2006; **91**:426–432

Carter MJ, Lobo AJ, Travis SP et al. on behalf of the British Society of Gastroenterology. Guidelines for the management of inflammatory bowel disease in adults. Gut 2004; **53**(Suppl V): v1–v16 available at www.bsg.org.uk)

Escher JC, Taminau JA, Nieuwenhuis EE et al. Treatment of inflammatory bowel disease: best available evidence. Inflammatory Bowel Dis 2003; **9**(1):34–58

European evidence based consensus on the diagnosis and management of Crohn's disease (ECCO). Gut 2006; **55**:1–58

Inflammatory bowel disease in children and adolescents: Recommendations for diagnosis—the PORTO criteria. Journal of Gastroenterology and Nutrition 2005; **41**:1–7

National Institute of Clinical Excellence (NICE). Guidance for the use of infliximab. www.nice.org.uk

Sawczenko A, Sandhu BK, Logan RF et al. Prospective survey of childhood inflammatory bowel disease in the British Isles. Lancet 2001; **357**:1093–1094

Patient Support Groups

National Association for Colitis and Crohn's Disease (NACC), 4 Beaumont House, Sutton Road, St Albans, Herts AL1 5HH. www.nacc.org.uk

Crohn's in Childhood Research Association (CICRA) Parkgate House, 356 West Barnes Lane, Motspur Park, Surrey KT3 6NB. www.cicra.org

Nutritional management of Crohn's disease

Crohn's disease in childhood has a significant effect on growth and development.

Enteral nutrition as a treatment for Crohn's disease was first introduced in the 1970s and is used as a primary therapy in children because of its proven efficacy, lack of side effects and positive impact on growth. The aim is to induce remission while promoting weight gain and subsequent height gain and pubertal development.

Enteral feeding can induce remission in 70–80% of children selected and if compliance is good. The enteral feed formula replaces a normal diet for a 6–8 week period.

Nutritional status

Nutritional status is compromised by:
- Malabsorption due to mucosal inflammation.
- Pro-inflammatory cytokine action leading to tissue catabolism.
- Nausea, anorexia, abdominal pain resulting in decreased nutrient intake.
- Gut losses of protein and micronutrients.

These factors can lead to significant weight loss and growth failure with delayed onset of puberty.

Nutritional status is assessed by the following:
- Diet history including normal (average) and recent intake (including assessment of appetite).
- Estimation of weight loss.
- Anthropometry including mid-arm circumference, subscapular skin thickness.
- Weight and height as plotted on standard growth charts.
- Estimation of requirements (including physical activity levels).

In the absence of other data on basal energy requirements in active Crohn's disease, the estimated average requirement (EAR) for age (reference nutrient intake, RNI) is used.

Treatment

Exclusive enteral nutrition

Enteral nutrition needs to be given exclusively as the complete feed source (with no other foods) over a 6–8 week period.

Nutritional requirement

This is usually 100–120% of the RNI. The aim is to achieve 100% of RNI within the first 2–4 days, as children often require increasing amounts particularly as physical activity levels increase. In cases of severe growth failure it may prudent to use the height age EAR value. A minimum of the RNI for protein, vitamins, and minerals should be provided in the full feed volume. Fluid requirements should be assessed based on body weight. Continued discussion of physical activity levels are needed in order to adjust requirements and therefore intake appropriately.

The most commonly used formulae are:
- Modulen IBD® (Nestlé): a polymeric feed designed specifically for use in inflammatory bowel disease
- Elemental 028® (SHS): an elemental feed.

Polymeric feeds have been found in numerous studies to be as effective as elemental feeds. They are also cheaper and more palatable.

A multidisciplinary approach in instigating treatment is essential. In our experience compliance has been shown to be better with a 3–5 day inpatient admission to access members of the team and establish a tailored enteral feed regimen. The feed can be established slowly, particularly if the child is very unwell and/or at risk of refeeding syndrome. During this time the following can be addressed:
- Spending time with the family promoting the benefits of enteral nutrition.
- Building up feed volumes as tolerated to meet requirements.
- Addressing practical issues such as school, holidays, and special occasions.
- Involve psychologist/psychiatrist input in cases of severe anorexia and depression.
- Parents / carers can observe the method of feed preparation and become familiar with their recipe.
- Arrange prescription for enteral feeds through contact with the GP and community pharmacist.
- Nursing support and encouragement.
- Adjustment of the recipe if necessary to optimize nutritional content within a manageable volume.
- Consider and establish exclusive or partial nasogastric feeding if the patients fail to take it orally.

In order to meet requirements large volumes are needed, but the recipe can be individualized. If calorific requirements are to be met within a specific volume, the feed may be concentrated. This is also aids compliance if the prescribed volume is more acceptable to the patient. The standard concentration of Modulen IBD® is 20% (1 kcal/mL) but in practice concentrations up to 30% (1.5 kcal/mL) are tolerated. If symptoms of abdominal discomfort or diarrhoea are reported then the concentrations should be reduced in 1–2% increments until tolerance is achieved.

Feeds should preferably be taken orally with the total volume divided into a minimum of six drinks per day given at regular intervals, for example at meal and snack times including one taken at bedtime. Modulen IBD® can be taken as it is or flavoured with Nestlé flavour sachets or other commercially available milkshake flavourings, such as Crusha™ which is a liquid flavouring that mixes well with Modulen IBD.® Elemental 028®/ Elemental 028 Extra® can be flavoured with flavour sachets, or Elemental 028 Extra® prescribed in ready-to-feed flavoured cartons.

Nasogastric feeding is an option if there are difficulties with taste and volumes. Feeds are given as boluses that are gravity fed unless the risk of refeeding syndrome or severe malnutrition warrants a continuous feeding regimen using a pump. Avoiding use of the pump allows easier and earlier discharge home. In such cases patients are strongly encouraged to try to take a proportion of the prescribed volume orally, and ideally weaned off the nasogastric feeding in the early weeks on enteral nutrition.

Once full volumes are established patients are allowed to take sugar-free chewing gum, sugar-free boiled sweets, and squash-type drinks with no added sugar if desired. It is advised that sugar-free boiled sweets are limited to 4–5 sweets per day because they contain sorbitol, a type of sweetener, which has a laxative effect if taken in excess.

Refeeding syndrome

Refeeding syndrome is the occurrence of severe fluid and electrolyte shifts with associated complications in malnourished patients undergoing enteral/ parenteral nutrition and is a risk in children with Crohn's disease who present in a poor nutritional state. Careful questioning is essential to establish recent dietary intake, amount of weight lost, and over what period of time. If the patient is at risk and dietary intake has been poor with rapid weight loss enteral feeds can be introduced at 50% of requirements (up to a maximum of 1000 kcal) for the first 48 h to avoid rapid electrolyte shifts. Patients at high risk may only tolerate 25% of requirements for the first 48 h. Feeding too quickly can result in severe drops in phosphate, potassium, and magnesium, which can lead to disturbances in body systems including cardiac arrhythmias Careful monitoring of serum electrolytes (including phosphate and magnesium) is essential, with supplementation if necessary, and feeds increased gradually over 5–7 days to meet requirements.

Monitoring

It is assumed that, as energy levels return and as patients resume normal activities, calorific requirements will increase further above EAR requirements. Weekly contact by telephone ensures that the feed recipe is optimized. Hunger is used as an indicator to increase quantity as either volume or concentration of feed. If a patient is getting hungry after taking the prescribed volume, compliance is more likely to be compromised.

Children who are particularly active and regularly participate in sport can be given an additional one-off drink recipe, e.g. 250–300 mL, to cover these periods of activity.
- Failure to respond clinically may be due to poor compliance.
- Insufficient follow-up can result in failure to gain expected weight if feed quantity is not being adapted to needs.

Patients are usually seen in clinic 4 weeks into treatment and then at 8 weeks to introduce the food reintroduction programme.

Food reintroduction

Food is reintroduced gradually over a 2–3 week period. There is no consensus or standardized protocol, but it is widely accepted that food should not be introduced too rapidly. During this period nutritional support needs to be maintained by a gradual weaning of the enteral feed.

The following is an example of a food reintroduction programme that has proved to be acceptable to patients, based on a variety of foods in the initial stages and length of time to return to a normal diet.

- Stage 1 Introduce 'bland' foods—wheat/gluten-free, milk and dairy-free, low fat and fibre, non-spicy—over 5 days.
- Stage 2 Introduce foods containing wheat and gluten over 5 days.
- Stage 3 Introduce milk and dairy foods over 5 days.
- Stage 4 Introduce high fibre, higher fat, spicy foods over 10 days.

Continued nutritional support following exclusive enteral nutrition

Children who have severe growth failure will continue to have greater nutritional requirements once returned to a normal diet. Optimizing nutritional intake in the immediate period following enteral nutrition and during remission can be aided with the use of various supplements. Many patients prefer to continue to take 250–500 mL of the enteral feed formula. Others, particularly those who had difficulties in accepting the enteral feed formula, prefer to take an alternative. A standard sip feed such as Fortini® (Nutricia), Paediasure® (Abbott), Fortisip,® Fortijuce® (Nutricia), Ensure Plus,® Enlive® (Abbott) can be used as indicated. If a high-energy supplement is needed to support a good nutritional intake Scandishake® (SHS) or Calshake® (Fresenius) are well accepted by children. Calogen® (SHS) can be used as an energy supplement if other drink-style supplements are refused. Multivitamin and mineral supplementation is recommended.

References and resources

Dietary reference values for food energy and nutrients for United Kingdom. Department of Health, London, 1991.

Ulcerative colitis

25% of inflammatory bowel disease presents in childhood, 1/3 as ulcerative colitis. Presentation can occur at any age and ulcerative colitis is the commonest cause of inflammatory bowel disease in the younger child. Family history of Crohn's disease or ulcerative colitis is common in index cases.

Clinical presentations

- Acute toxic colitis
- Pancolitis—mild, moderate or severe
- Left-sided disease/distal colitis.

Pancolitis is the most common presentation in children. Characteristic symptoms are abdominal pain, diarrhoea, and blood per rectum although atypical presentations can occur. There may be significant pain before or during bowel movement, relieved by the passage of stool (tenesmus). Night stools are common. A history of foreign travel should be excluded. Systemic disturbance can accompany more severe disease including tachycardia, fever, weight loss, anaemia, hypoalbuminaemia, leucocytosis, and raised inflammatory markers. The presentation can be more indolent with occult blood loss or non-specific abdominal pain. Constipation can be a feature, particularly in distal colitis.

- Extraintestinal manifestations include:
  - arthropathy (10%), usually knees, ankles
  - ankylosing spondylitis (rare in childhood)
  - liver disease (sclerosing cholangitis, auto-immune liver disease)
  - erythema nodosum
  - iritis and uveitis.
- Disease associations include:
  - pyoderma gangrenosum
  - ankylosing spondylitis and sacroileitis.
- Complications include:
  - toxic megacolon
  - osteoporosis
  - growth failure
  - colorectal cancer.
- There is an increased thrombotic tendency in severe disease.
- It is common to develop an 'irritable bowel type syndrome' as the colitis enters remission.
- Proximal constipation is common in distal colitis.

Investigation

Clinical presentation is generally with abdominal pain and bloody diarrhoea. It is important to give careful consideration to the differential diagnosis. Investigation is by careful history and examination with basic blood testing including blood count, differential, inflammatory markers including C-reactive protein and ESR, and liver function. Bloods tests can be normal. It is essential to culture the stool to exclude an infective cause. Further investigation is with upper and lower gastrointestinal endoscopy including ileoscopy with biopsies. This will help differentiate between ulcerative colitis and Crohn's disease. In children with indeterminate changes (not diagnostic of Crohn's disease or ulcerative colitis) on histology, pANCA status may be useful. pANCA is positive in 70% of ulcerative colitis and <10% of patients with Crohn's disease or controls.

If liver function is abnormal, then a more detailed auto-antibody screen and liver ultrasound should be performed with consideration of ERCP/liver biopsy. Family history of inflammatory bowel disease should lower the threshold for investigation.

Endoscopy is indicated in all cases in order to get a tissue diagnosis and assess disease extent unless disease is so severe (e.g. toxic megacolon) and empirical treatment required, in which case it can be deferred.

Clinical course

Ulcerative colitis runs a chronic relapsing and remitting course. A single episode of active disease followed by a sustained clinical remission is rare. Growth failure is a feature, particularly when high doses of corticosteroids are used or disease becomes steroid dependent. Many children will miss periods of schooling, and their illness may disrupt their social and psychological well-being. Major anxieties can occur about school toilets, for example. These are important issues that need to be addressed by the multidisciplinary team responsible for the management of this chronic condition.

Management

General principles

- The general principles are similar to those for Crohn's disease (Chapter 42) and involve careful assessment, follow-up, and input from the multidisciplinary team. Psychological factors are of particular importance.
- The aim of treatment is to induce and maintain a disease remission avoiding either disease or treatment-related complications. The choice of treatment is influenced by disease severity and extent (Fig. 44.1). The treatment regimens used in childhood are similar to those for adults, and the comprehensive guidelines from the British Society of Gastroenterology are useful and generally applicable to the management of children. Many of the therapies used have significant toxicity and the reader is referred to these guidelines and the paediatric BNF (see References and resources) for a fuller account of these including the specific monitoring regimens.
- The lifelong nature of the condition means that appropriate arrangements need to be put in place for transition to adult care.
- It is important to pay attention to general factors including the importance of good nutrition, educational strategies (e.g. access to the toilet in school, recognition of the impact of a chronic disease on learning) and management of psychological problems including anxiety. Milk exclusion or other elimination diets help a number of cases but need to be under careful dietetic supervision to maintain calorific and nutritional adequacy of the diet. Many patients claim benefit from fish oil supplements and probiotics.

Acute toxic colitis

This implies that in addition to colitic symptoms (pain, diarrhoea, and blood per rectum) the child has systemic upset with pyrexia, tachycardia, and abdominal tenderness/distension. **Toxic megacolon** (colonic dilation on plain abdominal radiograph) is a life-threatening complication of this, although fortunately rare in childhood. It is important to get multiple stool cultures to exclude infection which can be a trigger either for disease presentation or for disease flare-up, and is important in differential diagnosis. It is important to specifically request testing for *C. difficile* toxin, which can precipitate an acute exacerbation.

- It is important to remember that Crohn's disease can occasionally present as acute toxic colitis.
- Children with acute toxic colitis are best managed in specialist centres by paediatric gastroenterologists in conjunction with paediatric/adult surgeons.

Practical management

Practical management of acute toxic colitis

- **Fluid resuscitation** with saline bolus if required for reduced peripheral perfusion.
- **Blood transfusion** if Hb < 8 g/dL.
- **Intravenous fluids**—Initially 0.45% saline/dextrose with 20 mmol KCl per 500 mL modified depending on fluid balance and electrolyte results.
- **Intravenous hydrocortisone** 10 mg/kg in four divided doses— maximum 100 mg four times daily.
- **Broad-spectrum intravenous antibiotics if pyrexial** (e.g. ciprofloxacin, metronidazole).
- Intravenous ciclosporin can be considered.
- **Plain abdominal radiograph**—if toxic megacolon (colonic dilation) repeat every 12–24 h, or if deteriorates clinically.
- **Abdominal ultrasound** to look at bowel wall thickening.
- **Surgical review** (at presentation) as up to 50% with toxic megacolon will require colectomy, although most with an acute toxic colitis (not megacolon) will settle.
- **Consider subcutaneous heparin** for prophylaxis of venous thrombosis if the illness is prolonged.

- Once the child is stable, fluids and light diet can be allowed.
- Ciclosporin is occasionally used in the acute phase to induce remission in severe refractory colitis not responding to therapy in patients for whom colectomy is being considered. This can act as a bridge to azathioprine therapy, which is likely to take some weeks to take effect. There is significant toxicity, however. There has been limited recent experience using a single dose of the monocolonal antibody anti-TNF given acutely in children and adults with fulminant ulcerative colitis.

Pancolitis

Pancolitis—mild, moderate, severe but not toxic—is the more usual presentation in childhood.

Prednisolone and 5-ASA derivatives (sulfasalazine, mesalazine) should be started in most cases. In very mild disease 5-ASA derivatives can be used as sole therapy. Prednisolone is given as 1–2 mg/kg (usual maximum 40 mg) for 2–4 weeks weaned once remission is achieved over the subsequent 6–8 weeks. Soluble rather than enteric-coated preparations should used. Calcium and vitamin D supplements given as Calcichew D3 forte® should be given to children at risk of deficiency, particularly during the adolescent growth spurt. DEXA scanning of bone mineral density is useful, though needs to be interpreted in the context of height, weight, and pubertal status. Mesalazine preparations are generally given at high dose. Sulfasalazine, which is available as syrup, can be given to younger children. Higher doses of prednisolone are occasionally used. Intravenous steroids may be useful for 2–5 days in moderate to severe disease. It is sometimes necessary to use an antacid preparation in children with gastritis on upper gastrointestinal endoscopy. Exclusive enteral nutrition has no role. Milk exclusion is occasionally helpful. Dietetic input is useful, as most children with colitis will be in energy deficit with high calorific needs, and most children long-term should receive regular input.

The 5-ASA derivative should be continued long-term and will reduce the risk of relapse and of colorectal carcinoma. Toxic effects include headache, nausea, vomiting, and diarrhoea. Rare side effects include Stephen Johnson syndrome, pancreatitis, and agranulocytosis. Mesalazine preparations are general better tolerated than sulfasalazine.

There is no role for long-term steroids and these should be avoided where possible.

Disease severity in ulcerative colitis

- **Mild:** >4 stools per day ± blood. No systemic disturbance.
- **Moderate:** 4–6 stools per day with blood. Minimal systemic disturbance.
- **Severe:** 6+ stools per day, with systemic disturbance (fever, tachycardia, anaemia, hypoalbuminaemia).

Distal colitis

In children rectal treatments are not well tolerated and most will require systemic treatment. In older children local therapy should be considered, particularly if disease is distal involving sigmoid colon and rectum only. 5-ASA derivatives tend to be more effective than corticosteroids. Mesalazine preparations can be given as enema (usually in 100 mL) or suppository. Steroid preparations include Predfoam,® Predsol® (prednisolone), and Colifoam® (hydrocortisone).

It is important that children and families are adequately supported in the administration technique and positioning required. This will improve adherence and acceptability. Enemas are best given with the patient lying on their left side with the foot of the bed elevated and ample time given for the enema to act locally, i.e. 30–45 min before getting up and going to the toilet. Suppositories and small-volume enemas are easier to apply but are only effective for rectal disease. Proximal constipation is common in distal disease and should be treated with laxatives if present.

Thiopurine derivatives (azathioprine, 6 mercaptopurine)

- The main indication for azathioprine in ulcerative colitis, like Crohn's disease, is for steroid-sensitive, frequently relapsing disease (>2 flare-ups in 12 months), steroid-dependent disease (early relapse on weaning or discontinuation of steroids) and steroid-resistant disease (failure to respond to steroids).
- The aim of thiopurine therapy in children is to improve clinical well-being and reduce steroid requirements. There is an increasing tendency to give it at diagnosis in severe disease, particularly to those who don't respond rapidly to treatment. It can take 3–6 months to take effect. There is significant potential toxicity, with flu-like symptoms, gastrointestinal symptoms, leucopenia, hepatitis, pancreatitis, rash, and infection.
- Thiopurine methyl transferase (TPMT) is important in the metabolism of thiopurine derivatives. Genetic polymorphisms for this will increase the risk of toxicity and consideration should be given to checking this before starting.
- There is small increase in the risk of lymphoma with long-term use of thiopurine derivatives.
- Frequent blood monitoring is required. There are various suggested regimens. The BNF for children recommends a weekly full blood count for 4 weeks then 3 monthly. Parents/children should be told to report any symptoms or signs of bone marrow suppression (bruising, bleeding, infection) acutely.
- 6-Mercaptopurine is effective in a number of children either intolerant of or resistant to azathioprine.
- Dose of azathioprine is 2–2.5 mg/kg per day and 6-mercaptopurine 1–1.5mg/kg per day given as a single daily dose.
- There is no evidence base for the use of methotrexate in ulcerative colitis.

Surgical management

Surgery can be curative for ulcerative colitis. Surgery will be required in at least 15% within 5 years of diagnosis and 25% by 10 years. Subtotal colectomy and temporary ileostomy is the most commonly performed operation. This can be performed as an emergency (acute toxic colitis with failure to respond to medical treatment) or electively leaving a rectal stump as short as is practical. Indications for elective colectomy include disease resistant to medical treatment with morbidity either from the disease or complications of treatment, e.g. growth failure, high-grade dysplasia. Reconstruction is often timed after puberty to coincide with the holidays after school exams (aged 16+). This is usually in conjunction with the adult colorectal team.

Colectomy is curative from the point of view of the colitis. Following reconstruction, bowel frequency will be 10–12/day initially, reducing to 3–4/day by 1 year. However, there may be major long-term morbidity from faecal incontinence, defecation at night, adhesion obstruction, or problems with the rectal stump. Pouchitis affects at least 33% of all pouches, though antibiotics (metronidazole) may be helpful if given intermittently. Infertility can be a problem in women.

20% of patients prefer a permanent ileostomy combined with excision of the rectal stump, especially if there have been multiple complications following reconstruction.

Stoma management

This needs to be discussed before surgery where possible with the support of a stoma nurse who will advise about the practical management. Careful attention needs to be paid to stoma losses. The colon normally functions to reabsorb salt and water. Salt supplements may be required. Sodium status can be monitored by urine electrolytes, with low urinary sodium being suggestive of sodium depletion. If stoma losses increase significantly, e.g. during infection, there is a high risk of dehydration and IV fluid replacement may be required.

Cancer surveillance

Patient with colitis for >10 years, particularly if active, are at increased risk of colorectal cancer. Regular colonoscopic surveillance is indicated every 2–3 years. This is an issue for the paediatrician in children who have presented with disease at a young age. Risk factors for malignancy include young age at onset, longer duration of disease, and extent of colonic involvement. Colectomy is recommended if there is high-grade dysplasia or malignancy.

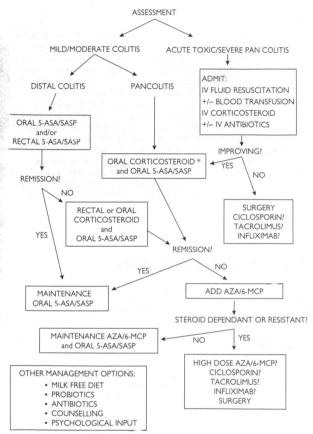

Fig. 44.1 Algorithm for the treatment of UC in children.

Abbreviations: 5-ASA, 5-aminosalicylates; AZA, azathioprine; 6-MCP, 6-mercaptopurine; SASP, sulfasalazine.

*Consider initial 2–5 days of IV therapy in moderate to severe pancolitis

Case study

An 10 year old girl presents with abdominal discomfort associated with frequent loose stools containing blood and mucus. Investigations show mild anaemia with thrombocytosis but no other abnormality. Stool cultures are negative. Colonoscopy shows a pancolitis with no normal mucosa. Histology is consistent with ulcerative colitis. She does well initially with corticosteroids and 5-ASA derivatives, but her disease relapses three times in the first year. Despite further course of steroids and a trial of milk exclusion, she becomes steroid dependent with poor growth and mood disturbance. She is started on azathioprine. This induces a more sustained remission, but 4 years later she is less well with steroid-dependent disease and significant toxicity. Repeat colonoscopy shows a featureless 'hosepipe' colon. After appropriate preoperative counselling she undergoes a subtotal colectomy with ileostomy and mucus fistula formation and does well with a symptom-free adolescence. She will be a good candidate for future reconstructive surgery after she has completed her schooling.

References and resources

Beattie RM, Croft NM, Fell JM, Afzal NA, Heuschkel RB. Inflammatory bowel disease. *Arch Dis Child* 2006;**91**:426–432

Bremner AR, Beattie RM. Therapy of ulcerative colitis in childhood. Expert opinion. *Pharmacotherapy* 2004;**5**(1):37–53

Carter MJ, Lobo AJ, Travis SP et al on behalf of the British Society of Gastroenterology. Guidelines for the management of inflammatory bowel disease in adults. *Gut* 2004;**53**(Suppl V): v1–v16

Collins P, Rhodes J. Ulcerative colitis, diagnosis and management. *BMJ* 2006; **333**:340–343

Escher JC, Taminau JA, Nieuwenhuis EE et al. Treatment of inflammatory bowel disease: best available evidence. *Inflammatory Bowel Dis* 2003;**9**(1):34–58

Eosinophilic disorders

This chapter discusses the wide spectrum of eosinophilic (allergic) disorders of the gut. They are generally not IgE mediated. Presentation is with the full spectrum of gastrointestinal symptoms and signs. Outside infancy the disorders may only become apparent on investigation of chronic gut symptoms by endoscopy to exclude oesophagitis, peptic ulceration, enteropathy, or colitis. Important disorders to consider are:

- Eosinophilic proctocolitis of infancy (dietary protein-induced proctocolitis of infancy)
- Eosinophilic enterocolitis of infancy (dietary protein-induced enterocolitis of infancy)
- Eosinophilic gastroenteropathies in the older child
- Eosinophilic oesophagitis.

Eosinophilic proctocolitis of infancy (dietary protein-induced proctocolitis of infancy)

- This is a common disorder and generally benign with a good prognosis.
- Most infants present while being breast- or formula-fed.
- Mean age at diagnosis of 2 months.
- Infants are generally healthy with visible specks or streaks of blood mixed with mucus in the stool. Blood loss is usually minimal, and anaemia is rare. There is a lack of vomiting, diarrhoea, or systemic symptoms. The infants are generally thriving.
- Differential diagnosis includes infection, constipation, anal fissures
- Cow's milk proteins and, less commonly, soy protein are the commonest triggers.
- Symptoms occur as a result of maternally ingested proteins excreted in breast milk or whole protein (casein)-based feeds.
- Endoscopic examination is usually deferred but if indicated will show a predominantly distal colitis with an eosinophilic infiltrate on biopsy. Endoscopic examination is indicated in infants in whom there is doubt about the initial diagnosis or a poor response to treatment.
- Blood work-up is usually unremarkable. Mild anaemia, thrombocytosis, and a low serum albumin may be seen. Peripheral eosinophilia is occasionally seen. Serum IgA may be low. IgE antibody skin prick testing and IgE RAST testing are often negative.
- The need to treat is dependent on the clinical symptoms.
- Diagnosis is secured by response to dietary elimination of the causal antigen. For breastfed infants, maternal restriction of cow's milk is required. This requires dietetic input. For cow's milk formula-fed infants or infants who have been breast-fed (with maternal dietary restriction) and want to switch to a formula feed, substitution with a protein hydrolysate formula (e.g. Nutramigen®, Mead Johnson) generally leads to cessation of bleeding. An amino acid-based formula (e.g. Neocate®, SHS) may be needed in those who have prolonged bleeding or persistence of other symptoms, e.g. colic, while taking an extensive hydrolysate. Bleeding is expected to resolve within 72 h of dietary exclusion. Continued bleeding may be an indication for referral for more invasive testing (i.e. biopsy).

- The condition generally resolves completely by age 1 or 2 years, and the causal food protein can be gradually added back to the diet at that time with monitoring.
- Delayed weaning until 6 months should be encouraged, with solids free of milk, soya, egg, and wheat in the first instance.
- It is usual to challenge first at 6–12 months. This is best done as a day case under supervision.
- The disorder is not IgE antibody mediated.

Eosinophilic enterocolitis of infancy (dietary protein-induced enterocolitis of infancy)

- This is part of a disease spectrum. Enterocolitis implies involvement of the small and large bowel and therefore the more severe end of the spectrum of eosinophilic proctocolitis of infancy.
- It can present with severe diarrhoea, dehydration, lethargy and acidosis with raised inflammatory markers and hypoalbuminaemia.
- Infants may require resuscitation if fluid losses are severe.
- Wide differential diagnosis, particularly sepsis.
- Cow's milk or soya are the proteins generally implicated.
- Upper and lower gastrointestinal endoscopy is indicated.
- Biopsy may show an enteropathy and/or a colitis both of which can be severe. Eosinophils are commonly seen.
- There may be a coexistent problem with immune tolerance.
- Treatment is by removal of the offending antigen. Amino acid-based formulas are generally required, with delayed introduction of other foods.
- Challenge can result in severe reactions (delayed), so should be done in hospital.
- A proportion of the most severe cases may require a period of bowel rest on total parenteral nutrition, anti-inflammatories/steroids, and/or other immunosuppression.
- Most infants outgrow the allergy by age 2–3 although may have a persistent hypersensitivity/dislike of the offending antigen.
- The disorder is not IgE antibody mediated.

Eosinophilic gastroenteropathies in the older child

- This is a spectrum of disorders which have in common eosinophilic inflammation of the gut.
- Different subtypes:
  - eosinophilic gastritis
  - eosinophilic oesophagitis
  - eosinophilic gastroenterocolitis
  - eosinophilic colitis.
- These conditions present with a full spectrum of gastrointestinal symptoms and presentations including nausea, dysphagia, pain, vomiting, diarrhoea, and blood per rectum.
- There is a wide differential diagnosis including gastroenteritis, parasitic infection, bacterial overgrowth, immunodeficiency, Inflammatory bowel disease, vasculitis.
- Diagnostic criteria is presence of:
  - gut symptoms
  - eosinophilic infiltrate in on or more areas from the oesophagus to the rectum
  - absence of other causes.
- Diagnosis is by biopsy and then clinicopathological correlation.
- Eosinophils are normally present in the lamina propria of the gut mucosa but not the submucosa, muscular or serosal layers.
- >20 eosinophills per high-power field with infiltration into the submucosa, muscular, or serosal layers is diagnostic in the presence of gut symptoms.
- Peripheral eosinophillia is common
- The condition is difficult to treat, and treatment decisions should be based on symptoms.
- A proportion of children are food sensitive. The usual offending food antigens are milk, egg, soya, and wheat. Exclusion of the presumed offending antigen should be on a trial basis with dietetic supervision (4–6 weeks) and careful observation of clinical symptoms. Skin-prick testing and IgE RAST antibody testing are most helpful in this food-sensitive group.
- Treatment of the non-food-sensitive group is very difficult, and immunosuppressive medication including corticosteroids may be required.

Eosinophilic oesophagitis

- Symptoms overlap with gastro-oesophageal reflux with a predominance in older atopic males.
- Dysphagia is common secondary to oesophageal dysmotility (this is an unusual symptom in children and should prompt consideration of further investigation).
- Skin-prick testing and IgE RAST antibody testing may be helpful.
- Acid reflux may be present on pH study (usually more prominent during the day than at night).
- Endoscopy in conjunction with the clinical picture is diagnostic.
- Diagnostic criteria on oesophageal biopsy are:
  - reflux oesophagitis >7 eosinophils per high-power field,
  - allergic eosinophilic oesophagitis >20 per high-power field.
- Treatments include those for gastro-oesophageal reflux, a trial of dietary elimination, corticosteroids, anti-inflammatories, and immunosuppression. Inhaled corticosteroids taken into the mouth then swallowed may be useful.
- Dietary elimination should be with milk and soya exclusion in the first instance. Wheat exclusion can be considered (second line). NB: Coeliac serology should be performed as a baseline if wheat exclusion is considered.
- The treatment can be difficult and response should be by clinical review and follow up endoscopy with repeat biopsies in difficult cases.
- The natural history not well defined, with relapse, remission, and chronicity.

Features suggestive of food allergy as a cause of gastrointestinal disease

- Temporal relationship between characteristic symptoms and ingestion of particular foods.
- Improvement in symptoms with removal of the implicated food.
- Confirmation of a relationship between ingestion of the specific dietary protein and symptoms by clinical challenge or repeated exposures.
- Evidence of specific IgE antibody/skin-prick test positivity in settings of IgE-mediated disease.
- Associated other atopic features including dermatitis, allergic rhinitis, asthma.

> **Specific clinical scenarios that may warrant evaluation for food allergy or intolerance**
>
> - Immediate gastrointestinal symptoms (oral, pruritus, vomiting, diarrhoea) after ingestion of particular food(s).
> - Mucous/bloody stools in an infant.
> - Faltering growth.
> - Malabsorption/protein-losing enteropathy.
> - Subacute/chronic vomiting, diarrhoea.
> - Dysphagia/food bolus obstruction in an older child.
> - Gastrointestinal symptoms in a patient with atopy.
> - Gastro-oeosophageal reflux disease refractory to standard therapies.
> - Infantile colic poorly responsive to behavioural interventions.
> - Chronic constipation refractory to conventional management.

References and resources

Khan S, Orenstein SR. Eosinophilic gastroenteritis: epidemiology, diagnosis and management. Pediatr Drugs 2002;4:563–70

Sampson HA, Anderson JA. Summary and recommendations: classification of gastrointestinal manifestations due to immunologic reactions to foods in infants and young children. J Pediatr Gastroenterol Nutr 2000;30:S87–S94

Sicherer SH. Clinical aspects of gastrointestinal food allergy in childhood. Pediatrics 2003;111:1609–1616

The pancreas

Congenital anomalies

These are rare. Most anomalies are sporadic. Only the gene coding for the homeodomain protein PDX1 is clearly demonstrated to be causal of pancreatic agenesis. Inactivation or inhibition of signalling molecule sonic hedgehog (Shh) could potentially lead to annular pancreas, pancreatic divisum, and pancreatic ectopia.

Pancreatic divisum

- Commonest anomaly.
- Pancreatic ducts from the dorsal and ventral pancreas drain separately into the duodenum by a main papilla and a smaller accessory papilla.
- The small accessory duct leads to functional obstruction of the pancreas and pancreatitis.
- Pancreatic divisum was identified in 7.4% of all children with pancreatitis and 19.2% of children with relapsing or chronic pancreatitis.
- Endoscopic retrograde cholangiopancreatography (ERCP) or magnetic resonance cholangiopancreatography (MRCP) can confirm the presence of the duct of Santorini draining via the accessory papilla.
- Transduodenal spincteroplasty via endoscopy may be beneficial in reliving the obstruction.

Annular pancreas

- Complete encirclement of the second part of the duodenum by a thin, flat band of pancreatic tissue.
- Occurs in 1 in 20 000 births.
- Associated with other congenital malformations in >75%.
- Result of hypertrophy of normal pancreatic tissue after the failure of atrophy of the left ventral bud and ventral pancreas becomes fixed before rotation.
- Pancreatic tissue often penetrates the muscularis of the duodenum.
- Variable degree of duodenal obstruction can result; 50% will present by 1 year of age.
- Double bubble sign on plain radiograph demonstrates duodenal obstruction, usually in the neonates. In older children, contrast-enhanced CT and MRCP can be useful in diagnosis.
- Definitive diagnosis is made at the time of laparotomy.
- A large duodenoduodenostomy is recommended as a bypass operation as direct dissection of the annular ring is not recommended due to the high risk of pancreatic peritonitis, postoperative pancreatitis, fistulae, and late fibrosis.

Ectopic pancreatic tissue

- Presence of pancreatic tissue lacking anatomic and vascular continuity with the main body of the pancreas.
- Located commonly in the pylorus, duodenum, Meckel diverticulum.
- Most cases are asymptomatic.
- Occasionally, it may present with gastrointestinal haemorrhage secondary to mucosal ulcerations, pain secondary to pancreatitis, intestinal obstruction (usually prepyloric region in newborns), intussusception or malignant transformation.
- Definitive diagnosis is made histologically.

Pancreatic hypoplasia/agenesis

- Pancreatic agenesis is lethal. Lack of insulin leads to intrauterine growth retardation, hyperglycaemia, coma, and death.
- Hypoplasia is unlikely to be symptomatic as endocrine and exocrine function continue to be normal.

Common channel syndrome

- The normal junction of the extrahepatic bile duct and main pancreatic duct is initially extraduodenal and then in the duodenal wall, surrounded by a sphincter mechanism.
- A long common pancreaticobiliary channel results from failure of the junction to be included in the duodenal wall.
- Reflux of pancreatic enzymes into the common bile duct occurs with resulting damage to the biliary tree and formation of choledochal cyst
- Occasionally, bile may also reflux into the pancreatic duct, causing pancreatitis.
- MRCP, ERCP, or percutaneous transhepatic cholangiography (PTC) can effectively demonstrate the anomaly.
- Excision of the choledochal cyst and hepaticoenterostomy is the treatment of choice.
- Choledocojejunostomy and/or endoscopic sphincteroplasty may be performed if there is no associated choledochal cyst

Pancreatitis

Acute pancreatitis

- Defined clinically as the sudden onset of abdominal pain associated with a rise in amylase or lipase of at least 3 times the upper limit in the blood or urine.
- Rare in children.
- Involves premature activation of trypsinogen, triggering an aggressive immune response.
- Presents typically with epigastric pain. Pain can also be located in right or left upper quadrant and back. The typical radiation of pain to the back is not seen in 60–90% of children.
- May have prominent nausea and vomiting, usually aggravated by food.
- Less commonly there may be fever, tachycardia, hypotension, jaundice, and abdominal signs such as guarding, rebound tenderness, and a decrease in bowel sounds.

Causes of acute pancreatitis (see Table 46.1)

- Trauma is the commonest cause of acute pancreatitis in children.
- Exhaustive evaluation in children <4 years is recommended as there usually is an underlying cause.

Recurrent acute pancreatitis

- Recurrent acute pancreatitis is seen in 10% of children after a first episode of acute pancreatitis and commonly associated with structural abnormalities, idiopathic or familial pancreatitis.
- Commonest cause of familial pancreatitis:
  - mutations in cationic trypsinogen gene (e.g. *PRSS1*) enhance trypsin activation
  - mutations in the *SPINK1* (serine protease inhibitor Kazal type 1) result in an abnormal pancreatic secretory trypsin inhibitor
  - mutations of *CFTR* (cystic fibrosis transmembrane conductance regulator). which reduces the pancreatic fluid secretion capacity, increase the risk of keeping activated trypsin in the pancreas for a longer period of time.

Diagnosis

Threefold rise in serum amylase and lipase levels is consistent with pancreatitis.

- Amylase:
  - rises within 2–12 h
  - remains elevated for 2–5 days
  - up to 40% of children with pancreatitis may have normal amylase levels
  - hyperamylasaemia is non-specific and can be caused by intra-abdominal disorders (appendicitis, intestinal obstruction, acute cholecystitis), salivary gland disease (mumps, Sjögren syndrome), renal insufficiency, and macroamylasaemia (chronic elevation of amylase resulting from amylase being bound to immunoglobulin, forming a complex too large to be filtered by the kidneys).

- Lipase:
  - greater sensitivity and specificity for pancreatitis than amylase
  - can also be elevated in patients with abdominal conditions.
- Measurement of both amylase and lipase together has a sensitivity of 94%. Both concentrations do not correlate with severity of disease.

Imaging

To confirm diagnosis of pancreatitis, identify the cause and assess complications.
- Abdominal ultrasound:
  - increased pancreatic size
  - decreased pancreatic echogenicity
  - sensitivity is ~65%
- Contrast-enhanced CT: the most useful method for evaluating severity and detecting complications. Indications are:
  - significant history of blunt trauma
  - to stage severe pancreatitis, particularly to look for necrosis
  - to determine significant intra-abdominal complications of pancreatitis (Table 46.2).
- There is limited experience in MRI of the pancreas in children.

Table 46.1 Aetiology of acute pancreatitis in children

Idiopathic	
Trauma	Blunt injury (handlebar, child abuse, etc.) Endoscopic retrograde cholangiopancreatography (ERCP)
Inflammatory / systemic disease	Haemolytic uraemic syndrome Reye's syndrome Kawasaki disease Inflammatory bowel disease Henoch–Schönlein purpura Systemic lupus erythematosus
Infections	Epstein–Barr virus Mumps Measles Cytomegalovirus Influenza A Mycoplasma Leptospirosis Malaria Rubella Ascariasis Cryptosporidium
Metabolic	α_1 antitrypsin deficiency Hyperlipidaemias Hypercalcaemia
Periampullary obstruction	Gallstones Choledochal cyst Pancreatic duct obstruction Congenital anomalies of pancreas (especially pancreas divisum) Enteric duplication cyst
Drugs	Salicylates Paracetamol Cytotoxic drugs (e.g. L-asparaginase) Corticosteroids Immunosuppressives (e.g. azathioprine, 6-mercaptopurine) Thiazides Sodium valproate Tetracycline (particularly if aged) Erythromycin
Toxin	Scorpion Gila monster Tropical marine snakes
Miscellaneous	Refeeding pancreatitis

Table 46.2 Complications of pancreatitis

Local	Systemic
Oedema	Shock
Inflammation	Pulmonary oedema
Fat necrosis	Pleural effusions
Pancreatic necrosis	Acute renal failure
Sterile	Coagulopathy
Infected	Haemoconcentration
Abscess	Bacteremia, sepsis
Fluid collections	Distant fat necrosis
Pseudocysts	Vascular leak syndrome
Duct rupture and strictures	Haemorrhage
Extension to nearby organs	Multiorgan system failure
	Hypermetabolic state
	Hypocalcemia
	Hyperglycemia

Prognosis

The acute pancreatitis scoring system for children of DeBanto et al (2002), which predicts severity of disease and mortality, includes the following parameters:

- Age (<7 years)
- Weight (<23 kg)
- Admission white blood cell count (>18.5 × 109/L)
- Admission lactate dehydrogenase (>2000 IU/L)
- 48-hour trough Ca^{2+} (<8.3 mg/dL)
- 48-hour trough albumin (<2.6 g/dL)
- 48-hour fluid sequestration (>75 mL/kg)
- 48-hour rise in urea (>5 mg/dL)

Each criterion is assigned a value of 1 point. Cumulative score predicts the outcome of patients:

- 0–2 points: 8.6% severe, 1.4% death
- 2–4 points: 38.5% severe, 5.8% death
- 5–7 points: 80% severe, 10% death.

Chronic pancreatitis

- Defined as a complex process beginning with acute pancreatitis and progressing to end-stage fibrosis as the result of recurrent and chronic inflammatory processes.
- It is the final common pathologic pathway of a variety of pancreatic disorders: necrosis–fibrosis theory (see Table 46.3).
- Usually associated with genetic conditions like cystic fibrosis or hereditary pancreatitis, or is idiopathic.
- Diagnosis of this condition is based on a combination of clinical features (abdominal pain, weight loss, diabetes mellitus) and functional (documented exocrine pancreatic insufficiency) and imaging studies.

Causes

Cystic fibrosis is the most important cause of chronic pancreatitis in children. CFTR mutation-associated pancreatitis can be divided into four mechanistic subtypes:

- Type 1   CFTRsev/CFTRsev genotype
- Type 2   CFTRsev /CFTRm-v genotype
- Type 3   CFTRsev or CFTRm-v plus a second pancreatitis modifier or susceptibility gene (e.g CFTRsev /SPINK1)
- Type 4   CFTRsev or CFTRm-v plus a strong environmental risk factor such as alcohol.
  - CFTRsev : severe CFTR mutation phenotype
  - CFTRm-v : mild or variable CFTR mutation phenotype.
- Hereditary pancreatitis.

Functional testing

Pancreatic insufficiency is a sign of chronic pancreatitis but is not diagnostic (see Pancreatic insufficiency, p. 000).

Imaging

- Chronic pancreatitis with calcifications can be identified on abdominal radiography or by transabdominal ultrasonography. When present, the diagnosis of chronic pancreatitis can be made with 90% confidence.
- Other abdominal imaging methods used include CT, ERCP, endoscopic ultrasonography (EUS), and MRI or MRCP.

Genetic testing

- Diagnostic testing for *PRSS1*, *SPINK1*, *CFTR* and other mutations can be performed if the patient has symptoms of pancreatitis and the genetic test is done to determine the underlying cause.
- Predictive testing (i.e. testing in subjects without evidence of pancreatic disease) is not recommended in children.

Indications for genetic testing

- Recurrent (2 or more) attacks of acute pancreatitis for which there is no explanation (e.g. anatomic anomalies, ampullary or main pancreatic strictures, trauma, viral infections, gallstones, alcohol drugs, hyperlipidaemia).
- Unexplained (idiopathic) chronic pancreatitis.
- A family history of pancreatitis in a first-degree (parent, sibling, child), second-degree (aunt, uncle, niece, nephew), or third-degree (grandparent, first cousin) relative.

Management
- The mainstay of current treatment is analgesia, intravenous fluids, pancreatic rest, and monitoring for complications.
- Nutrition:
  - mild acute pancreatitis—normal diet, enteral nutrition is only required if unable to consume normal food for >5 days
  - severe necrotizing pancreatitis—continuous gastric or jejunal feeding with peptide-based formula, may need supplementation with parenteral nutrition
  - chronic pancreatitis—80% can be treated adequately with normal diet supplemented by pancreatic enzymes. 10–15% will require whole protein oral nutritional supplements and 5% may need tube feeding.
- Surgical management is limited to debridment of infected necrotic pancreas or cholecystectomy or endoscopic sphincterotomy in the presence of gallstones.
- Antibiotics are usually not necessary unless in severe pancreatic necrosis (Bassi et al. 2003).
- Octreotide infusions may reduce pancreatic secretions in those with pancreatic fluid sequestration.
- Antioxidants such as vitamin E may be beneficial.

Table 46.3 Aetiologic risk factors for chronic pancreatitis (TIGAR-O system)

Toxic–metabolic	Alcoholic
	Tobacco smoking
	Hypercalcaemia
	Hyperparathyroidism
	Hyperlipidaemia
	Chronic renal failure
	Medications
	Phenacetin abuse
	Toxins
	Organotin compounds (e.g di-n-butyltin dichloride)
Obstructive	Pancreas divisum
	Sphincter of Oddi disorders (controversial)
	Duct obstruction (e.g. tumour)
	Periampullary duodenal wall cysts
	Post-traumatic pancreatic duct scars
Idiopathic	Early onset
	Late onset
	Tropical
	Tropical calcific pancreatitis
	Fibrocalculous pancreatic diabetes
	Other
Genetic	Autosomal dominant
	Cationic trypsinogen (codon 29 and 122 mutation)
	Autosomal recessive / modifier genes
	CFTR mutations
	SPINK1 mutations
	Cationic trypsinogen (codon A16V, D22G, K23R)
	α_1-antitrypsin deficiency
Autoimmune	Isolated autoimmune chronic pancreatitis
	Hyper IgG4 associated pancreatitis
	Syndromic autoimmune chronic pancreatitis
	Sjögren syndrome-associated pancreatitis
	Inflammatory bowel disease-associated chronic pancreatitis
	Primary biliary cirrhosis-associated pancreatitis
Recurrent and severe acute pancreatitis associated chronic pancreatitis	Post-necrotic (severe acute pancreatitis)
	Recurrent acute pancreatitis
	Vascular disease / ischaemia
	Post-irradiation

Source: Etemad and Whitcomb (2001).

Pancreatic insufficiency

The pancreas has marked functional reserve and has to be severely damaged (>98%) before functional loss can be clinically recognized.

Exocrine insufficiency

- Pancreatic exocrine function includes the secretion of digestive enzymes, fluids, and electrolytes.
- Steatorrhoea, weight loss, failure to thrive (fat and protein malabsorption), night blindness, rickets, haemolytic anaemia, peripheral neuropathy, ataxia, ophthalmoplegia (deficiencies of fat-soluble vitamins), and dermatitis (lack of essential fatty acid) can result.
- For causes, see Table 46.4.

Classification
- *Mild*: pathologic volume and bicarbonate secretion, normal secretion of enzymes, no steatorrhoea.
- *Moderate*: pathologic volume and bicarbonate secretion, pathologic enzyme secretion, no steatorrhoea.
- *Severe*: pathologic volume and bicarbonate secretion, pathologic enzyme secretion, steatorrhoea.

Patients are classified according to their faecal fat excretion:
- Pancreatic sufficient (PS): without steatorrhoea.
- Pancreatic insufficient (PI): with steatorrhoea.

Tests
Functional tests (Table 46.5) do not give information of the underlying pancreatic process.
- **Indirect tests** have limited sensitivity and specificity, especially in cases of mild to moderate exocrine pancreatic insufficiency. They mainly examine for:
  - absorption of markers that are hydrolysed from conjugates by
  - pancreatic enzymes and subsequently appear in urine or serum
  - undigested and unabsorbed food components in the faeces or oxidation products of digested and absorbed fat in expired air
  - measurement of pancreatic enzymes in the serum or stool.
- **Faecal elastase** has the highest sensitivity in detecting pancreatic insufficiency:
  - <150 micrograms/g is quite specific for exocrine pancreas insufficiency
  - there is no interference of results from pancreatic enzyme supplements
  - however, it does not differentiate between primary exocrine pancreatic deficiency and exocrine dysfunction secondary to intestinal villous atrophy
  - false positives may occur with acute diarrhoea.
- **Invasive pancreatic stimulation tests** are gold standard for assessment of pancreatic insufficiency but are not usually indicated as they are time consuming, expensive, uncomfortable, and not well standardized in children.

Table 46.4 Causes of exocrine pancreatic insufficiency in childhood

Pancreatitis	Idiopathic
	Traumatic
	Viral
	Drug-induced
	Nutritional
	Autoimmune
Inherited diseases	Cystic fibrosis
	Shwachmann–Diamond syndrome
	Johanson–Blizzard syndrome
	Pearson syndrome
	Hereditary pancreatitis
	Isolated enzyme deficiencies (lipase, colipase)
Insufficiency secondary to other disorders	Pancreatic resection
	Coeliac disease and other cases of villous atrophy
	Malnutrition
	Primary sclerosing cholangitis
	Allagille's syndrome
	Diabetes
	Enterokinase deficiency
Anatomical abnormalities	Pancreatic agenesis
	Pancreatic hypoplasia
Neoplastic disease	

Table 46.5 Tests of exocrine pancreatic function

Indirect tests	Direct tests
Urinary and plasma markers Bentiromide Pancreolauryl Dual-label Schilling	Exogenous hormonal stimulants Secretin Cholecystokinin (CCK)
Breath test Carbon-14-lipids Carbon-13-lipids and starch	Nutrient stimulants Lundh test meal Fatty acids Amino acids Hydrochloric acid
Stool Microscopy for fat globules 72 h faecal fat excretion Faecal chymotrypsin Faecal elastase	

Treatment
- Diet plan:
  - frequent small meals
  - diet should be rich in protein (1–1.5 g/kg) and carbohydrates
  - 30% of calories should be given initially as fat (vegetable fat is well tolerated)
  - if adequate weight gain cannot be achieved and steatorrhoea is persistent, then medium-chain triglycerides can be administered
  - low-fibre diet, as fibres absorb enzymes
  - supplementation with fat-soluble vitamins if clinical deficit is apparent
  - enteral nutrition is indicated if patient cannot ingest sufficient energy, has acute complications, or prior to surgery.
- Pancreatic enzyme replacement therapy (PERT) (see box, p. 000):
  - dose of PERT varies with age and amount of fat intake and should not be based solely on weight
  - drug availability is affected by lipase level, shelf life, and conditions of storage
  - absorption is influenced by gastric and intestinal motility, gut pH (decreases with acid environment)
  - common side effects include mouth ulcers, perineal irritation, hyperuricaemia, and allergic reactions, including anaphylaxis
  - fibrosing colonopathy is a complication associated with doses >10 000 U/kg of lipase
  - patients with persistent symptoms despite adequate doses of PERT need to be investigated
  - stool chymotrypsin can be used to monitor compliance.

Pancreatic endocrine insufficiency

- Glucose intolerance occurs in 40–90% of all cases with severe pancreatic insufficiency.
- Diabetes occurs in 20–30% of all patients, associated with impaired glucagon release.

References and resources

Bassi C, Larvin M, Villatoro E. Antibiotic therapy for prophylaxis against infection of pancreatic necrosis in acute pancreatitis. Cochrane Database Syst Rev 2003:CD002941 (PMID 14583957)

DeBanto JR, Goday PS, Pedrose MRA et al. Acute pancreatitis in children. *Am J Gastroenterol* 2002;**97(7)**:1726–1731

Etemad B, Whitcomb DC. Chronic pancreatitis: diagnosis, classification, and new genetic developments. *Gastroenterology* 2001;**120**(3):682–707.

Pancreatic enzyme replacement therapy in cystic fibrosis: Australian guidelines. *J Pediatr Child Health* 1999;**35**;125–129

Things to evaluate before increasing PERT doses

Distribution
Check that PERT is correctly distributed over the day's meals based on the fat content of individual meals, snacks, and fluids e.g. milk.

Administration
- Capsules should be swallowed whole or the granules inside the capsules mixed with an acidic fruit purée. e.g. apple. Granules should not be chewed/
- Enzymes should be taken before and/or during a meal or snack. Enzymes are effective for 30 min after consumption and thus additional enzymes are required if eating or drinking milk 30 min after the last dose.

Storage
- Store capsules in an airtight container in a cool, dry place.
- Check that the enzyme capsules have not exceeded the expiry date.

Adherence
- Administer PERT with all meals, snacks, and fluids containing fat.
- If non compliant, avoid increasing dose; develop strategies to improve adherence.

Efficacy
Implement and evaluate the following if PERT appears to be ineffective:
- Measure faecal fat excretion (%FFE).
- Increase PERT by small doses but avoid exceeding the maximum safe daily 'dose' of 10 000 U/kg lipase
- Consider the use of adjunctive therapies, e.g. H_2 blockers, synthetic prostaglandins.
- Refer to gastroenterologist for review of PERT and/or GI investigations

Before using acid-suppressing agents:
- Document %FFE and usual PERT intake and distribution.
- Add adjunctive agent.
- Repeat measurement of %FFE and assessment of PERT intake and distribution.

Adapted from the Australian Guidelines for Pancreatic Enzyme Replacement Therapy

Neonatal jaundice

Epidemiology

- 30–50% of normal term newborns are jaundiced after birth.
- Physiological and breast milk jaundice account for the majority of cases.
- 1 in 2500 infants has conjugated hyperbilirubinaemia.
- The recommended current practice is to exclude conjugated hyperbilirubinaemia in any infant clinically jaundiced at 14 days.

Unconjugated hyperbilirubinaemia

Bilirubin metabolism

- Unconjugated bilirubin is a product of haem metabolism and is transported by albumin.
- Conjugation is with glucuronic acid by esterification to make it water soluble (enzyme—bilirubin uridine diphosphate glucuronyltransferase UGT1A1).
- Secretion occurs against a concentration gradient through the canalicular membrane into the bile.

Causes (Table 47.1)

Most common:
- Physiological jaundice
- Breast milk jaundice
- Haemolysis
- Congenital defects of bile conjugation.

Kernicterus may result from high levels of unconjugated bilirubin.
Management strategy is with phototherapy (if serum bilirubin >250 µmol/L in term babies; standard charts available for the preterm), adequate hydration, identifying and treating the underlying causes.

Table 47.1 Causes of neonatal unconjugated hyperbilirubinaemia

Increased production of unconjugated bilirubin from haem	Haemolytic disease (hereditary or acquired)
	Isoimmune haemolysis (neonatal; acute or delayed transfusion reaction; autoimmune)
	Rh incompatibility
	ABO incompatibility
	Other blood group incompatibilities
	Congenital spherocytosis
	Hereditary elliptocytosis
	Infantile pyknocytosis
	Erythrocyte enzyme defects
	Glucose-6-phosphate dehydrogenase deficiency
	Pyruvate kinase deficiency
	Hemoglobinopathy
	Sickle cell anaemia
	Thalassaemia
	Others
	Sepsis
	Microangiopathy
	Haemolytic–uraemic syndrome
	Haemangioma

Table 47.1 Causes of neonatal unconjugated hyperbilirubinaemia (*Continued*)

	Ineffective erythropoiesis
	Drugs
	Infection
	Enclosed haematoma
	Polycythemia
	Diabetic mother
	Fetal transfusion (recipient)
	Delayed cord clamping
Decreased delivery of unconjugated bilirubin (in plasma) to hepatocyte	Right-sided congestive heart failure
	Portacaval shunt
Decreased bilirubin uptake across hepatocyte membrane	Presumed enzyme transporter deficiency
	Competitive inhibition
	Breast milk jaundice
	Lucy–Driscoll syndrome
	Drug inhibition (radiocontrast material)
	Miscellaneous
	Hypothyroidism
	Hypoxia
	Acidosis
Decreased storage of unconjugated bilirubin in cytosol (decreased Y and Z proteins)	Competitive inhibition
	Fever
Decreased biotransformation (conjugation)	Physiologic jaundice
	Inhibition (drugs)
	Hereditary (Crigler–Najjar):
	type I (complete enzyme deficiency)
	type II (partial deficiency)
	Gilbert disease
	Hepatocellular dysfunction
Enterohepatic recirculation	Intestinal obstruction
	Ileal atresia
	Hirschsprung's disease
	Cystic fibrosis
	Pyloric stenosis
	Antibiotic administration
Breast milk jaundice	

Specific conditions

Physiological jaundice
- 50% of term and 80% of preterm babies are jaundiced in the first week.
- Jaundice within the first 24 h of life is always pathological and cannot be attributed to physiological jaundice.
- Aetiology of physiological jaundice is not precisely known but probably reflects immaturity of bilirubin uridine diphosphate glucuronyl transferase (UGT) activity.
- Jaundice peaks on day 3 of life.

Breast milk jaundice
- Occurs in 0.5–2% of newborn babies.
- Develops after day 4 (early pattern) or day 7 (late pattern).
- Jaundice peaks around the end of second week.
- May overlap with physiological jaundice or be protracted for 1–2 months.
- Diagnosis is supported by a drop in serum bilirubin (≥50% in 1–3 days) if breastfeeding is interrupted for 48 h.

Haemolysis
- Commonly due to isoimmune haemolysis (Rh, ABO incompatibility), red cell membrane defects (congenital spherocytosis, hereditary elliptocytosis), enzyme defects (glucose-6-phosphate dehydrogenase or pyruvate kinase deficiency), or haemoglobinopathies (sickle cell anaemia, thalassaemia).
- Finding of jaundice in the presence of anaemia and a raised reticulocyte count necessitate further investigation for cause of haemolysis.

Inherited disorders of unconjugated hyperbilirubinaemia
- This spectrum of disease depends on the degree of bilirubin uridine diphosphate glucuronyl transferase (UGT) deficiency.
- Liver function tests and histology are normal.
- Autosomal recessive inheritance. Gilbert syndrome and Crigler–Najjar type II can also have autosomal dominant transmission.

Gilbert syndrome
- Mild, 7% of population
- Polymorphism with TA repeats in the promoter region (TATA box) in whites compared to exon mutations in Asians on chromosome 2q37
- Higher incidence of neonatal jaundice and breast milk jaundice
- Usually presents after puberty with an incidental finding of elevated bilirubin on blood tests or jaundice after a period of fasting or intercurrent illness
- More common in males
- No treatment required, compatible with normal life span.

Crigler–Najjar type I
- Severe deficiency of UGT
- High risk of kernicterus
- Require life-long phototherapy or even liver transplantation.

Crigler–Najjar type II
- Moderate deficiency
- May require phototherapy and phenobarbitone.

Conjugated hyperbilirubinaemia

Definition
- Conjugated (direct) bilirubin >15% of total serum bilirubin level.
- Conjugated jaundice is always pathological and needs prompt diagnosis and therapy.

Pathophysiology
The defect lies at the hepatocyte level or in the biliary drainage system. Disorders affecting the major bile ducts are usually amenable to surgical correction while the management of the defects at the hepatocyte or bile canalicular level is mainly medical. Liver transplantation may be necessary for those who progress to end-stage liver disease.

Causes of conjugated jaundice (Table 47.2)
Common causes:
- 'Idiopathic' neonatal hepatitis (40%).
- Biliary atresia (25–30%).
- Intrahepatic cholestasis syndromes (20%), e.g. Alagille, progressive familial intrahepatic cholestasis (PFIC).
- α_1-antitrypsin deficiency (7–10%).

If biliary atresia is suspected the child should be referred to a liver unit for further investigation.

Clinical features
- Jaundice.
- Dark urine.
- Pale stools (not always).
- Hepatomegaly or hepatosplenomegaly.
- Variable degree of liver failure - hypoglycaemia, ascites, acid-base imbalance, electrolyte imbalance, coagulopathy.

Investigation (see box, p. 000)
- Confirm conjugated hyperbilirubinaemia
- Look for evidence of sepsis or liver failure
- Look for cause of conjugated jaundice

Perform an extended metabolic screen if there is evidence of:
- Hypoglycaemia
- Increased lactate or pyruvate
- Steatosis on liver biopsy.

Table 47.2 Causes of neonatal conjugated hyperbilirubinaemia

Biliary tree disorders	Biliary atresia
	Biliary hypoplasia (non-syndromic)
	Mucous plug
	Bile duct stenosis/stricture
	Spontaneous perforation of common bile duct
	Neonatal sclerosing cholangitis
	Caroli's disease
	Compression of bile duct by a mass
	Inflammatory pseudotumour at porta hepatis
Infections	Bacterial
	Urinary tract infection
	Septicaemia*
	Syphilis
	Listeriosis
	Tuberculosis
	Parasitic
	Toxoplasmosis
	Malaria
	Viral
	Cytomegalovirus
	Herpes simplex*
	Human herpes virus type 6*
	Herpes zoster
	Adenovirus
	Parvovirus*
	Enterovirus
	Reovirus type 3
	Human immunodeficiency virus
	Hepatitis B*
	?Hepatitis A
	? Rotavirus
Metabolic disorders	Carbohydrate metabolism
	Galactosemia*
	Fructosemia*
	Glycogen storage disease type 4
	Carbohydrate deficient glycoprotein*
	Protein metabolism (amino acid)
	Tyrosinemia*
	Hypermethioninemia
	Urea cycle defects (arginase deficiency)
	Lipid metabolism
	Niemann–Pick disease (type C)
	Cholesterol ester storage disease (Wolman's disease)*
	Gaucher disease
	Bile acid metabolism disorders (primary/secondary)
	Zellweger syndrome
	Bile acid transport disorder
	Rotor syndrome
	Dubin Johnson syndrome
	Fatty acid oxidation defects*
	Disorders of oxidative phosphorylation*
	Other mitochondrial disorders*

Table 47.2 Causes of neonatal conjugated hyperbilirubinaemia (*Continued*)

Endocrine disorders	Hypothyroidism Hypopituitarism (with or without septo-optic dysplasia)
Chromosomal disorders	Trisomy 21 (Down syndrome) Trisomy 18 (Edward syndrome) Trisomy 13 (Patau syndrome) Cat-eye syndrome Leprechaunism
Other genetic metabolic defects	α_1-Antitrypsin deficiency Cystic fibrosis
Familial cholestasis syndromes	Alagille syndrome Byler's syndrome (PFIC1) Bile salt export protein defect (BSEP defect, PFIC2) Multidrug resistant 3 deficiency (MDR3, PFIC3) Hereditary cholestasis with lymphoedema (Aagenaes syndrome)
Metals and toxins	Neonatal haemochromatosis* Copper related cholestasis* Parenteral nutrition Fetal alcohol syndrome Drugs
Haematological disorders	Haemophagocytic lymphohistiocytosis* Langerhan's cell histiocytosis Inspissated bile syndrome
Immunological disorders	Neonatal lupus erythematosis Giant cell hepatitis with Coomb's positive haemolytic anaemia* Graft versus host disease Adenosine deaminase deficiency
Vascular anomalies	Haemangioendothelioma Budd Chiari syndrome Congenital portocaval anomalies
Idiopathic	Familial Non-familial (good prognosis)
Miscellaneous	Hypoperfusion of liver* ARC syndrome (arthrogryposis, renal tubular dysfunction and cholestasis)

* Conditions that can present as acute liver failure.

Urgent investigations at first contact

- Liver function tests
- Prothrombin time
- Blood sugar
- Serum electrolytes, urea and creatinine
- Full blood count, reticulocyte count, peripheral blood smear, and direct Coomb's test if evidence of haemolysis
- Blood and other body fluid cultures if indicated (unwell baby)
- Urine culture
- Urine for reducing substances (Clinitest).

Subsequent investigations to consider

- α_1-Antitrypsin phenotype*
- Galactose-1-phosphate uridyl transferase*
- Urine succinyl acetone
- Serum TSH and T_4
- Serum cortisol (short synacthen test if cortisol low)
- Immunoreactive trypsin (<4 weeks of age)
- Serum and urine amino acid
- Urine organic acids
- Urine bile acids (child must be off ursodeoxycholic acid for 2–3 weeks)
- Serum triglyceride
- Serum fibrinogen
- Serum ferritin
- TORCH screen, VDRL
- Serology for HIV, HHV6, and parvovirus B19
- Hepatitis B antigen, hepatitis C antibody
- Ultrasound of liver and biliary tree
- Radiograph long bones and spine
- Ophthalmic examination (anterior chamber, lens and retina)
- Liver biopsy
- Endoscopic/percutaneous/MRCP, hepatobiliary scintigraphy (depending on local expertise) to demonstrate biliary tree patency
- Bone marrow examination (to excluded storage disorders particularly Niemann–Pick type C, haemophagocytic lymphohistiocytosis or other haematological conditions)
- Exploratory laparotomy and operative cholangiography.

* Test should be carried out on parents if baby received blood products in last 6 weeks.

Management

- Identify treatable cause urgently and institute treatment
- Manage vitamin K deficiency
- Manage acute liver failure
- Optimize nutrition.

Coagulopathy

Prothrombin time (PT) can be prolonged due to:

- Vitamin K deficiency leads to deficient γ-carboxylation of factors II, VII, IX, and X, resulting in the failure to trigger the clotting cascade. Administer 1 mg/year of age (max. 5 mg) of intravenous vitamin K and recheck PT 4–6 h later. PT should normalize.
- Acute liver failure results in decreased synthesis of factors II, V, VII, IX, and X. Deficiency of factord VII and V is the most prominent as they have the shortest half-lives. Administration of vitamin K does not correct this coagulopathy.

Special dietary requirements

- Exclude galactose from diet until galactosaemia is excluded.
- If baby not thriving while awaiting investigations, start feed based on medium-chain triglycerides.
- Give fat-soluble vitamins (A, D, E, and K), twice recommended daily allowance. Can be a combination of Ketovite® liquid 5 mL and 3 tablets with 1 mg of Konakion MM® once daily, or Abidec® 1.2 mL and vitamin E 100 mg/kg daily with 1 mg Konakion MM®.

Idiopathic neonatal hepatitis

- Diagnosis of exclusion (see Table 47.3).
- Associated with low birth weight or prematurity.
- Histology:
  - hepatocellular swelling (ballooning), focal hepatic necrosis and multinucleated giant cells
  - bile duct proliferation and bile duct plugging are usually absent.
- Factors predicting poor prognosis:
  - severe jaundice beyond 6 months
  - acholic stools
  - familial occurrence
  - persistent hepatosplenomegaly.
- 90% do well with no long-term liver disease.

Table 47.3 Clinical clues to the diagnoses

Signs	Conditions
Cleft lip/palate, micropenis, optic nerve hypoplasia	Septo-optic dysplasia
Peripheral pulmonary stenosis, triangular facies, posterior embryotoxon	Alagille syndrome
Cataract	Galactosaemia
Cutaneous hemangioma	Haemangioendothelioma
White hair	Haemophagocytic lymphohistiocytosis (HLH)
Rickets	Tyrosinaemia
Coagulopathy	Tyrosinaemia, galactosaemia, HLH
Inverted nipples, lipoatrophy	Congenital disorders of glycosylation

Biliary atresia

Definition

Biliary atresia (BA) is a progressive cholangiopathy of unknown aetiology affecting extra- and intrahepatic biliary system presenting within the first several weeks of life.

Incidence

BA is a sporadic condition with an estimated worldwide incidence of around 1/12 000–15 000 live births. It has been described in isolation in twin and triplet pregnancies, with no seasonal pattern. Children are typically born at term, with no gender predominance.

Types

There are three macroscopic types of BA:
• Type I, affecting the distal part of the common duct.
• Type II, affecting the common hepatic duct, common bile duct and gallbladder.
• Type III, affecting right and left hepatic ducts and the gallbladder.

Some 10–20% of patients with BA have other congenital anomalies, including splenic abnormalities (asplenia, polysplenia, lobulated spleen), partial or complete situs inversus, mediopositioned liver, intestinal malrotation, atretic inferior vena cava, preduodenal portal vein, and congenital heart defects. These 'syndromic' children may represent a separate aetiologic subgroup, which has been termed biliary atresia splenic malformation (BASM) syndrome because of the consistent presence of splenic pathology.

Pathogenesis

The cause of BA is unknown. Several viruses have been suspected of triggering inflammatory response in this condition, including reovirus, rotavirus type C, cytomegalovirus (CMV), human papilloma virus (HPV) and human herpes virus type 6 (HHV6). It is conceivable that BA may represent a final phenotypic pathway of neonatal liver injury caused by diverse aetiologies, including developmental, infectious, or vascular factors, which could be operational antenatally or within the first several weeks of life. It is also tempting to speculate that aberrant host immune reactivity, related to physiologically impaired immune competence at this age, may play a role in this condition, unique to early infancy.

Clinical presentation

Most children with BA have clinical features indistinguishable from other causes of conjugated hyperbilirubinaemia in infancy. These include jaundice, mild hepatosplenomegaly, dark urine, and acholic stools, which could initially contain some pigment. Blood tests indicate non-specific elevation of conjugated (direct) bilirubin, transaminases, gamma-glutamyl-transpeptidase, and alkaline phosphatase. Ascites or cutaneous signs of chronic liver disease are rarely detected. Coagulopathy, if present, readily responds to intravenous vitamin K. The initial good general condition and appropriate weight gain of the infant with BA could often be misleading, resulting in late referral to specialist centres.

Diagnosis

Expert ultrasonography could point to BA by demonstrating an irregularly shaped or absent gallbladder. A skillfully performed and interpreted percutaneous liver biopsy under local anaesthesia using the Menghini technique is diagnostic in up to 90% of cases. Histological features of BA include expansion of portal tracts, cholestasis, and bile duct damage and reduplication with various degree of increased fibrosis. In ambiguous cases endoscopic retrograde cholangiopancreatography (ERCP) may be required.

Treatment

If untreated, BA leads to complete biliary obstruction, cirrhosis, and death in infancy. The treatment of biliary atresia is surgical. The complete excision of the atretic biliary tree is followed by re-anastomosis, using ~40 cm of the patient's bowel to form a Roux-en-Y loop, connecting viable bile ducts at the resected surface of the liver with proximal jejunum (portoenterostomy or Kasai procedure). Because of the progressive nature of BA, the earlier operation has better chances of establishing the effective bile flow. Approximately 50–60% of the patients will have a successful operation, completely clear the jaundice, and avoid liver transplantation in the short term; 11% of children operated on at a specialist centre have no clinical signs of liver disease after a 10 year follow-up.

The operated patients receive initial antibiotic prophylaxis to minimize likelihood of ascending infection from the gut and long-term fat-soluble vitamin supplements. Development of portal hypertension and blood supply to the liver are monitored by regular ultrasound Doppler studies.

Liver transplantation in patients with BA should be complementary to Kasai portoenterostomy. Primary transplantation should be reserved for infants in whom decompensated cirrhosis has already developed because of delayed diagnosis.

Complications

The main complications of BA are:
- Ascending cholangitis
- Portal hypertension
- Synthetic hepatic failure
- Chronic encephalopathy
- Hepatopulmonary syndrome.

The successful management of these complications by standard means such as intravenous antibiotics or banding and sclerotherapy of oesophageal varices, when necessary, contributes to improved long-term outcome.

Prognosis

Around 20–30% of operated children will require liver transplantation during the first 2 years of life. Another 20–30% have established compensated chronic liver disease and may need liver transplantation later in childhood, particularly peripubertally. An unknown but small proportion of long-term survivors may need consideration for liver transplant in adulthood. Overall, combined surgicomedical management with sequential Kasai portoenterostomy and liver transplantation provides long-term survival with a good quality of life for 95% of the patients treated at the specialized centres.

α_1-antitrypsin deficiency

α_1-Antitrypsin (α_1-AT) is a 55 kD glycoprotein produced predominantly by hepatocytes, alveolar macrophages and intestinal endothelial cells. It acts as a protease inhibitor during an acute-phase response. It can be electrophoretically differentiated into four main variants: PiM (normal), PiZ, PiS, and Pi Null (abnormal). There are >80 other rare, clinically irrelevant, variants. α_1-AT deficiency affects predominantly people of white European ancestry. The estimated prevalence of PiMZ (carrier) state is 1/30 in this group. The inheritance is autosomal co-dominant.

- α_1-AT deficiency is the commonest genetic indication for liver transplantation in children.
- Aberrant polymerization leads to retention of the abnormal PiZ protein in the liver and, in ~10–15% progression to chronic liver disease of a varying severity. The liver damage ranges from a mild non-specific hepatitis to advanced fibrosis and cirrhosis. In the most severe cases the cirrhosis may decompensate during first 2 years of life, necessitating liver transplantation.
- PiZ, PiS, and Pi Null variants can induce chronic obstructive pulmonary disease (COPD) in the third or fourth decade of life (particularly in smokers).
- Other conditions described in association with α_1-AT are vasculitis, glomerulonephritis, and panniculitis.

Clinical features

- The typical presentation of liver disease secondary to PiZ α_1-AT deficiency is prolonged neonatal jaundice (pale stools, dark urine, elevated liver enzymes, vitamin K-responsive coagulopathy). These features are clinically indistinguishable from other hepatic disorders presenting early in infancy such as biliary atresia, progressive familial cholestasis, neonatal hepatitis, and others. The remaining symptomatic PiZ cases present later during childhood with the signs of established liver disease, including impaired liver synthetic function, hepatosplenomegaly, and portal hypertension.
- The liver histology usually demonstrates non-specific hepatitis with variable cholestasis, mild biliary features, and slender fibrosis; these appearances can mimic biliary atresia.
- Of the symptomatic PiZ children (presenting with conjugated jaundice in newborn period), ~25% will progress to end-stage chronic liver disease and require liver replacement during childhood. Another 25% may decompensate in the second decade. Presence of fibrosis in the liver biopsies and jaundice after 6 months of age are associated with higher risk of developing end-stage liver disease. Alpha-fetoprotein negative hepatocellular carcinoma can occur.

Management

- There is no effective medical treatment for α_1-AT deficiency, other than liver transplantation. Standard therapy for complications of the chronic liver disease such as banding ligation or sclerotherapy for bleeding varices, diuretics, albumin, and vitamin supplementation may temporarily control the disease.
- It is sensible not to drink alcohol or smoke, the latter in view of the risk of early-onset COPD.
- Overall liver transplant results are similar to other indications for elective liver replacement, approaching >90% 5 year patient survival. Transplant recipients may be at risk of developing hypertension in the immediate postoperative period and calcineurin inhibitor-related nephrotoxicity long term due to the subclinical α_1-AT deficiency-related renal involvement.

Liver disease in other forms of α_1-AT deficiency

- PiS and PiMS α_1-AT deficiency are not associated with liver disease
- Homozygous and heterozygous forms of PiZ α_1-AT deficiency are increasingly recognized in adults with cryptogenic liver disease or associated with other co-morbid conditions such as alcoholism, iron overload, autoimmunity, or chronic viral hepatitis. It is conceivable that possession of one PiZ allele may represent an initial risk factor in the 'multiple hit' pathogenesis of the liver injury. Family screening is therefore important in order to highlight appropriate lifestyle modifications, such as avoiding active and passive smoking and heavy drinking.

Alagille syndrome

Alagille syndrome is a complex multisystem disorder with a prevalence of 1:40 000–1:100 000, characterized by hepatic, cardiac, renal, and ocular involvement. At least three of the following five major criteria are required to establish the diagnosis:

- **Cholestasis** (typically presenting as neonatal jaundice).
- **Characteristic facies:** broad forehead, deep-set eyes, straight nose with a bulbous tip, and a pointed chin giving the face a triangular appearance.
- **Heart disease:** most commonly peripheral pulmonary artery stenosis followed by Fallot's tetralogy, ventricular septal defect, atrial septal defect.
- **Posterior embryotoxon:** a prominent ring at the junction of cornea and sclera best seen with a slit lamp. It does not affect visual acuity and is seen in 8–15% of normal eyes.
- **Vertebral anomalies:** characteristically butterfly vertebrae.

More recently, renal disease (renal tubular acidosis or structural abnormalities-dysplastic kidney, renal cysts, ureteropelvic obstruction) has been included as a diagnostic criterion.

Growth retardation, pancreatic exocrine insufficiency, and intracranial bleeding are other important manifestations

Genetics

- Autosomal dominant with variable penetrance.
- Jagged 1 mutation can be identified in 70%. Only 30–50% of mutations are inherited. Others are de novo mutation or defects in notch signalling pathways. The mutations are unique to each pedigree and clinical features are highly variable, even within families.

Clinical features

- Jaundice; mainly conjugated hyperbilirubinaemia
- Pale stools
- Hepatomegaly
- Splenomegaly (40%)
- Intrauterine growth retardation
- Failure to thrive
- Pruritus (rare before 3–5 months of age)
- Heart murmur
- Triangular facies
- Short stature
- Steatorrhoea (fat malabsorption)
- Rickets
- Xanthomas
- Delayed puberty
- Intracranial bleeding.

Differential diagnosis

- Biliary atresia
- Other causes of neonatal cholestasis:
  - sepsis, UTI
  - galactosaemia
  - tyrosinaemia
  - choledochal cyst
  - α_1-antitrypsin deficiency
  - peroxisomal disorders
  - intrauterine infection
  - congenital hypothyroidism
  - congenital hypopituitarism
  - cystic fibrosis
  - progressive familial intrahepatic cholestasis.

Investigations

- Liver function tests: raised total and conjugated bilirubin, AST, gamma GT, alkaline phosphatase, INR.
- Raised serum bile acids.
- Raised serum cholesterol and triglycerides
- Vitamin A, D, E concentrations
- Serum bicarbonate (renal tubular acidosis).
- Radiography of thoracolumbar spine.
- Slit lamp examination of eyes for posterior embryotoxon.
- Ultrasound of liver, gallbladder, spleen (small, contracted, or absent gallbladder in 28%).
- Ultrasound of kidneys for structural abnormalities.
- A full cardiac evaluation, including echocardiogram.
- MRI/MRA of head and/or angiography for symptomatic intracranial bleeding. Head injuries and neurological symptoms should be evaluated aggressively.
- DISIDA (di-isopropyl iminodiacetic acid) scan : non-excretion of the isotope after 24 h seen in ~60% (potential false positive for biliary atresia).
- Liver biopsy: closed needle biopsy typically shows paucity of bile ducts in 75–90%.
- Percutaneous transhepatic cholangiography (PTC) or endoscopic retrograde cholangiopancreatography (ERCP) to distinguish from biliary atresia where there is a diagnostic uncertainty.
- Laparotomy and operative cholangiography to differentiate from biliary atresia. Inappropriate Kasai porto-enterostomy may worsen the outlook.
- Molecular testing is expensive and not routinely recommended.

Management: multidisciplinary approach

- Medium-chain triglyceride feeds.
- Nasogastric feeding/gastrostomy may be necessary to optimize nutrition.
- Fat-soluble vitamin supplementation.
- Antipruritic agents: ursodeoxycholic acid, colestyramine, rifampicin and naltrexone.
- Management of cardiac condition.
- Management of renal anomalies.
- Routine immunizations along with hepatitis A and B vaccines.
- Liver transplantation—indications are:
  - severe failure to thrive
  - intractable pruritus affecting quality of life
  - end-stage liver disease or portal hypertension
  - severe xanthomas
  - severe metabolic bone disease.

Prognosis

- Mortality is ~10% with cardiac disease, vascular accidents, and liver disease accounting for most of the deaths.
- Estimated 20 year survival rates are 80% for those not requiring liver transplantation.
- Liver transplantation has an 80% 5 year survival rate and 60% 20 year survival rate.

Familial and inherited intrahepatic cholestatic syndromes

Definition

The presence of persistent cholestasis or remitting cholestasis that has relapsed on at least one occasion with:

- Direct or indirect evidence of an inherited aetiology (or a single remitting episode with direct evidence of heredity).
- Supportive histological features.

Onset may be at any time from the neonatal period into adolescence. Early-onset cases typically present as neonatal cholestasis; later-onset cases may present as unexplained or drug-related cholestasis.

Nomenclature

Several of the conditions falling within this spectrum have names derived from their description, with characteristic syndromic features. Among these are Aagenes syndrome and North American Indian cholestasis. Others have names derived from their pathophysiological mechanisms such as bile salt export pump (BSEP) deficiency or from their gene markers, PFIC1 disease. Table 51.1 shows a classification of familial intrahepatic cholestasis variants that combines clinical features with available genetic knowledge.

Because definitive tests even for the variants of PFIC with accepted markers are not generally clinically available, allocation of patients to this classification may be approximate or impossible, and in practice diagnostic and therapeutic uncertainty compromises patient care.

Epidemiology

Recent attention to cholestatic syndromes facilitated by understanding of their genetics and pathophysiology has revealed that they are more common than previously recognized, and has shed light on the pathophysiological mechanisms of cholestasis. Inheritance and gene markers are in favour of autosomal recessive aetiology in most types. Clearer understanding of the breadth of possible phenotypes has shown that cases of neonatal hyperbilirubinaemia, particularly those that recur or have a poor prognosis for chronic liver disease, or some patients with cryptogenic chronic liver disease, fall within this spectrum. Obstetric cholestasis, although genetically and pathophysiologically related to some variants, is not considered in this paediatric text.

Table 51.1 Classification of PFIC types

Phenotype	Current condition name	Previous names	Gene marker/defect
Infantile cholestasis			
low γGT—may have diarrhoea, short stature, and short digits	PFIC1 disease	Byler disease	*FIC1*—ATP8B1
low γGT	BSEP deficiency	PFIC2	ABCB11
high γGT ± cholangiopathy	MDR3 deficiency	High γGT neonatal intrahepatic cholestasis	ABCB4
Neonatal sclerosing cholangitis	NSC	–	Unknown
Neonatal sclerosing cholangitis with icthyosis	NISCH syndrome	–	CLDN1
Infantile cholestasis	EPHX1 deficiency	Hypercholanaemia	*EPHX1*
(Benign) recurrent cholestasis			
low γGT ± pancreatitis	BRIC1	Summerskill–Walshe–Tygstrup syndrome	ATP8B1
low γGT	BRIC2	Summerskill–Walshe–Tygstrup syndrome	BSEP mutations of ABCB11 E186G, V444A
high γGT	–	–	ABCB4
Severe cholesterol gallstone formation	MDR3 deficiency	–	ABCB4
Pregnancy/OC induced cholestasis	Cholestasis of pregnancy	–	ABCB4, ATP8B1 D2S1374

Pathophysiology

Primary pathophysiologic mechanisms of cholestasis may occur at hepatocellular, basolateral membrane, or canalicular levels. A key, common mechanism in the progress of liver disease appears to be local concentration of free bile acids with detergent effects on hepatocyte and/or biliary canalicular cell and intracellular membranes. Remitting or benign recurrent variants have inducible or suppressible critical enzymes or steps within the bile acid transport pathway.

Most patients with liver disease progress towards end stage either progressively or with variable episodes of remission. Even in cases initially identified as benign, a contentious concept considered later, fibrosis tends to accumulate insidiously over time. Patients proceed towards either biliary cirrhosis or a reticulate porto-portal fibrosis. Copper-associated protein is frequently seen in periportal areas as evidence of chronic cholestasis.

Aetiologies and subtypes

Low serum values of gamma-glutamyl transpeptidase (γGT) in the setting of cholestasis usually allude to the diagnosis of progressive familial intra hepatic cholestasis. The aetiology of the cholestasis must lie up-stream of the canalicular membrane since γGT was not being released and circulated in the blood. They also showed that the low γGT subgroup had a worse prognosis, with 50% dying or coming to liver transplantation within 5 years.

Some subtypes are associated with syndromic features that may be helpful in making the diagnosis and indicating the prognosis. Among these are PFIC1 associated with short stature, diarrhoea, short fingers with lichenification of skin, and renal tubular acidosis. Aagenes syndrome is associated with lymphoedema that may develop over months or years. North American Indian cholestasis is associated with pancreatitis and 'paper-money skin'.

Disease pathophysiology

Deficiency of the bile salt export pump (BSEP) results in rapid onset of cholestasis, typically with aggressive liver disease. Remitting or recurrent types are described but the condition presents as progressive intrahepatic cholestasis complicating neonatal hepatitis/cholestasis. The condition PFIC1 results from deficiency of an ATP-dependent membrane transporter, accounting for later-onset cholestasis requiring the accumulation of synthesized bile salts within hepatocytes. The various extrahepatic manifestations and the persistence of features, particularly diarrhoea, renal tubular acidosis, and fatty liver after liver transplantation are accounted for by transporter defects expressed in other organs. BSEP deficiency results in failure of bile salt transport across the canalicular membrane. A third defect, MDR3 deficiency, is explained by relative absence of phospholipid to protect the canalicular membrane from detergent effects of biliary bile acids. Canalicular membrane and bile duct damage with cholestasis and possible cholangiopathy result. Undoubtedly other important mechanisms for low and high serum γGT cholestasis remained to be discovered with approaching 30% of low-γGT variants still lacking a gene marker.

Clinical features

Presentations

- **Progressive intrahepatic cholestasis** as a complication of neonatal cholestasis or neonatal hepatitis syndrome. High and low serum γGT types can present in this way. At presentation, stools may have a variable degree of pallor, occasionally mimicking biliary atresia. Histology of low γGT subtypes such as BSEP deficiency is more likely to be giant cell hepatitis whereas that of high γGT types such as MDR3 deficiency or neonatal sclerosing cholangitis may have giant cell hepatitis but is more likely to have portal tract expansion with bile ductular reduplication. Other known causes of progressive cholestasis complicating neonatal cholestasis not falling within this definition must be excluded.

- **Cholestasis of later onset in infancy.** Patients may present for the first time with jaundice at 3–6 months of age or later. Histology may be of bland cholestasis with little inflammation or giant cell transformation. 'Byler bile' may be present on electronmicroscopy, suggestive of PFIC1 disease.

- Patients may present with a **first or second episode of acute cholestasis** with jaundice, pale stools, and dark urine and ultimately itch at any age in childhood or adolescence. Precipitating factors such as drugs, particularly penicillin antibiotics and oestrogens, may be recorded up to 2 months before the onset of jaundice. Puberty may be a contributing factor. Previous episodes may have been misinterpreted as viral hepatitis including hepatitis A. Low serum γGT types predominate. Drugs associated with cholestasis are shown in Table 51.2.

- **Cholestasis in pregnancy** can present at any time from late in the first trimester onwards, although it is commoner in the second and third trimesters. Itch is the predominant symptom and jaundice follows (if present) by ~2 weeks. Serum transaminases are usually minimally elevated or in the normal range. Glucose intolerance may be associated. Histological features typically show bland cholestasis with occasionally bile plugs but little inflammation. There is an increased risk of premature delivery and fetal death. The reader should look to an adult text for further information on this topic.

- **Benign recurrent cholestasis.**

- Patients with full clinical, biochemical and histological remission after two or more cholestatic episodes may be said to have **benign recurrent cholestasis (BRIC)**. Serum γGT is usually low. Drug cholestasis may be suspected initially and drugs may be a trigger as above. This diagnosis requires extreme caution as many cases prove not to be benign with progression insidious, or precipitate after long periods without apparent progression.

Natural history

Occasional cases of both high and low γGT intrahepatic cholestasis complicating neonatal cholestasis follow an unremitting course with nutritional impairment, fat-soluble vitamin deficiency, portal hypertension and its complications, and finally decompensation of liver synthetic function sometimes at an age as early as 8 months to 2 years comparable with deterioration following missed biliary atresia.

Later onset infantile cases, those presenting as drug-related cholestasis but with a poor prognosis, and apparent benign recurrent cholestasis cases who have subsequently declared themselves as having progressive disease all tend to have a remitting and relapsing course. Pruritus, failure to thrive, and fat-soluble vitamin deficiencies require close monitoring and vigorous treatment. Loose stools or diarrhoea often complicate classical PFIC1 disease and short stature is particularly problematic.

Management

Extrahepatic consequences of cholestasis, particularly nutritional, including failure to thrive and essential fat-soluble vitamin deficiencies, are frequent. Vitamin D and E deficiencies are common, but vitamin A deficiency is less so. Supplementation is mandatory even among patients without jaundice. Medications for treatment and prophylaxis of deficiency are shown in Table 51.3. Essential fatty acid deficiency may be detected following prolonged cholestasis. Its significance for neurodevelopment is unclear.

Our institutional regimen for the management of pruritus is shown in Table 51.4. Non-cirrhotic patients with residual bile flow may respond to external or internal biliary diversion. Both of these methods involve interrupting the intrahepatic recirculation of bile salts at a point between the extrahepatic biliary system and the point of a bile salt re-uptake in the terminal ileum. External diversion may be by the insertion of a loop of ileum between the gallbladder brought out as a stoma usually in the right iliac fossa. Alternatively the preterminal ileum may be brought out as a double-barrel stoma. Internal diversion involves the formation of distal ileum to colon fistula with the terminal ileum in a blind loop. This latter diversion avoids a stoma but may cause bile-salt-related diarrhoea and has a theoretical increased risk of colonic carcinoma in the long term. The second and third methods will require regular provision of vitamin B_{12} since its terminal ileal uptake will be interrupted. Excellent results for improvements of pruritus, jaundice, and liver histology have been described. Our institutional experiences have been less good, probably because of selection of patients who were cirrhotic and with very poor bile flow.

Liver transplantation

Indications for liver transplantation include:
- Management of poor quality of life
- Failure to thrive
- Intractable pruritus
- Dysplastic hepatic nodules with raised alphafetoprotein
- Risk of hepatic cellular carcinoma
- Established hepatocellular carcinoma <5 cm
- Failure of synthetic function.

Patients with PFC1 disease may have very severe intra- and extrahepatic complications after transplantation. Their longitudinal growth improves initially after transplantation but very short stature may persist. Diarrhoea may worsen considerably and tacrolimus or ciclosporin treatment may unmask severe renal tubular acidosis and risk of dehydration with electrolyte disturbance. A prolonged and intractable hepatic steatosis is frequently seen in the early months to years after successful transplantation.

Monitoring for hepatocellular carcinoma

Intrahepatic cholestasis due to BSEP deficiency has a risk of hepatocellular carcinoma in excess of other causes of PFIC or biliary cirrhosis. Many patients continue to have raised alpha-fetoprotein levels suggesting hepatocyte dysplasia. Patients require regular monitoring of alpha-fetoprotein and liver ultrasound 6 monthly for early recognition.

Benign recurrent cholestasis

Cases with more than one episode of cholestasis where symptoms recede fully and liver function tests, ultrasonography, and liver biopsies return entirely to normal between episodes maybe considered benign. Episodes of cholestasis may last up to several months and treatments for pruritus and fat-soluble vitamin deficiency should be given as described above. There is no evidence that earlier treatment with choleretics cuts short the duration of the episodes. However, temporary biliary diversion by nasal biliary intubation and drainage has been shown to cut short episodes very rapidly. Patients should be labelled benign with extreme caution as they may have low-grade chronic liver disease that can take years to declare itself. Recognized precipitants such as antibiotics or oestrogens should be avoided in such patients.

Table 51.2 Drugs associated with cholestasis

Group	Examples
Antibiotics	Amoxicillin, flucloxacillin, macrolides, rifampicin
Steroids	Glucocorticoids, oestrogens, androgens
Psychtropic/neurology	Chlorpromazine, phenothiazines, methyldopa
Cardiology	Verapamil, nifedipine, amiodarone
Antimetabolites	Methotrexate
Immunosuppressant	Ciclosporin

Table 51.3 Nutritional supplements—vitamins and minerals

Nutritional element	Daily requirement	Means of administration	Comments/ monitoring
Vitamin A	<10 kg 5000 IU >10 kg 10000 IU IM–50 000 IU	Oral	IM supplement only in severe refractory deficiency Serum retinol/ RBP ≥ 0.8
Vitamin D	10 000–40 000 units per day IM–30 000 IU 1–3 monthly	Oral/IM	Supplementation with oral products containing calciferol may suffice. Refractory cases may require 25-OHD or IM preps 25-OHD serum levels >20 ng/mL
Vitamin E	TPGS* 25 IU/kg IM 10 mg/kg (max. 200 mg) every 3 weeks	Oral	Vit E/total lipids ≥0.6 mg/g Vit E <30 g/mL Look for reflexes!
Vitamin K	2 mg/d Weekly 5 mg 5–10 kg 10 mg >10 kg IM—5–10 mg every 2 weeks	Oral IM	Prothrombin time PIVKA II <3 ng/mL
Water-soluble vitamins	Twice RDA	Oral	Supplement as needed
Minerals Calcium Selenium Zinc Phosphate	25–100 mg/kg 1—2 µg/kg 1 mg/kg 25—50 mg/kg	Oral	Supplement as needed

Table 51.4 The sequence of medical management of pruritus of cholestasis

Number	Medicine	Dose range
1	Colestyramine	4 g sachets (1–4/day)
2	Ursodeoxycholic acid	15–30 mg/kg/day in 2 doses
3	Rifampicin	7–10 mg/kg/day in 2 doses
4	Naltrexone	0.3–0.6 mg/kg/d in 1 dose
5	Ondansetron	2–8 mg/day in 2 doses as for anti-emetic treatment
6	UVA light treatment or acupuncture may be offered with benefit for some patients.	

Drug-induced liver injury

Drug induced liver injury (DILI) is a variable and complex diagnosis of exclusion, as it can present in different ways. Because of the liver's central role in drug metabolism, most prescribed drugs can cause liver injury. Liver damage can occur through drugs in a predictable, intrinsic dose-related way or in a unpredictable, idiosyncratic dose-unrelated fashion.

Epidemiology

Drug induced liver injury is a relatively rare but heterogeneous condition. About 2–3% of all hospital admissions are due to drug toxicity.

There is variable severity from unrecognized self-limiting presentations and transient elevation of liver enzymes to acute liver failure. Transient elevations of liver transaminases occurs frequently, but the incidence of severe liver failure is about 100: 100 000 users for offending drugs, like isoniazid, phenytoin, valproic acid, and chlorpromazine; 10:100 000 users for amoxicillin-clavulanic acid, ketoconazole, sulfasalazine, and cimetidine, and 1:100 000 users for NSAIDs, 6-mercaptopurine, carbamazepine, and itraconazole.

Pathophysiology

The liver plays a pivotal role in the metabolism of drugs through a variety of metabolic pathways. There are two principal enzymatic pathways: the phase 1 oxidases (cytochrome P-450 system), reductases, and hydrolases and the phase 2 transferases. Drugs do not necessarily need to go through the phase 1 pathway first, they can be metabolized through the phase 2 pathway independently. Drug toxicity can be induced or inactivated by the above pathways. It can be acute or chronic.

Patterns of drug induced liver injury can be divided into
• Direct hepatotoxicity
• Immune-mediated hepatotoxicity.

Both can present with either cholestasis or a hepatocellular picture, or both.

Direct hepatotoxicity leads to impaired cellular function and ultimately cell death. This also lead to responses of the innate and adaptive immune system with the release of pro-inflammatory mediators, causing further hepatocyte damage and leading to acute or chronic failure. Hepatocellular injury can lead to steatosis, degeneration, fibrosis, cirrhosis, and necrosis of the liver (Table 52.1 and box on p. 376).

Table 52.1 Patterns and causes of drug-induced hepatic injury

Acute	
Hepatocellular	
Steatosis	Methotrexate, tetracycline, valproic acid
Degeneration	Many hepatotoxic drugs in low doses
Necrosis	Paracetamol (acetaminophen), isoniazide, halothane, methyldopa
Granulomas	Sulfonamides, allopurinol
Cholestatic	
Pure cholestasis	Anabolic steroids
Cholestatic hepatitis	Isoniazid, erythromycin, chlorpromazine, ciclosporin
Chronic	
Hepatocellular	
Steatosis and fibrosis	Methotrexate, alcohol
Lipid storage disease	Amiodarone
Chronic persistent/active hepatitis	Nitrofurantoin
Cirrhosis	Alcohol
Cholestatic	
Chronic intrahepatic cholestasis	
Biliary cirrhosis	Chlorpromazine, testosterone
Vascular disorders	
Veno-occlusive disease	Tioguanine, busulfan, cyclophosphamide
Occlusion of large hepatic veins	Contraceptive steroids (oestrogens, androgens)
Sinusoidal dilatation/peliosis hepatis	Contraceptive/anabolic steroids
Biliary sludge	Ceftriaxone
Hepatoportal sclerosis/perisinusoidal fibrosis	Vitamin A, arsenicals
Tumours	
Hepatocellular adenoma	Anabolic and contraceptive steroids
Hepatocellular carcinoma	
Cholangiocarcinoma	
Angiosarcoma	

Reproduced with permission from Hepatology.

Drugs causing liver injury

Dose related-injury
- amiodarone
- ciclosporin
- methotrexate
- oral contraceptives
- paracetamol (acetaminophen)
- tetracycline.

Dose-unrelated injury
- amoxicillin/clavulanic acid
- chlorpromazine
- diclofenac
- erythromycin/macrolides
- ibuprofen
- isoniazide
- methotrexate
- methyldopa
- minocycline
- oral contraceptives
- phenytoin
- valproic acid.

Herbal drugs and alternative medicines

Herbal drugs and alternative medicines have gained huge popularity over the last few years. As with other drugs and toxins, the clinical picture can vary from a self-limiting unnoticed clinical picture to fulminant liver failure (Table 52.2). Because of the adulteration of herbal medicines with chemical substances such as steroids, diuretics, salicylates, NSAIDs, hormones, and heavy metals (mercury, lead, cadmium, arsenic), even herbal drugs that seem safe to use can precipitate liver injury.

Table 52.2 Examples of herbal drugs causing DILI

Herbal drug	Adverse effect
Chaparral	Nausea, emesis, hepatitis
Cinnamon oil	Abuse syndrome (?)
Comfrey	Hepatic veno-occlusive disease
Echinacea	CNS stimulation, anaphylaxis
Ginseng	Agitation, anxiety, insomnia
Heliotropium	Hepatic veno-occlusive disease
Jin bu huan	Hepatitis
Kava kava	Hepatitis, cirrhosis
Liquorice	Hypertension, hypokalemia, arrhythmias
Ma huang	Hypertension, arrhythmias, stroke, seizures
Pennyroyal	Centrilobular liver necrosis
Poke root	Hepatotoxicity
Sassafras	Hepatotoxicity, hepatocarcinogen
Valerian	Hepatotoxicity

Risk factors

Patients with a positive family history to the offending drug may be less able to metabolize or eliminate the toxins because of a genetic predisposition to DILI. Also, lack of enzymes in the individual may increase the risk of adverse reaction to the offending drug.

Clinical features

The diagnosis of DILI is clinical and should be considered and suspected if no underlying other cause of abnormal liver function can be found. A diagnostic tool can be helpful in scoring the patient and determining whether the likelihood of DILI definite, probable, possible, unlikely or excluded (Table 52.3). The patients may present with very non-specific clinical symptoms, such as abdominal pain, fever, skin rash, and general malaise. Some patients may not have any clinical symptoms at all, but are being picked up by regular screening, e.g. when taking sodium valproate.

Underlying liver conditions like sepsis, viral hepatitis, biliary tree obstruction, and pre-existing liver disease have to be excluded.

Acute hepatocellular injury

Laboratory
- Most common type of DILI, with up to 90% of cases.
- ALT and AST elevation >3 times the upper normal limit.
- Bilirubin can be elevated or normal.
- Alkaline phosphatase (ALP) normal or slightly elevated.
- No upper limits in hepatic enzyme elevation.

Clinical picture
Non-specific, e.g. anorexia, nausea, and fatigue. If acute liver failure occurs, then signs of encephalopathy, jaundice, and coagulopathy, with poor prognosis.

Drugs
Methyldopa, paracetamol, sodium valproate.

Acute cholestatic injury

Laboratory
- Elevated bilirubin, ALP and gamma glutamyltranspeptidase (gGT).
- Takes longer to resolve, but has good prognosis.

Clinical picture
Jaundice and pruritus, pale stools, dark urine.

Drugs
Anabolic steroids, amoxicillin/clavulanic acid, chlorpromazine, oral contraceptives.

Acute mixed injury

Laboratory
Raised ALT and AST >8 times the upper limit, ALP raised >3 times the upper limit.

Clinical picture
Usually good prognosis.

Drugs
Amoxicillin/clavulanic acid, carbamazepine, ciclosporin, erythromycin and other macrolides, tricyclic antidepressants, nitrofurantoin, NSAIDs, sulfonamides.

Chronic hepatitis

Laboratory
Majority female patients, with positive autoantibodies.

Clinical picture
Hepatosplenomegaly, ascites, coagulopathy, and jaundice

Drugs
Diclofenac, methyldopa, minocycline.

Chronic steatosis

Clinical picture
Most patients without symptoms, methotrexate steatosis can lead to liver cirrhosis.

Drugs
Amiodarone, glucocorticoids, methotrexate, sodium valproate.

Others (veno-occlusive disease, hepatic vein thrombosis)

Laboratory
Clinical signs
Depending on underlying pathomechanism, hepatosplenomegaly, ascites and jaundice

Drugs
Anabolic steroids, azathioprine, cyclophosphamide, etoposide, methotrexate, mitomycin, oral contraceptives, vincristine.

Investigation

- Bilirubin conjugated/unconjugated
- AST, ALT, gGT, ALP
- Total IgE
- FBC with film, including eosinophils
- Drug levels where appropriate
- Hepatitis A, B, C serology
- Autoantibodies and immunoglobulins
- Liver ultrasound
- MRCP

A liver biopsy should be considered, but it is only necessary and indicated in patients where the diagnosis is not clear cut and other underlying hepatic conditions are suspected or need to be excluded.
- Paediatric patients should not be re-challenged with the suspected drug as this is unhelpful and unethical.
- DILI may unmask other underlying liver pathology like autoimmune hepatitis and mitochondrial cytopathies.

Management

The most important treatment is to suspect and to withdraw the offending drug. Patients should be treated supportively according to their presentation. In clinically well patients with abnormal LFTs, the withdrawal of the offending drug should be sufficient. Patients who present with acute liver failure should be treated according to tertiary referral centres guidelines and should always be referred to a liver unit.

Paracetamol overdose treatment protocol at King's College Hospital, London

If a paracetamol overdose is suspected or known, the child must be treated immediately with N-acetylcysteine, at the local hospital whatever the time between the alleged overdose and the visit to the hospital. The 'high-risk treatment line' is used in all cases once a level is known. The N-acetylcysteine should be continued until the INR is normal (<1.2). Indication for treatment after known time since ingestion by plasma level corresponding to the high-risk treatment line is shown in Fig. 52.1.

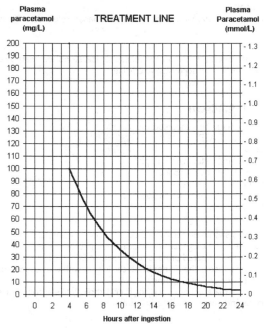

Fig. 52.1 High-risk treatment line.

Investigations

- Liver function tests, paracetamol level, INR, blood sugar, renal function tests and blood gases including lactate. Blood sugar must be closely monitored (hourly BM stix).
- INR, blood sugar, renal function and blood gases must be repeated at least twice a day and, if abnormal, 3 times a day. Start immediately broad-spectrum antibiotics if INR abnormal (amoxicillin and cefuroxime), and in the presence of abnormal renal function, itraconazole or liposomal amphotericin IV.
- Hypoglycaemia has to be avoided and the child should be maintained on 10% dextrose. Higher concentrations of dextrose may be needed.
- The most important prognostic parameter is acidosis on day 2. If, despite N-acetylcysteine treatment and good rehydration, the child becomes acidotic, the prognosis is poor. Acidosis is the best prognostic factor independent of all other factors. Even in the presence of a very prolonged INR, a patient who is not acidotic will have 80% chances of surviving. If the pH is <7.25, there is a 95% mortality and the child should be emergency listed for transplantation.
- Other factors predicting a poor outcome are the development of grade III hepatic encephalopathy with oliguric renal failure (which usually occurs 3–4 days after ingestion), and/or a prothrombin time of >100 s, and raised plasma lactate.

Prevention/prognosis

- Liver function tests should be routinely performed on a regular basis in drugs known to cause DILI.
- Patients should be informed about the side effects of the drugs they are taking and patients should be made aware of the clinical signs of DILI.
- Suspected DILI cases should be reported to a central database.
- Recognition and identification of DILI and the removal of the offending drug is paramount in preventing further liver injury.
- Avoid re-challenging the patient with the offending drug or drugs from the same family as this can cause fatal hepatic necrosis.
- Drug levels should be monitored to avoid toxic levels causing liver injury.
- The prognosis of DILI depends on the severity and the pattern of the insult but is usually completely reversible when the offending drug is withdrawn.
- Presentation as acute liver failure predicts poor outcome.

Table 52.3 DILI diagnostic scale

I. Temporal relationship between drug intake and onset of clinical picture

A. Time from drug intake until onset of first clinical/laboratory manifestations

4/7 to 8/52	3
<4/7 or >8/52	1

B. Time from withdrawal of drug until onset of manifestations

0–7/7	3
8–15/7	0
>15/7	−3

C. Time from withdrawal of drug until normalization of lab values

<6/12 cholestatic/mixed picture	3
<2 hepatocellular	3
>6/12 cholestatic/mixed picture	0
>2 hepatocellular	0

II. Exclusion of alternative causes

Viral hepatitis

Biliary tree obstruction

Pre-existing liver disease

Others

Complete exclusion	3
Partial exclusion	0
Possible cause detected	−1
Probable cause detected	−3

III. Extrahepatic manifestations

Rash, fever, arthralgia, eosinophilia (>6%), cytopenia

>4	3
2	
1	1
None	0

IV. Intentional/accidental exposure to drug

Positive re-challenge	3
Negative/absent re-challenge	0

V. Previous report in literature of cases of DILI associated with drug

Yes	2
No (<5 years marketed)	0
No (>5 years marketed)	−3

Total score in points

Scoring: Definite >17, Probable 14–17, Possible 10–13, Unlikely 6–9, Excluded <6

Drugs that may cause liver damage

- amitriptyline
- amoxicillin
- amphotericin
- anabolic steroids
- anaesthetics
- analgetics
- anti-acne drugs
- anticonvulsants
- antifungals
- antimicrobials
- antineoplastic drugs
- antituberculous drugs
- azathioprine (6-mercaptopurine)
- capsofungin
- ciclosporin
- erythromycin
- Fansidar
- griseofulvin
- halothane
- hormones
- ibuprofen
- immunosuppressant drugs
- indometacin
- isoflurane
- isoniazid
- itraconazole
- ketoconazole
- mebendazole
- methotrexate
- naproxen
- oral contraceptives
- paracetamol (acetaminophen)
- penicillamine
- phenoburbital
- ranitidine
- rifampicin
- sodium valproate
- tetracycline
- total parenteral nutrition
- tricyclic antidepressants
- vincristine

Autoimmune liver disease

In paediatrics, two forms of autoimmune liver disease are recognized:
- Autoimmune hepatitis (AIH)
- AIH/sclerosing cholangitis overlap syndrome (autoimmune sclerosing cholangitis, ASC).

Autoimmune hepatitis (AIH)

- Progressive inflammatory liver disorder, preferentially affecting females, characterized serologically by high levels of transaminases and IgG and presence of autoantibodies, and histologically by interface hepatitis in the absence of a known aetiology.
- AIH is divided into two types according to the autoantibody profile:
  - type 1 is positive for anti-nuclear (ANA) and/or anti-smooth muscle (SMA) antibody
  - type 2 is positive for anti-liver kidney microsomal antibody type 1 (anti-LKM-1).
- Type 1 AIH represents 2/3 of the cases. Severity of disease is similar in the two types. Anti-LKM-1 positive patients are younger and have a higher tendency to present with acute liver failure, but the duration of symptoms before diagnosis and the frequency of hepatosplenomegaly are similar in the two groups. Both have a high frequency of associated autoimmune disorders (~20%) and a family history of autoimmune disease (40%).
- The presentation of AIH is variable. Up to 40–50% of patients present with symptoms of acute hepatitis, some 40% with an insidious onset, characterized by progressive fatigue, relapsing jaundice, headache, anorexia, and weight loss, and some 10% with complications of portal hypertension, such as splenomegaly, haematemesis from oesophageal varices, bleeding diathesis, chronic diarrhoea, and weight loss. The disease should therefore be suspected and excluded in all children with symptoms and signs of prolonged or severe liver disease. The course of disease can be fluctuating, with flares and spontaneous remissions, a pattern that may result in delayed referral and diagnosis.
- On physical examination clinical signs of an underlying chronic liver disease, i.e. cutaneous stigmata (spider naevi, palmar erythema, leukonychia, striae), firm liver, and splenomegaly are common.
- On USS the liver parenchyma is often nodular and heterogeneous.
- Anti-LKM-1-positive children have higher levels of bilirubin and transaminases at presentation than those who are ANA/SMA positive and present more frequently with fulminant hepatic failure. Most patients have increased levels of IgG, but ~20% do not, indicating that normal IgG values do not exclude the diagnosis of AIH. Partial IgA deficiency is significantly more common in LKM1-positive than in ANA/SMA-positive patients.
- Histologically, the severity of interface hepatitis at diagnosis is similar in both types, but cirrhosis on initial biopsy is more frequent in type 1 than in type 2 AIH, suggesting a more chronic course of disease in the former. Progression to cirrhosis during treatment is also more frequent in type 1 AIH.

- AIH is exquisitely responsive to immunosuppression except from the children presenting with acute liver failure with encephalopathy, in which case liver transplantation is the only option.

Standard treatment at King's College Hospital

- **Prednisolone** is started at a dose of 2 mg/kg per day (max. 60 mg daily), which is gradually decreased over the next 4–8 weeks to a minimum dose of 2.5–5 mg depending on the age. It is important to monitor the blood tests (liver function tests, full blood count and clotting profile) weekly and aim to an 80% transaminase decrease in 6 weeks to avoid steroid side effects.
- **Azathioprine** can be introduced as a steroid-sparing agent but should not be used as first line treatment because of its hepatotoxicity. Because of the myelosuppressive effect, a starting dose of 0.5 mg/kg is used, to be increased to maximum 2 mg/kg per day. Blood tests will need to be continued. Daily treatment is advisable and should not be discontinued just before or during puberty because the risk of relapse.

Alternative management

- Mycophenolate mofetil has been used both in children and adults who were intolerant to azathioprine, with good response.
- Ciclosporin has been used to induce remission and both ciclosporin and tacrolimus have been used in patients who did not respond to standard treatment.

Cessation of treatment can be discussed when liver function tests and serum IgG have been within normal limits for at least 1 year with negative or low-titre auto antibodies. A liver biopsy should be performed to assess the degree of inflammation. If there is no inflammation present, first the dose of azathioprine and subsequently the dose of prednisolone should be discontinued under frequent monitoring of the blood tests. In our experience, children with type 2 AIH all relapsed and had to be restarted on treatment, and only 20% with type 1 disease could stay off immunosuppression.

- Despite the efficacy of standard immunosuppressive treatment, severe hepatic decompensation may develop even after many years of apparently good biochemical control, leading to transplantation 10–15 years after diagnosis in 10% of the patients. In our analysis bilirubin levels and INR at diagnosis were found to be independent risk factors of death and/or transplantation.

Autoimmune hepatitis/sclerosing cholangitis overlap syndrome (ASC)

- A prospective study at our centre was conducted over a period of 16 years, in which all children with serological (i.e. autoantibodies, high IgG levels) and histological (i.e. interface hepatitis) features of autoimmune liver disease underwent a cholangiogram at the time of presentation. Approximately 50% of these patients had alterations of the bile ducts characteristic of sclerosing cholangitis, though generally less advanced than those observed in adult primary sclerosing cholangitis. A quarter of the children with ASC, despite abnormal cholangiograms, had no histological features suggesting bile duct involvement and the diagnosis of sclerosing cholangitis was only possible because of the cholangiographic studies.
- Virtually all patients (55% of whom were female) were seropositive for ANA and/or SMA. The mode of presentation was similar to that of typical AIH.
- Inflammatory bowel disease was present in about 45% of children with ASC compared to about 20% of those with typical AIH.
- Increased serum IgG levels were found in 90% of children with ASC. At the time of presentation, standard liver function tests did not help in discriminating between AIH and ASC, though the alkaline phosphatase/aspartate amino transferase ratio was significantly higher in ASC. Perinuclear anti-neutrophil nuclear antibodies (pANCA) were present in 74% of patients with ASC compared to 45% of patients with AIH type 1 and 11% of those with AIH type 2.
- Children with ASC respond to the same immunosuppressive schedule used in AIH, liver test abnormalities resolving within a few months after starting treatment in most patients. Steroids and azathioprine, although beneficial in abating the parenchymal inflammatory lesion, appear to be less effective in controlling the bile duct disease. Ursodeoxycholic acid is usually added at a dose of 20–30 mg/kg per day, although its usefulness in arresting the progression of ASC has not been proved.
- The medium-term prognosis is good, with a reported 7 year survival of 100%, though 15% of the patients required liver transplant during this period of follow-up. Evolution from AIH to ASC has been documented but whether the juvenile autoimmune form of sclerosing cholangitis and AIH are two distinct entities, or different aspects of the same condition, remains to be elucidated.

Metabolic liver disease

Background

The diagnostic approach to a child with metabolic liver disease requires a high degree of suspicion, detailed history and physical examination, and extensive blood and urine tests; liver, skin, and muscle biopsy are usually necessary to establish the diagnosis.

Important features in the history
- Family history of metabolic condition or genetic disorder
- Unexplained early neonatal deaths, stillbirths, and recurrent miscarriages
- Consanguinity
- Developmental delay or neurological regression
- Recurrent episodes of vomiting of unknown aetiology
- Episodes of encephalopathy.

There are seven major clinical presentations in a patient with liver disease of metabolic origin:
- Neonatal ascites
- Infantile cholestasis
- Acute liver failure
- Hepatomegaly and/or splenomegaly
- Abnormal liver enzymes or fatty liver reported on USS performed incidentally
- Hyperammonaemia
- Acidosis.

Clinical features

There are a wide variety of clinical signs and symptoms strongly associated with specific metabolic disorders affecting the liver including::
- Coarse facies:
  - gangliosidosis
  - mucopolysaccharidosis (MPS)
  - sialidosis.
- Corneal clouding:
  - MPS I, IV, VI.
- Macroglossia:
  - GM1
  - gangliosidosis.
- Diarrhoea:
  - Wolman's disease
  - cystic fibrosis
  - mitochondrial disorders.
- Lymphadenopathy:
  - Wolman's disease
  - Gaucher's disease.
- Cherry-red spot
  - Niemann–Pick
  - GM1 gangliosidosis.
- Ichthyoids or collodion skin:
  - Gaucher's disease.

- Hypotonia, seizures:
  - urea cycle defect
  - long chain acyl co-enzyme A dehydrogenase deficiency
  - carbohydrate deficient glycoprotein syndrome type Ia and Ib
  - mitochondrial disorders.
- Hypertonia:
  - short-chain acyl co-enzyme A dehydrogenase deficiency
  - mitochondrial disorders.
- Hypertrophic cardiomyopathy in newborn:
  - glycogen storage disorder II, IV
  - gangliosidosis mucolipidosis II.
- Abnormal fat distribution:
  - carbohydrate-deficient glycoprotein syndrome.
- Sweaty feet:
  - glutaric acidaemia
  - isovaleric acidaemia.
- Rancid, fishy, or cabbage-like smell:
  - tyrosinaemia.

Investigation

First line investigations

Blood
- Full blood count, urea and electrolytes, liver function
- Blood gas and electrolytes
- Glucose, ammonia, uric acid
- lactate and pyruvate (L:P ratio)
- Ketones.

Urine
- Ketones
- Reducing substances
- pH
- Electrolytes, calcium, phosphate for tubular dysfunction.

Blood film
- Vacuolated white blood cells on blood film:
- Wolman's disease
- GM1 gangliosidosis
- Sialidosis type II
- Niemann–Pick disease
- Glycogen storage disease II
- MPS VI

Disease-specific enzyme assays
- Wolman's disease:
  - acid lipase levels in white blood cells or cultured fibroblasts
- Gaucher's disease:
  - β-glucocerebrosidase activity in white blood cells, cultured fibroblasts, or the placenta
- Sialidosis type II:
  - neuraminidase activity in white blood cells and cultured fibroblasts
- Infantile sialic storage disease:
  - elevated sialic acid levels
- GM1 gangliosidosis:
  - acid β-galactosidase deficiency in white blood cells and cultured fibroblasts.

Histologic clues
- Skin biopsy:
  - Laffora body disease, GM1 gangliosidosis storage cells
- Bone marrow:
  - Wolman's disease, Gaucher's disease, sialidosis type II, Niemann–Pick type C, haemophagocytic lymphohistiocytosis
- Liver biopsy:
  - PAS+/diastase resistant granules: α_1-antitrypsin deficiency, GSD type IV, afibrinoginaemia
  - iron deposition: neonatal haemochromatosis, Zellweger's syndrome
  - fatty changes: non-specific finding in metabolic disorders
  - glycogen and plant like cells: glycogen storage disease

- Copper:
  - Wilson's disease, Indian childhood cirrhosis, other copper toxicity states

Radiology

- Stippled epiphyses, periosteal cloaking of long bones and ribs:
  - sialidosis II, GM1, gangliosidosis
- Dysostosis multiplex:
  - advanced glycoprotein storage disorder
- Calcified adrenal glands:
  - Wolman's disease

Clinical presentations of metabolic disorders

Neonatal ascites

Neonatal ascites can be a presenting feature in the following conditions:

Storage diseases

- **Wolman's disease:** Autosomal recessive (AR) lysosomal storage disease caused by deficiency of the acid lipase and the accumulation of cholesterol esters and triglycerides in histiocytic cells of most visceral organs. Other salient features are diarrhoea, fat malabsorption, and adrenal calcification.
- **Gaucher's type II (acute neuronopathic disease):** AR disease caused by β-glucosidase deficiency, which results in the accumulation of glucosylceramide-laden macrophages. It can present with hypersplenism, gross hepatosplenomegaly, bone marrow infiltration, and skeletal disease.
- **GM1(gangliosidosis):** AR lysosomal storage disorder characterized by the generalized accumulation of GM1 ganglioside, oligosaccharides, and the mucopolysaccharide keratan sulfate (and their derivatives). There are three clinical subtypes classified according to the age of presentation: the infantile, juvenile, and adult types.
- **Muccopolysaccharidosis VII (Sly):** AR disorder that results from the β-glucuronidase enzyme deficiency and presents with a somatic phenotype similar to Hurler's disease with dysostosis multiplex but normal intelligence.
- **Sialidosis II:** AR disorder caused by the α-neuraminidase enzyme deficiency, categorized into congenital, infantile, and juvenile subtypes.
- α$_1$-*Antitrypsin deficiency:* See Chapter 49.
- *Neonatal haemochromatosis:* Syndrome defined by the coexistence of liver disease of antenatal onset with excess iron deposition at extrahepatic sites but with the reticuloendothelial components remaining iron free. Liver disease is usually apparent at birth or shortly after. Lower lip mucosa biopsy can be supportive of the diagnosis. Liver transplantation is the treatment of choice. Pregnant mothers with a previous affected child are offered weekly IV immunoglobulin infusions, with reassuring results.
- *Niemann–Pick types A, B, and C:*
  - Types A and B result from the deficient activity of sphingomyelinase, a lysosomal enzyme encoded by the gene 11p15.1-p15.4. Sphingomyelin accumulates in the monocyte-macrophage system.
  - Type C is characterized by an abnormality in cholesterol transport, causing accumulation of sphingomyelin and cholesterol in the lysosomes and a secondary reduction in sphingomyelinase activity. Patients can present with massive hepatosplenomegaly in severe cases, a cherry-red spot on retinal examination, vertical supranuclear gaze palsy in type C and neurological disorder later in life in types A and C. Diagnosis can be established on bone marrow aspirate storage cells and also on rectal biopsy ganglion storage cells (type C).

Infantile cholestasis

- α_1-antitrypsin deficiency (see Chapter 49)
- **Progressive familial intrahepatic cholestasis** (PFIC) I, II, and III (see Chapter 51).
- **Cystic fibrosis** (see Chapters 21 and 22). There are two chapters on CF one general and the other on liver disease.
- **Neonatal haemochromatis** (See Chapter 63, acute liver failure).
- **Hypothyroidism:** Thyroxine can affect bile flow and prolonged unconjugated hyperbilirubinameia with cholestasis is a common presentation of hypothyroidism. Patients will have a suboptimal TRH response test and symptoms usually resolve within a few weeks of supplementation with levothyroxine.
- **Congenital hypopituitarism:** Presenting usually within the first few weeks of life and is associated with dysmorphic facial features (frontal bossing, depressed nasal bridge), hypotelorism and nystagmus indicating septo-optic dysplasia, and micropenis. Patients can present with hypoglycaemia, hypothermia, hypotension and conjugated hyperbilirubinaemia. Biochemical findings include low early morning cortisol level and abnormal short Synacthen® test. Patients can also have a suboptimal TRH response. Treatment is with hydrocortisone and levothyroxine where appropriate. Patients may require growth hormone supplementation after the first year. Cholestasis usually resolves within 6 months of treatment.
- **Galactosaemia (galactose-1-phosphate uridyltransferase deficiency):** AR inherited disorder; patients can present with failure to thrive, vomiting, diarrhoea, renal tubular aminoaciduria, coagulopathy and bleeding. There is exacerbation of jaundice in the neonate after lactose ingestion. Cirrhosis may be evident at birth, with cerebral oedema and cataracts;patients demonstrate a predisposition to gram-negative sepsis. The management is lactose exclusion from the diet, usually a soya based formula with appropriate calcium supplementation is given.
- **Fructosaemia (fructose-1, 6-diphosphatase deficiency):** Presentation is usually before 6 months of age with enlarged and fatty liver, muscle hypotonia, severe ketotic hypoglycaemia and hyperventilation with severe metabolic acidosis. All infant formulas (except Galactomin 19® and Isomil®) can be used, and all feeds (except Pediasure®). Main aim is to eliminate all sources of fructose from their diet, but an intake of 1–2 g per day is acceptable. Supplementation is required for vitamin C, folic acid and fibre due to dietary restrictions.
- **Tyrosinaemia type I:** AR inherited disorder caused by deficiency of fumarylacetoacetate hydrolase, the last enzyme of tyrosine degradation. It can also present as ALF with hypoglycaemia, coagulopathy and a raised serum AFP. Can also present with porphyric crises, renal tubular acidosis, FTT and rarely with hypertrophic cardiomyopathy. It is diagnosed by hypertyrosinaemia, hypermethioninaemia and raised urinary succinylacetone and δ-aminolaevulinic acid. Raised incidence of hepatocarcinoma. Restriction of dietary protein intake (1 g/kg per day) to maintain tyrosine and phenylalanine levels within range. Ensure adequate intake of other essential amino acids (special metabolic protein mix). Administration of 2-(2-nitro-4-trifluoromethylbenzoyl)-1,3-cyclohexanedione (NTBC) has revolutionized the outcome of tyrosinaemia.
- **Niemann–Pick disease types A, B, and C:** See p. 394.

- *Glycogen storage disease type I:*
  - Patients present during infancy with a doll face, fatty buttocks and protruding abdomen, massive hepatomegaly, hypoglycaemia, metabolic acidosis, coagulopathy and growth failure; there is also raised cholesterol, triglycerides, liver enzymes and uric acid.
  - Enlarged kidneys, glomerular hyperfiltration, proteinuria and renal calcification; there is risk of developing hepatic adenomas.
  - General management guidelines (see p. 402), plus continuous overnight nasogastric feed is usually required in GSD types 1 and 3 and is continued until the child reaches puberty or established on uncooked corn starch (UCCS).
  - UCCS will need to be introduced as soon as possible to improve compliance.
- *Glycogen storage disease type III (debrancher enzyme deficiency)*:
  - Usually presents in first year of life with massive hepatomegaly, abnormal liver function tests, muscle enzyme elevation and hyperuricaemia. Progressive muscle weakness, cardiac failure and hypoglycaemia. Risk of hepatic adenoma in up to 25% of patients.
  - Abnormal ECG or EMG in most patients.
- *Glycogen storage disease type IV (1, 4 glucan-6-glycosyl transferase deficiency):* AR inherited disorder presenting with hydrops fetalis, hepatomegaly, FTT, liver cirrhosis with associated complications, cardiac failure, skeletal muscle weakness, hypoglycaemia, metabolic acidosis, raised cholesterol and triglycerides. Diagnosis confirmed by branching enzyme deficiency in leucocytes and cultured fibroblasts. Liver transplantation has been performed but neurological prognosis remains guarded.
- *Glycogen storage disease type VI (liver phosphorylase deficiency):* Patients present with hepatomegaly, FTT, and mild hypoglycaemia. Progression to cirrhosis is uncommon.
- *Wolman's disease:* See p. 394.
- *Gaucher's disease:* See p. 394.
- *Generalized peroxisomal disorders:* Diagnosis is made by skin fibroblast studies, plasma assays of VLCFAs, phytanic acid, L-pipecolate, and bile acid intermediates by gas chromatography/mass spectrometry.
  - **Zellweger's syndrome:** An AR inherited disorder characterized by wide anterior fontanelle, prominent forehead, anteverted nostrils, low nasal bridge, epicanthic folds, flattened philtrum, clinodactyly, talipes equinovarus, hypotonia, areflexia, mental retardation and seizures. The liver involvement includes hepatomegaly, jaundice and eventually cirrhosis. Average age at death is 5 months.
  - **Neonatal adrenoleucodystrophy:** An X-linked inherited disorder associated with dysmorphic features, deafness, developmental delay, hypotonia, seizures, and characteristic hepatomegaly. Survival is greater that in Zellweger's syndrome.
  - **Infantile Refsum's disease:** An AR disorder with a milder clinical picture than in Zellweger's syndrome with sensorineural deafness and pigmentary retinopathy (Leber's congenital amaurosis). Hepatomegaly and cholelithiasis have been reported.
  - **Primary hyperoxaluria type I:** Secondary to the deficiency of the enzyme alanine–glyoxylate aminotransferase, characterized by a

continuous high urinary oxalate excretion and progressive bilateral oxalate urolithiasis and nephrocalcinosis. No characteristic craniofacial features. Liver transplantation is the treatment of choice with renal transplantation at a later stage in patients with end-stage renal disease.

- **Inborn errors of bile acid metabolism:** Present with cholestasis usually within the first week of life, rickets and pruritus later on in life. Normal serum gGT. Diagnosed by urine and bile spectrometry of bile acids, fast atom bombardment ionization mass spectrometry (FAB-MS), and liquid–gas chromatography. On liver biopsy there is giant cell transformation with bile duct proliferation and canalicular plugging progressing to cirrhosis. Supplementation with cholic and/or ursodeoxycholic acid; patients may require liver transplantation.

- **Haemophagocytic lymphohistiocytosis:** There is a sporadic and a familial form (AR) presenting at various ages. Associated with Epstein–Barr virus infection. Can present with fever, hepatosplenomegaly, jaundice, lymphadenopathy, encephalopathy, seizures, and a maculopapular rash. There is evident hypertriglyceridemia, hypofibrinogenaemi,a and diagnosis is established with histiocyte erythrophagocytosis evident in bone marrow aspirate. Treatment includes immunoglobulins, dexamethasone, and chemotherapy; prognosis generally poor.

Organic acidaemias

β-Glucosidase deficiency

- -Presents with hypersplenism, gross hepatosplenomegaly, bone marrow infiltration, and skeletal disease. There is a predisposition (type I) in the Ashkenazi Jewish population and there is also the progressive neurovisceral storage disease (type II, III).
- -Management is with enzyme replacement therapy, symptomatic treatment, allogenic bone marrow transplantation, and selective splenectomy.

Methylmalonic acidemia

- -Episodic metabolic ketoacidosis with the most severe defect presenting in the first week of life; hyperammonemia in up to 80% of patients, hypoglycaemia in 40% of patients. These episodes are possibly associated with neutropenia and thrombocytopenia. Some patients can develop a severe extrapyramidal disorder.
- -Elevated plasma glycine levels and raised plasma and urine methylmalonate levels. There is low free carnitine level accompanied by a larger percentage of short-chain acylcarnitine levels.

Propionic acidemia

- -Patients present with episodic metabolic ketoacidosis. In the newborn period the ammonia levels may simulate urea cycle defects; episodes possibly associated with neutropenia and thrombocytopenia.
- -Investigations: Elevated plasma glycine, propionic acid, and methylcitrate levels. Low free carnitine levels accompanied by a larger percentage of acylcarnitine; fatty liver.

Isovaleric acidemia

- Recurrent episodes of metabolic ketoacidosis progressing to coma, with 50% of patients presenting at 3–14 days of age. Characteristic odour of sweaty feet during these episodes from sweat, urine, blood, and saliva. Refusal to eat; possible alopecia; some patients may develop pancreatitis during acute episodes.

- Investigations: during an acute episode there could be hyperglycaemia or hypoglycaemia, neutropaenia, thrombocytopaenia, or pancytopaenia with elevated urinary isovaleryglycine.

Acute liver failure

Table 54.1 illustrates the clinical presentation and diagnostic tests for conditions presenting as acute liver failure.

Table 54.1 Clinical presentation and diagnostic tests for metabolic conditions presenting as acute liver failure

Diagnosis	Coagulopathy	Encephalopathy	Tubulopathy	Jaundice	Age	Features	Diagnostic tests
Fatty acid oxidation	+	+	±	-	<10 yr	↓ketones	
Zellweger's syndrome	+	+	-	+	0–3 yr	Dysmorphic features Hypotonia	VLCFA
CDGS 1A	+	±	-	±	0–1yr	FTT Dysmorphic features Hypotonia	Phosphomannose mutase deficiency
CDGS 1B	+	+	-	+	Any	Cyclic vomiting Protein losing enteropathy	Phosphomannose isomerase deficiency
NH	+++	+	-	+++	0–2 wk	Hepatocellular loss	Ferritin Buccal biopsy
Wilson's disease	+	±	+	++	>5 yr	Kayser–Fleischer rings	Copper studies
Lysosomal disorders	+	±	-	+	0–4 wk	Ascites	BMA WBC enzymes
Bile acid defects	++	±	-	+	>2 mo	Rickets Steatorrhea	Urine bile acid analysis

BMA, bone marrow aspirate; CDGS, carbohydrate deficient glycoprotein syndrome; NH, neonatal haemochromatosis; VLCFA: very-long-chain fatty acids.

Hepatosplenomegaly

The following metabolic disorders can present as hepatosplenomegaly:
- Wolman's disease (see p. 394)
- Gaucher's disease (see p. 394)
- MPS VII (see p. 394)
- Gangliosidosis (see p. 394)
- Sialidosis II (see p. 394)
- Haemophagocytic lymphohistiocytosis 395.

Incidental abnormal liver enzymes

Incidental abnormality of liver transaminases should be further investigated to exclude metabolic liver disorders. It is important to measure creatine kinase to exclude muscle as source of transaminase elevation. However, elevation of gGT and conjugated bilirubin are specific to liver pathology. Conditions that are commonly picked up in this manner are Wilson's disease, paediatric fatty liver disease, fatty acid oxidation defects, and mitochondrial cytopathies. Age-appropriate and disease-specific investigations are recommended.

Hyperammonaemia

Urea cycle defects usually present within first day of life with irritability, poor feeding, vomiting, lethargy, and respiratory distress leading to hypotonia, seizures, and coma. There are five enzyme defects affecting the liver, all AR inherited apart from ornithine transcarbamylase (OTC) which is X-linked. The other four affected enzymes are carbamyl phosphate synthetase, arginosuccinic acid synthetase, arginosuccinic lyase, and arginase. They all present with raised ammonia levels, absent acidosis, and ketosis, and come after the first day of life. The treatment in suspected cases is haemodialysis within a few hours after birth and limited protein intake diet. Liver transplantation could be beneficial but is associated with a high mortality and morbidity. Poor neurological outcome once patients suffer hyperammonaemic coma.

Acidosis and ketosis

Organic acidaemias (see under Infantile cholestasis 395):
- Propionic acidaemia
- Methylmalonic acidaemia
- Isovaleric acidaemia
- Glutaric acidaemia.

Fatty acid oxidation defect
Medium-chain acyl coenzyme A dehydrogenase deficiency
- The presenting features include Reyes-like syndrome or sudden infant death (SID) syndrome, usually within the first 2 years of life, with hypoketotic hypoglycaemia secondary to poor oral intake. Possible mild hepatomegaly.
- The levels of ammonia and liver enzymes may be elevated. Raised levels of urinary N-hexanoglycine, 3-phenylpropionyl glycine, suberyl glycine, and C6–12 dicarboxylic acid during episodes. Acylcarnitine profiles also reflect increased medium chain fatty acid coenzyme A thioesters.

Short-chain acyl coenzyme A dehydrogenase deficiency
- In the neonatal period patients can present with altered consciousness, hypertonicity, and metabolic acidosis. Later in life there are signs of failure to thrive and muscle weakness.
- There is lipid deposition in muscle and liver tissue. Low muscle carnitine with low normal plasma carnitine levels. Raised short-chain acyl carnitine levels. Ethylmalonate in the urine is highly elevated and so are ethylmalonic acid, methylsuccinic acid, butyryl glycine, and butyryl carnitine.

Long-chain acyl co-enzyme A dehydrogenase deficiency
- Reyes or SID-like syndrome with hypoketotic hypoglycaemia, hepatomegaly, cardiomegaly, hypotonia in the first 6 months of life, and muscle cramps.
- Diagnosed by acetylcarnitine profile in plasma and blood spots and skin fibroblast studies.

Glutaric acidemia II
- Presents with non-ketotic hypoglycaemia and acidosis. Fat deposition in the liver, renal tubular epithelium, and myocardium. There are three types according to time of presentation: neonatal onset with congenital anomalies, mild, or late onset.

General management

Avoidance of catabolic states

- Avoid fasting—can be fatal.
- Strict feeding regimen (timing, prescribed diet).
- Every patient should have an individual feeding plan.

Early detection of catabolic states

- Vomiting is an alarming symptom; fluid losses may need to be replaced or administer emergency regimen.
- Assess an odd-smelling child (? catabolites).

Detecting loss of metabolic control

This could be associated with any of the following conditions:
- Unexplained abnormal behaviour
- Hypo- or hyperglycaemia
  - regular testing of blood glucose is essential especially at the initial presentation until the patient is established on a structured diet
- Metabolic acidosis
- Hepatic encephalopathy
- Cerebral oedema
- Abnormal coagulation studies and subsequent bleeding
- Seizures
- Hyperammonaemia
- Dehydration and severe electrolyte imbalances
- Cardiac arrhythmias
- Loss of temperature control
- Respiratory depression
- Renal impairment
- Pancytopaenia
- Myocardial insults.

Managing acute illness and regaining metabolic control

- Close monitoring of TBR, BP, oxygen saturation.
- Check blood sugars regularly.
- Some patients may require neuro-observations.

Emergency regimen

- This consists of a high energy, protein-free, and fat-free drink which should be offered frequently and in small amounts either orally or via a nasogastric tube.
- High concentration in carbohydrates for energy (e.g. Maxijul®) but more tolerable substitutes can also be used (e.g. Lucozade®).
- If the oral regime is not tolerated or the child has persistent ketoacidosis an IV infusion of 10% or higher concentration glucose will be required.
- Patients with protein metabolism disorders should not stay off protein for a prolonged time as this may cause an endogenous release of protein.
- Working closely with an experienced dietitian in the field is advisable.

Acute hypoglycaemic event

- Prompt treatment is essential in order to avoid subsequent neurological damage.
- Initially in a conscious child, who is feeding glucose 10–20 g is given by mouth in a liquid form (GlucoGel®, milk, etc.). This may need to be repeated after 10–15 min.
- Alternatively 5 mL/kg of IV 10% glucose (500 mg/kg of glucose) may be given IV into a large vein, following a saline flush as the preparation is a potential irritant and may cause an extravasation injury or even lead to venous thrombosis.
- Hypoglycaemia that is not responding to the above measures, or hypoglycaemia that causes loss of consciousness or fitting, requires IM or IV administration of glucagon.
- No response to glucagon should raise the suspicion of glycogen storage disease types I, VI, X, XI or fatty acid oxidation defect.

Management of other systems

- Invasive monitoring of the acutely unwell patient is recommended.
- Patients may develop an oxygen requirement and some may also need to be intubated and ventilated.
- Peritoneal dialysis, haemofiltration, or exchange transfusions may be required in order to remove harmful metabolites and restore haemostasis.

Fatty liver disease in children

Fatty liver disease is now increasingly recognized in children, particularly in the setting of obesity.

The term non-alcoholic steatohepatitis (NASH) was first coined in 1980 by Ludwig to describe a pattern of liver injury in adults in which the liver histology was consistent with alcoholic hepatitis, but in whom significant alcohol consumption was denied. NASH can be considered as part of a broader spectrum of non-alcoholic fatty liver disease that extends from simple steatosis through steatohepatitis that is characterized by the potential to progress to fibrosis, cirrhosis and subsequent end stage liver disease.

In childhood, as alcohol is less of an issue, the more appropriate definition is 'steatosis with or without inflammation and fibrosis, in the absence of a known inherited metabolic defect or toxins, and associated in the majority with obesity and insulin resistance' and should be termed paediatric fatty liver disease (PFLD).

Demographics

- Overall, a male predominance has been reported.
- Several studies have reported the mean age at presentation as 11.6 years to 13.5 years, although the diagnosis of PFLD can be made in children as young as 2 years (Rashid & Roberts 2000).
- Data from the National Health and Nutrition Examination Survey (NHANES) suggest a tripling of the prevalence of obesity among adolescents in the US population, from 5% in 1960 to 15% in 2000. In conjunction with this rise, 7% of US adolescents exhibit impaired glucose tolerance.
- Similar data is now available from the UK, where obesity incidence in children aged 5–10 years has increased from 1.5% in 1974 to 6% in 2003 (Stamatakis et al. 2005).

Pathophysiology

The exact pathophysiology is not yet completely understood. However the accepted paradigm of the pathogenensis is the 'two-hit' theory, where fat accumulates in the hepatocytes by increased transport of fatty acids from the adipose tissue due to insulin resistance. There is also de novo fatty acid synthesis that further adds to the intrahepatocytic fatty acid load. Fatty acid export in the form of VLDL is also impaired further increasing the fatty acid load. Increased hepatocyte fatty acid load is considered the first hit. Hepatocellular injury results from oxidative stress induced lipid peroxidation and cytokine-mediated injury. Several genetic and environmental factors have been proposed to trigger this second hit which is considered to be responsible for inflammation and fibrosis that can lead to cirrhosis and sometime end-stage liver disease.

Differential diagnoses

- Metabolic liver disease (Wilson's, cystic fibrosis, mitochondrial and per-oxisomal defects of fatty acid oxidation, α_1-antitrypsin deficiency)
- Autoimmune liver disease
- Chronic viral infection (hepatitis B, C)
- Drug toxicity (steroids, amiodarone, valproate)
- Other metabolic disorders are particularly important to consider when investigating PFLD in non-obese children.

Presenting features

- Most common in the setting of obesity
- Usually asymptomatic, no liver specific symptoms
- May present with malaise, fatigue or vague recurrent abdominal pain (50%)
- Incidental finding of raised transaminases (usually less than 4× normal)
- Incidental finding of fatty liver on USS
- Acanthosis nigricans (velvety brown/black pigmentation in skin folds and axillae, related to hyperinsulinaemia), reported in as many as 50% of children with fatty liver disease, particularly those who have steatohepatitis.

Investigation

PFLD is a diagnosis of exclusion, other causes of chronic liver disease should be sought:

- FBC, LFT, U&E, INR
- Serum lactate, pyruvate, urate
- Serum Cu, caeruloplasmin, 24 h urinary Cu
- HBV, HCV serology
- α_1-Antitrypsin phenotype
- Plasma fatty acids and acyl carnitine
- Oral glucose tolerance test
- Tests for insulin resistance:
  - (HOMA, QUICKI HOAM-IR =(fasting insulin[uU/Ml yes])(fasting glucose[mmol/L]/22.5)
  - Insulin resistance HOMA-IR>2
  - QUICKI1/[(log[fasting insulin(μU/mL)+log(fasting glucose[mg/dL])]
  - Impaired SI is defined as QUICKI <0.339
- Liver USS
- MR imaging and MR spectroscopy are currently being evaluated by research as non-invasive tools for the assessment of hepatic steatosis.

Liver biopsy

This is the gold standard for confirmation of diagnosis and to establish the severity of fibrosis and the presence of cirrhosis, and exclude other coexisting conditions that can cause fatty liver disease. The histological findings differ from those in adults. In children the changes of steatosis, fibrosis, and inflammation are predominant around the portal spaces, whereas adults have changes centred around hepatic veins. This suggests that there may be important pathophysiological differences between adult and paediatric fatty liver disease.

Management

The only treatment that has been shown to be effective is gradual and sustained weight loss. Weight loss has produced improvement in liver transaminases and fat content in the liver as measured by various radiological techniques. High incidence of obesity and type 2 diabetes in the family members calls for a family-centred approach with counselling to support a sustained weight reduction programme and long-term lifestyle modification.

Pharmacological agents

Metformin, ursodeoxycholic acid, vitamin E, and several other drugs have been used in small clinical studies but without substantial long-term benefits. Results of ongoing prospective trials are awaited.

References and resources

Ludwig J, Viggiano TR, McGill DB, Ott BJ. Nonalcoholic steatohepatitis: Mayo Clinic experiences with a hitherto unnamed disease. *Mayo Clin Proc* 1980;**55**:434–438.

Rashid M, Roberts EA. Non-alcoholic steatohepatitis in children. *J Ped Gastroenterol Nutr* 2000;**30**:48–53.

Stamatakis E, Primatesta P, Chinn S, Rona R, Falascheti E Overweight and obesity trends from 1974 to 2003 in English children: what is the role of socioeconomic factors? *Arch Dis Child* 2005;**90**:999–1004

Wilson's disease

- Wilson's disease (WD) is an autosomal disorder of copper metabolism. The gene *ATP7B* codes for a copper carrier which both exports copper from hepatocyte to bile, and enables caeruloplasmin synthesis.
- WD occurs worldwide with reported incidences of 5–30 per million population. WD may present with almost any variety of liver disease in the age group 3–12 years, with psychiatric and/or neurological disease in adolescence or young adults, with combined hepatic and neurological problems, or less commonly with haemolysis or arthritis.
- Low plasma caeruloplasmin, a positive penicillamine challenge test, and raised hepatic copper concentration suggest the diagnosis. There are numerous diagnostic pitfalls.
- If diagnosed early, it is readily treatable with zinc or chelators, and has a good long-term prognosis.
- Fulminant hepatic disease has a poor outcome without transplantation. Molecular methods now aid diagnosis, but pose new management dilemmas.

Clinical features

WD has protean clinical presentations. Approximately 40% present with liver disease, usually between the ages of 3 and 12 years. Approximately 50% have a psychiatric or neurological presentation, usually in adolescence or early adult life. Approximately half of this group will have clinically detectable liver disease. The remainder present with skeletal, renal, or haemolytic disease, and these features may also be present in the other clinical categories. Younger siblings should be detected by screening

Liver disease in Wilson's disease

The first indication of liver disease in WD may be acute liver failure, acute hepatitis, chronic hepatitis, asymptomatic enlargement of the liver, the serendipitous finding of abnormal liver function tests, variceal haemorrhage from unsuspected portal hypertension, or signs of decompensated chronic liver disease. Therefore, since WD may present with almost any clinical variety of hepatic abnormality, the important message is to suspect WD in any child with undiagnosed liver disease. Other patients are discovered to have liver disease having presented with neurological, ophthalmic, haemolytic, skeletal or, rarely, renal problems. Clinical awareness of Wilson's is therefore all-important.

In all of these hepatic presentations, the absence of Kayser–Fleischer rings means that the diagnosis of WD will rest upon laboratory tests.

Diagnosis

The first essential in making the diagnosis of WD is to think of it.

A biochemical diagnosis is made by finding two of the following three abnormalities:

- Low plasma caeruloplasmin, <200 mg/L
- Raised urinary copper, >25 μmol/24 h following penicillamine—the penicillamine challenge
- Raised hepatic copper, >250 mg/g dry weight.

Alternatively, the diagnosis may be made on one of the following molecular grounds:

- Haplotypic identity with a biochemically proven sibling
- 2 WD mutations.

Studies may clarify the diagnosis in difficult patients.

Penicillamine challenge

Basal urine copper is an unreliable parameter, showing both poor sensitivity and poor specificity, though values >5 μmol/24 h are highly suggestive. A penicillamine challenge test gives greater discrimination. Following penicillamine 0.5 g 12 hourly × 2, urine copper >25 μmol/24 h in 88% patients with WD and 2% of those with other liver disorders.

Management

Diet

There is no clinical evidence that copper content of the diet influences the age of onset or the severity of WD, but there is some circumstantial evidence that it affects the severity of liver disease in animal models of WD. It is therefore appropriate to avoid excessive use of high-copper foods such as chocolate, shellfish, and liver.

Drugs

Three drugs are available to treat WD: D-penicillamine, trientine, and zinc. Both penicillamine and trientine may cause initial deterioration of neurological function on commencement of treatment. A fourth agent, ammonium tetrathiamolydate, remains under clinical investigation.

Penicillamine

Penicillamine 'detoxifies' the copper possibly by inducing metallothionein by augmenting the bile pool or by a direct anti-inflammatory action. Toxic effects include: skin rash, usually urticarial occurring soon after commencing treatment, and responding to cessation of treatment; proteinuria, in most cases mild and not requiring cessation of treatment but in a small number of patients proceeding to immune complex nephrotic syndrome; and bone marrow depression. Pyridoxine deficiency is a theoretical risk in childhood. A more serious and fortunately rare side effect is systemic lupus erythematosus.

Trientine

Trientine was initially introduced as a second line drug for patients intolerant of D-penicillamine. The most commonly reported side effect is sideroblastic anaemia.

Zinc

- Zinc, by inducing metallothionein in intestinal cells, reduces absorption and, by inducing metallothionein in hepatocytes, binds copper. It is of low toxicity and cheap, but its principal disadvantage is poor palatability.
- The initial management of WD must be tailored to the clinical presentation.
- Patients with fulminant hepatic failure (patients with encephalopathy) have a poor prognosis, and must be transferred to a centre where they can be offered liver transplantation. A prognostic score can help to predict the need for urgent liver transplantation in patients who present with decompensated liver disease (see Table 56.1).
- Treatment of young children identified on screening. There is no consensus on the best drug or the age when treatment should be instituted. Our practice is to treat children older than 2 years with zinc acetate only.

Indications for liver transplantation

Liver transplantation is indicated for patients with fulminant liver failure with adverse prognostic score (Table 56.1) and for those patients who do not respond to therapy, or who have advanced liver failure and/ or intractable portal hypertension.

Table 56.1 Revised King's Wilson Disease Index for predicting mortality (reprinted with permission from Liver Transplantation)

Score	Bilirubin (µmol/L)	INR	AST (IU/L)	WCC (10⁹/l)	Albumin (g/L)
0	0—100	0—1.29	0—100	0—6.7	>45
1	101—150	1.3—1.6	101—150	6.8—8.3	34—44
2	151—200	1.7—1.9	151—300	8.4—10.3	25—33
3	201—300	2.0—2.4	301—400	10.4—15.3	21—24
4	> 301	> 2.5	> 401	> 15.4	<20

Score of 11 or more indicates high mortality and need for liver transplantation.

Hepatitis B

Epidemiology

- About 2 billion people (1/3 of the world population) show evidence of exposure to hepatitis B virus (HBV) infection, with 300–400 million showing evidence of chronic HBV infection.
- There are 7 genotypes, A–G. A and G predominate in Europe and USA, B and C in Asia, E in Africa).
- HBV carrier rate varies from 1 to 20% of normal population worldwide (Table 57.1).

Transmission

HBV infection is commonly transmitted by percutaneous (i.e. puncture through the skin) or mucosal (i.e. direct contact with mucous membranes) exposure to infectious blood or to body fluids containing blood. Serum, semen, and saliva have been demonstrated to be infectious.

Perinatal transmission remains the most common route of transmission in children, followed by horizontal transmission from infected household contacts. Adolescents are at risk of HBV infection primarily through unprotected high-risk sexual activity and IV drug use.

The risk for chronic HBV infection in a newborn infant born to an HBsAg and HBeAg positive mother is 90% in the absence of postexposure immunoprophylaxis. The risk decreases to <10% in the absence of postexposure immunoprophylaxis if the mother is HBsAg positive but HBeAg negative. Rarely HBV infection can present as acute liver failure in perinatally infected infants born to a mother who is HBsAg positive but HBeAg negative.

Clinical features

- Incubation period 50–150 days.
- *Acute hepatitis B:* Mostly asymptomatic. If symptomatic, mainly constitutional symptoms like anorexia, nausea, vomiting, low grade fever, myalgia, fatiguability, right upper quadrant pain, and/or jaundice. Although acute liver failure has been reported in 2% of cases, viral clearance occurs in >95% of infected adolescents and adults.
- *Chronic hepatitis B:* Defined by presence of HBsAg in serum for >6 months. Usually patients are healthy carriers without any evidence of active disease. Sometimes they can present with constitutional symptoms as described for acute hepatitis B. The risk of chronicity depends on the age of acquiring infection (90% in infants, 25–50% in children, 5% in adults).

Interpretation of HBV serology

- HBV core antigen (HBcAg):
  - not detected in serum.
- HBc antibody (anti-HBc):
  - presence of anti-HBc IgM indicates early acute infection/reinfection
  - anti-HBc IgG can be detected in both acute and chronic HBV infection.
- HBV early antigen (HBeAg):
  - 'early' appearance during acute HBV infection
  - marker of a high degree of HBV infectivity
  - correlates with a high level of HBV replication.
- HBe antibody (anti-HBe):
  - often associated with decreasing levels of HBV DNA and liver enzymes in the blood marking the end of the replicative phase of the disease
  - high HBV DNA with positive HBeAb suggests precore mutants.
- HBV surface antigen (HBsAg):
  - presence in serum for at least 6 months indicates chronic infection.
- HBs antibody (anti-HBs):
  - indicates an immune response to HBV infection or vaccination, or the presence of passively acquired antibody (HBIg).
- HBV DNA (viral load):
  - best indicator of active viral replication.

The pattern of HBV infection and HBV serology is shown in Table 57.2.

Complications

- Cirrhosis: high risk in patients who continue to be HBeAg +ve; usually takes several years before decompensation
- Hepatocellular carcinoma
- Membranous glomerulonephritis
- Polyarteritis nodosum
- Panniculitis.

Table 57.1 Geographical distribution and the mode of transmission of HBV infection

	Rate	Areas	Mode of transmission
Low	0.1–2%	Canada, Western Europe, Australia, New Zealand	Sexual and parenteral
Intermediate	3–5%	Eastern Europe, Mediterranean basin, Middle East, South America, Central Asia	Sexual and parenteral
High	10–20%	South-east Asia, China, sub-Saharan Africa	Perinatal

Table 57.2 Pattern of HBV infection and HBV serology

	Acute infection	Chronic HBV		Precore mutant	Vaccinated	Resolved infection
		Low infectivity	High infectivity			
HBsAg	+	+	+	+	–	–
HBeAg	+/–	–	+	–	–	–
Anti-HBc IgM	+	–	–	–	–	–
Anti-HBc IgG	+/–	+	+	+	–	+
Anti-HBs	–	–	–	–	+	+
Anti-Hbe	+/–	+	–	+	–	+/–
HBV DNA	+/–	+	+++	++	–	–
Serum ALT	↑↑	N	N/↑	↑	N	N

Table 57.3 Prevention in term babies born to mother with hepatitis B infection

Hepatitis B status of mother	Hepatitis vaccine	HBIG
Mother is HBsAg +ve and HBeAg +ve	Yes	Yes
Mother is HBsAg +ve, HBeAg –ve but anti-HBe -ve	Yes	Yes
Mother is HBsAg +ve but e-markers unknown	Yes	Yes
Mother had acute hepatitis B infection in pregnancy	Yes	Yes
Mother is HBsAg +ve, HBeAg –ve and anti-HBe +ve	Yes	No

Prevention

Hepatitis B immunoprophylaxis
- Universal immunization against HBV in recommended.

Post-exposure prophylaxis
- Term babies born to mother with hepatitis B infection: see Table 57.3.
- Babies with a birthweight of 1500 g or less, born to mother infected with hepatitis B, should receive HBIG in addition to the vaccine regardless of the e-antigen status of the mother.
- Recommended vaccine schedule is the accelerated immunization schedule with vaccine at birth, 1 and 2 months, and 1 year of age.
- Children should be tested for HBsAg at 1 year of age at the time of the 4th dose to check if the vaccination has been successful or not.
- Response to vaccine (done 1–4 months after completing the schedule):
  - anti-HBs concentration >100 mIU/mL—responder, no further dose required
  - anti-HBs concentration >10 but <100 mIU/mL—responder but requires an additional dose at that time
  - anti-HBs concentration <10 mIU/mL—non-responder, repeat course of vaccine followed by another test to check the response
- Accidental exposure/contamination from blood from a known HBsAg +ve person
  - previously immunized and responder: booster dose
  - previously immunized but non-responder: HBIG and a booster dose with 2nd dose of HBIG after 1 month
  - previously unimmunized: accelerated course of HBV vaccine with HBIG 1 dose.
- Individuals at continuing risk of infection should be offered a single booster dose of vaccine, once only, ~5 years after primary immunization.
- Patients with chronic renal failure on haemodialysis should have antibody levels checked annually and if anti-HBs concentration <10 mIU/mL, they should receive a booster dose.

Management of chronic HBV infection

- Therapy currently recommended only for patients with chronic active disease (HBsAg +, HBeAg +, high HBV DNA and abnormal AST/ALT).
- Patients with HBeAg seroconversion and low/undetectable HBV DNA have improved outcome with prolonged survival without complications, reduced rate of HCC and clinical and biochemical improvement.

Antiviral therapy

Interferon alpha
- Antiviral and immunomodulatory protein
- About 30–40% adults achieve HBeAg seroconversion.
- High pre-treatment AST/ALT levels, low pretreatment HBV DNA, late acquisition of HBV infection and hepatocellular inflammation are the factors predicting good response.
- Side effects—flu-like symptoms, depression, bone marrow suppression, autoantibody induction, anorexia and weight loss, hair loss.
- If a severe reaction occurs, dose should be halved or discontinued.

Lamivudine
- Nucleoside analogue which inhibits DNA synthesis.
- Rapidly reduces HBV DNA levels to undetectable, however comes back to pretreatment levels after cessation of the medications.
- Side effects—GI symptoms (nausea, vomiting, abdominal pain, diarrhoea), malaise, fatigue, pancreatitis, cough, headache, dizziness, neutropenia, elevation of transaminases, myalgia, urticarial rash.
- Development of YMDD mutants increases with duration of the therapy (17% after 1 year to 63% after 5 years).

Adefovir
- Nucleoside analogue and a potent inhibitor of viral polymerase
- Effective in YMDD mutations
- Side effects: nephrotoxicity
- Currently in phase III trial.

Future potential therapies
- Pegylated interferon alone
- Pegylated interferon + nucleoside analogue
- Nucleoside analogue: entecavir, emtricitabine
- Gene therapy: antisense oligonucleotide, ribozyme, interfering proteins
- Immunomodulatory therapy: thymosin, DNA vaccine.

Hepatitis C

Epidemiology

- Hepatitis C virus (HCV) is an RNA virus of the flaviviride family.
- More than 150 million people are infected with HCV worldwide.
- UK prevalence of chronic HCV is 0.4%.
- There are 6 main genotypes (1–6) with subtypes (A–C):
  - genotype 1: Europe and USA
  - genotype 4: Egypt and Middle East
  - genotypes 2 and 3—South-east Asia, Europe, USA.
- In England and Wales, genotypes1 and 3 are most prevalent.

Risk of transmission

- Vertical transmission is the most common.
- Transmission from mother to child is ~5% but it increases if the mother is co-infected with HIV.
- Risk is negligible if mother is HCV antibody positive but HCV RNA negative.
- Mode of delivery does not affect the risk of transmission unless the mother is co-infected with HIV, when Caesarian section may have a protective role.
- Though HCV RNA can be detected in breast milk and colostrum, breast-feeding does not appear to increase the rate of HCV transmission.
- Other routes of transmission include parenteral, sexual, or blood-product transfusion.

Clinical features

- Incubation period: Average 6 weeks, range 2–26 weeks.
- Symptoms: Usually asymptomatic, non-specific illness like fatigue, headache present in 30–40%, 20–30% may develop jaundice.
- Extrahepatic manifestations: Membranous glomerulonephritis, autoimmune hepatitis, thyroiditis, polyarteritis nodosa, polymyositis, cryoglobulinemia.
- Chronic HCV infection is defined by persistence of HCV RNA in serum for >6 months.
- Patients with chronic HCV have intermittent abnormalities of liver enzymes.
- 75% of adults with HCV develop chronic infection with increased lifetime risk of cirrhosis (10–20% after 20 years) and hepatocellular carcinoma (1%).
- Children with transfusion-acquired chronic HCV infection have a higher chance of spontaneous resolution (27–48%) as compared to the vertical transmission (5.6–10%).
- Severe fibrosis leading to cirrhosis is very rare in the paediatric population.

Specific viral tests

- Anti-HCV antibody: positive ELISA test confirms exposure to HCV but not persistence of infection; in infancy it can represent transplacental passage of maternal anti-HCV antibodies.
- HCV RNA positivity confirms ongoing infection.
- HCV genotype influences the treatment regimen, with genotypes 2 and 3 responding best to treatment

Diagnosis of HCV infection in infants born to HCV +ve mother

- Check HCV RNA at 2–3 months of age:
  - if HCV RNA –ve, infection is unlikely; confirm by repeating at 6–12 months of age
  - if HCV RNA +ve, most likely the child is infected; confirm by repeating test in 6–12 months.

Management

- Currently combination of pegylated interferon + ribavirin is the recommended treatment for adults and the same combination has shown good response in the paediatric population with sustained viral clearance in about 50–60% in genotype 1, 80–100% in genotypes 2 and 3.
- Duration of treatment:
  - genotypes 1, 4, 5, 6: 12 months (check HCV RNA at 24 weeks, continue treatment only if HCV RNA becomes negative)
  - genotypes 2 and 3: 6 months.
- Side effects:
  - pegylated interferon: neutropenia, thrombocytopenia, hypothyroidism, autoimmune disorder, mood swings, depression, etc.
  - ribavirin: haemolytic anaemia.
- Good prognostic factors for antiviral treatment are absence of cirrhosis, young age at acquisition, and absence of co-morbidity (HBV and/or HIV).
- Newer antiviral medications include protease inhibitors and albuferon.

Bacterial, fungal, and parasitic infections of the liver

Infectious agents can affect the liver either via direct invasion or by release of toxins. The liver's dual blood supply renders it uniquely susceptible to infection, receiving blood from the intestinal tract via the hepatic portal system, and from the systemic circulation via the hepatic artery. Because of this unique perfusion, the liver is frequently exposed to systemic or intestinal infections or the mediators of toxaemia. The biliary tree provides a further conduit for gut bacteria or parasites to access the liver parenchyma.

Infections of the liver with a wide range of organisms present variously from asymptomatic biochemical abnormalities to symptomatic hepatitis, or space-occupying lesions (e.g. abscesses), or granulomata producing biochemical cholestasis but rarely significant jaundice. Some of these infections have a high mortality if not treated promptly.

Bacterial sepsis

Bacterial sepsis precipitating jaundice is well recognized particularly in neonates and infants.

Etiology and pathologic changes

- Diverse group of organisms are responsible for hepatic dysfunction following bacteremia:
- Gram negative organisms: *Escherichia coli*, *Klebsiella pneumoniae*, *Pseudomonas aeruginosa*, *Proteus species*, *Paracolon bacteria*, *Bacteroides*, *Salmonella typhi*
- *Haemophilus influenzae*
- Aerobic and anaerobic streptococci
- *Staphylococcus aureus*
- *Streptococcus pneumoniae*

The exact pathogenesis of hepatic insult is not known, but may be multifactorial;
- Direct invasion of liver parenchyma by blood borne pathogens
- Nonspecific injury secondary to hypoxia, fever and malnutrition
- Endotoxin induced cholestasis (see Fig. 59.1)

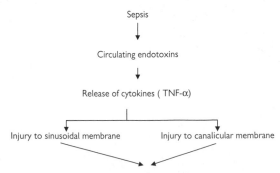

Fig. 59.1 Sepsis-induced cholestasis.

Laboratory diagnosis and treatment

Clinical evaluation and microbiological investigation may identify the source of sepsis and antimicrobial therapy usually results in complete resolution. Cytology and biopsies should be performed where indicated.

Liver abscess

Pyogenic liver abscess (PLA) in infancy and childhood is rare, with up to 40–50% occurring in immunocompromised children.

Pyogenic bacteria can reach the liver through various routes:
- Portal: Secondary to gut pathologies such as appendicitis, inflammatory bowel disease
- Biliary: Caused by extrahepatic biliary tract disease such as stricture, calculus, or malignancy
- Blood borne, from an infected focus anywhere in the body
- Contiguous extension from gallbladder or perinephric abscess
- Following penetrating wounds of liver
- Cryptogenic.

PLA may present as a single large lesion or multiple abscesses, the latter often secondary to biliary tract infection.
- *Staphylococcus aureus* is the most common isolate in children but Gram-negative aerobes, anaerobes, and microaerophilic streptococci are also common. Less frequent causes include *Pseudomonas* spp., *Clostridium* spp., *Salmonella typhi*, *Yersinia enterocolitica*, and *Pasteurella*.

Clinical presentation
- The classic presentation is pyrexia, chills, right upper quadrant abdominal pain, hepatomegaly, and leucocytosis, but may be non-specific.
- Unusual presentations include an abdominal mass or acute abdomen secondary to rupture into the peritoneal cavity or portal hypertension secondary to portal pyaemia and portal vein thrombosis.

Diagnosis
- Liver function tests may be unhelpful, with non-specific changes.
- USS, CT, and MRI are all sensitive but cannot always differentiate abscesses from other lesions such as cysts, tumours, or haemorrhage.
- USS- or CT-guided drainage of as much pus as possible (from as many abscesses as possible) confirms diagnosis, and is central to management.

Treatment and prognosis
- Aspiration under USS guidance is helpful.
- Initial treatment is conservative with broad-spectrum antibiotics (e.g. cephalosporins plus metronidazole or clindamycin) and should be adjusted when culture results are available. Duration of treatment is usually 3–6 weeks.

Cholangitis

The normal biliary tract is sterile and, in children, acute cholangitis rarely occurs in the absence of congenital abnormalities or interventions in the biliary tract.

Aetiology and pathogenesis

The children at highest risk include:

- Those with porto-enterostomy or choledochal cyst, and those who have non-operative biliary manipulations such as transhepatic cholangiography or endoscopic retrograde cholangiography with stent placement.
- Risk of cholangitis in children after Kasai operation is 40–50%.

Diagnosis and treatment

- Clinical diagnosis is based on fever, abdominal pain, jaundice, pale stools, or hepatic tenderness.
- Leucocytosis is common, but changes in liver function tests are non-specific; the serum bilirubin may be normal.
- In recurrent cholangitis liver biopsy may be indicated for confirmation and microbiological examination.
- Treatment requires supportive care and an urgent USS or CT to help establish whether obstruction requires drainage. Broad-spectrum antibiotics should be administered, such as an acylureidopenicillin (piperacillin, mezlocillin, or piperacillin-tazobactam) or late-generation cephalosporin (e.g. ceftazidime), plus an aminoglycoside. Duration of treatment is generally 3 weeks, but prolonged therapy for recurrent cholangitis.

Tuberculosis (TB)

Liver involvement alone by *Mycobacteria* is common in endemic areas. TB of the liver is almost invariably a complication of miliary disease, and occurs in 50% and 75% of patients with pulmonary or extrapulmonary TB respectively. The site of primary focus usually dictates presentation. Rarely the liver appears to be the sole site of infection such as in congenital TB acquired via the placenta.

Brucellosis

Granulomatous hepatitis may occur in acute or chronic disease and manifests as non-specific changes in liver function tests.

Listeriosis

Listeria monocytogenes may cause liver disease as part of systemic intrauterine infection of the fetus (granulomatosis infantiseptica) at birth or later in the neonatal period and in older immunocompromised children after ingestion of contaminated food or water. The major hepatic manifestation is granuloma; jaundice is rare.

Tularemia

Francisella tularensis: in some cases a hepatitis-like picture follows with raised aminotransferases. Hepatomegaly is rare and biopsy may show necrosis. Diagnosis is usually serological as the bacterium is difficult to recover in culture. Treatment with streptomycin or gentamicin is effective.

Spirochaetal infections

The spirochaetal infection which affect the liver are:

- Leptospirosis
- Borreliasis
- Congenital syphilis.

Leptospirosis

Epidemiology and clinical manifestations

- Human infection follows exposure to leptospires excreted in the urine of chronically infected animals including rats, cattle, and dogs, or water contaminated with urine.
- The incubation period is 5–15 days and in 90% of patients there is a self-limiting anicteric disease but 5–10% develop jaundice (Weil's disease).
- Weil's disease is characterized by hepatic, renal, and vascular dysfunction with persistent fever, profound jaundice, abdominal pain, renal failure, confusion, epistaxis, haematuria, GI bleeding, and other haemorrhagic phenomena.
- Death may follow cardiovascular collapse, renal failure, and GI or pulmonary haemorrhage, though with supportive therapy mortality should be <10%.

Diagnosis and treatment

- Liver histology and culture; leptospires may be recovered from blood, urine, or CSF during the first week of illness, and from urine thereafter.
- Diagnosis is usually serological, however; PCR can detect leptospiral DNA in blood, serum, CSF, urine, or aqueous humour.
- Penicillin or doxycycline are recommended and most beneficial if started early in the disease.

Borreliosis

- Also known as Lyme disease; caused by *Borrelia burgdorferi*, a tick-borne spirochaete.
- The hepatic involvement is part of systemic disease, abnormal liver function tests are seen in up to 19% of patients, particularly serum transaminases are raised. Rarely there is hepatomegaly and right upper quadrant tenderness.
- Diagnosis is based on clinical suspicion, positive serology, and histopathology.
- In the early stages of disease amoxicillin for children <9 years and tetracycline for children >9 years of age are the treatments of choice. In late stages of the disease, IV cefotaxime or ceftriaxone are recommended.

Congenital syphilis

- Hepatomegaly is seen in 50–90% of symptomatic infants. Neonatal death is caused by liver failure, severe pneumonia, or pulmonary haemorrhage.
- The diagnosis is made by detecting IgM specific antibodies and detection of antigen.
- Penicillin is the drug of choice and is risk free in the neonate; alternatively, ceftriaxone can be used.

Rickettsial infections

Q fever

- The causative organism is *Coxiella burnetii*.
- Infection results from inhalation of dust from infected animals, consumption of raw milk, or via transplacental transmission or blood transfusion.

Clinical manifestations

- The incubation period is 1–2 weeks, usual course is self limiting. There are three major presentations:
  - atypical pneumonia
  - flu like syndrome
  - hepatitis.
- Hepatitis occurs in 3–4% of cases, jaundice in 1/3 of cases, and fever and hepatomegaly in >70% of cases. The abnormal liver function tests are noted in up to 70–80% of patients. Commonest abnormality of liver function test is an elevation of the alkaline phosphatase.

Diagnosis

- History of contact with an animal host is a vital clue.
- Diagnosis is made by detection of phase I and phase II antibodies of *Coxiella burnetii*.
- Seroconversion usually detected 7–15 days after onset of clinical symptoms; 90% of patients have detectable antibodies by third week.

Treatment

- Treatment with tetracycline and chloramphenicol is effective.

Fungal infections

- Fungal infections of the liver are usually seen in the immunocompromised, including those with acute liver failure.
- Although *Candida albicans* predominates, other *Candida* spp. and *Aspergillus* spp. infections are increasingly reported.
- Other rare fungal infections of the liver include cryptococcosis, mucormycosis, histoplasmosis, blastomycosis, coccidioidomycosis, and paracoccidioidomycosis.

Parasitic infections

Hepatic amoebiasis

- *Entamoeba histolytica* is most commonly encountered in the tropics and subtropics.
- Hepatic abscess is a major complication of invasive amoebiasis and seen in 3–9% of adult cases but is less common in children.
- Amoebic trophozoites reach the liver via the portal vein, induce hepatocyte apoptosis and a leukocyte response resulting in abscesses containing viscous brown pus.

Clinical manifestations and diagnosis

- The hepatic lesion can manifest as multiple or single.
- Multiple abscesses may be associated with more severe disease.
- The abscess is commonly seen in the right lobe of liver.
- A typical presentation is with pyrexia (75%) and right upper quadrant pain radiating to the right shoulder.
- Tenderness in the hypochondrium (85%), tender hepatomegaly (80%), and localized swelling over the liver (10%) may be elicited.
- Less specific symptoms include nausea, vomiting, concurrent diarrhoea or dysentery (10%), and loss of weight.
- Jaundice is present in up to 8% of cases. The white blood cell count is usually elevated.
- Hepatic abscesses can be demonstrated by USS or CT scanning.
- Demonstrating cysts in stool may contribute to diagnosis, but serum antibodies are present in >95% of patients.
- Aspiration under USS guidance may yield 'anchovy sauce' pus; rarely amoebae are seen in necrotic abscess wall or adjacent parenchyma.

Complications

- Abscesses may rupture in to the peritoneal cavity, pleural cavity or lungs, pericardium, portal vein, or biliary tract, intraperitoneal rupture being more common than intrathoracic.

Treatment

- Extraintestinal amoebiasis should be treated with metronidazole or dehydroemetine for at least 2 weeks.
- To prevent continued intraluminal infection, a luminal amoebicide, such as paromomycin or diloxanide furoate, should be given.
- Percutaneous needle aspiration along with medical treatment is recommended if the abscess is large (>6 cm), or does not respond to medical treatment within 72 h, if there is imminent risk of abscess rupture.
- Surgical intervention is required in cases complicated with abscess rupture.

Schistosomiasis

Patients present with pyrexia, urticaria, eosinophilia, hepatosplenomegaly or upper GI tract bleeding from oesophageal varices.

- The diagnosis is made by demonstrating ova in stool and urine and may be identified in liver or rectal mucosal biopsy. Serological tests cannot distinguish past from active infection but a negative ELISA excludes the diagnosis.

- Praziquantel is the drug of choice; oxamniquine an alternative for
  S. mansoni.

Hydatid disease
- The liver is the most common site for cyst formation and in 60–85% of
  cases the cyst is located in the right lobe.
- The signs and symptoms of hepatic echinococcosis may include hepatic
  enlargement, with or without a palpable mass, epigastric pain, nausea,
  and vomiting.
- Rare presentations secondary to pressure effects or rupture of the
  cyst include portal hypertension, inferior vena cava compression or
  thrombosis, secondary biliary cirrhosis, biliary peritonitis, or pyogenic
  abscess.
- USS of the liver reveals round, solitary or multiple, cysts of variable size
  with multiple internal daughter cysts; calcification may be noted.
- Diagnosis requires demonstration of specific antibody.
- The primary treatment is surgical removal of the cysts. Both mebendazole and albendazole can cross the cyst wall and have the potential to
  treat small uncomplicated cysts.

Ascariasis
- Rarely ascariasis can invade the biliary tree and cause biliary obstruction.
- Ultrasonography may show worms in the common duct, or abscess
  formation may be noticed. Endoscopic retrograde cholangiography
  (ERCP) shows the adult worms as a filling defect or a worm protruding
  through the papilla.
- Treatment is with anthelmintic drugs, but endoscopic removal of the
  worm may be necessary in patients with persisting biliary symptoms.

Toxocariasis
- Hepatosplenomegaly, lymphadenopathy or pruritic skin lesions may be
  present.
- Serodiagnosis is available by ELISA technique.
- The treatment is thiabendazole 50 mg/kg per day in two divided doses
  for 5 days.

Liver flukes (*Fasciola hepatica*)
- Hepatic invasion is by penetration of the hepatic capsule by metacecariae
  which migrate through liver parenchyma and enter bile ducts causing
  cholangitis and hepatomegaly.
- The diagnosis is made by demonstrating ova in stool and on basis of
  positive serology.
- ERCP shows filling defects due to the inflammatory response; worms
  can also be aspirated.

Toxoplasmosis
Congenital toxoplasmosis
- Severely infected neonates present with cholestasis, purpura, and
  hepatosplenomegaly.
- Other associated symptoms and signs can be hydrocephalus,
  retinochoroiditis, intracranial calcification, and hydrops fetalis.

- The diagnosis of acute infection in the newborn is made on the basis of presence of IgA and IgM antibodies from peripheral blood of newborn. *Toxoplasma gondii* specific DNA is detected in body fluids (blood, urine, and CSF) by using PCR. Histologically liver biopsy shows giant cell hepatitis and extramedullary haematopoiesis.
- Pyrimethamine plus sulfadiazine twice daily plus folinic acid supplement for 3 weeks, alternating with spiramycin daily in two divided doses for 3 weeks. Continue the alternating therapy for 1 year.

Granulomatous hepatitis

Common infectious causes of granuloma in liver

- Bacterial causes:
  - tuberculosis
  - brucellosis
  - listeriosis
  - yersiniosis
  - *Mycobacterium avium intracellulare*
  - BCG infection
  - tularemia
  - rickettsia
  - Q fever
  - chlamydia
  - psittacosis
- Fungal infections:
  - candidiasis
  - histoplasmosis
  - nocardiosis
  - blastomycosis
  - coccidioidomycosis
- Parasitic infections:
  - schistosomiasis
  - visceral larva migrans
  - visceral leishmaniasis
  - toxoplasmosis

Liver tumours

Liver tumours in children are rare, accounting for 0.5–2% of all neoplasms in the paediatric age group.

Infantile haemangiomata

- Benign vascular tumour.
- Occurs almost exclusively in the first year of life.
- Relatively common in the skin and mucous membranes but can affect any organ system.
- In the liver, two histological types of lesions have been described:
  - capillary haemangioma (or haemangioendothelioma)
  - cavernous haemangioma.
- Presenting features are hepatomegaly and abdominal distension.
- Involvement can be as a single tumour or multifocal.
- Complications include high-output cardiac failure, often life threatening, due to the presence of significant shunting; Kasabach–Merrit syndrome (anaemia, consumptive coagulopathy, cholestasis); vascular malformation involving other organs, and rarely intraperitoneal haemorrhage secondary to rupture. Hypothyroidism can occur associated with increased activity of type 3 iodothyroxindiiodinase within the tumour.
- Diagnosis is made on imaging including USS with Doppler, CT, and MRI. Needle liver biopsy is contraindicated because of the high risk of bleeding. Liver tissue can be obtained at laparotomy in selected cases, when malignancy cannot be excluded on imaging.

Management

- Asymptomatic: does not warrant treatment because of the spontaneous resolution of the lesion over time.
- Symptomatic: depends on its severity.
- Medical treatment consists of symptomatic treatment of high-output cardiac failure with digoxin, diuretics, and ACE inhibitors. Other treatments to promote the involution of the lesions include radiotherapy, corticosteroids, interferon, and chemotherapy with vincristine.
- Surgical management includes resection of the lesion by hepatic lobectomy or hepatic artery ligation, depending on the size and localization of the lesion.
- Liver transplantation should be reserved for cases that do not respond to any of the above treatment options.

Mesenchymal hamartoma

- Rare benign tumour.
- Multicystic appearance.
- Typically affects children during the first 2 years of life.
- Presentation can be with symptoms of abdominal distension but is often an incidental finding on clinical examination or imaging and is rarely symptomatic.
- Biochemically, AFP can be mildly raised, liver function tests usually normal.
- Imaging with USS, CT, and MRI.
- Final diagnosis is made on the basis of histology, usually obtained at the time of resection. Spontaneous regression has been described.

Focal nodular hyperplasia (FNH)

- Benign epithelial tumour.
- The lesion, typically well circumscribed and lobulated, can vary in size and be single or multiple.
- Seen in all age groups, more common in females, has been reported in older patients with GSD type 1.
- Presentation with abdominal pain is common.
- Imaging with USS, CT, and MRI are usually diagnostic.
- Three treatment strategies are employed:
  - conservative management with regular clinical and radiological follow-up
  - surgical excision of the mass
  - interventional treatment with embolization or ligation of the hepatic artery.
- No reports of malignant transformation.

Nodular regenerative hyperplasia (NRH)

- Rare in paediatric age group.
- Usually asymptomatic; hepatosplenomegaly is detected fortuitously.
- CT and MRI usually suggest the diagnosis.
- Can involve the whole liver and lead to portal hypertension and its complications.
- Treatment is management of the complications.

Hepatoblastoma

- Embryonic tumour derived from the epithelial cells of the fetal liver and characterized by a rapid growth.
- Most frequent malignant liver tumour in children, most commonly diagnosed in the first 3 years of life.
- Male preponderance.
- Spreads by vascular invasion, typically in the lungs.
- Presentation usually with abdominal distension, abdominal pain, and failure to thrive.
- Anaemia and thrombocytosis are common; very high AFP levels are characteristic and are a marker of response to therapy.
- CT or MRI is necessary for an accurate differentiation between tumour and normal liver tissue.
- Diagnosis is by liver biopsy.
- Treatment consists of chemotherapy and complete tumour resection by partial hepatectomy or, if the tumour is unresectable, by liver transplantation.
- Adverse prognostic factors are low serum AFP (<100 ng/mL), lack of response to chemotherapy, and presence of metastases at diagnosis.

Hepatocellular carcinoma (HCC)

- Rare in paediatric age group, but when present, is typically seen in older children/teenagers.
- Most commonly, HCC develops in the presence of an underlying liver disease such as chronic viral hepatitis (e.g. hepatitis B) or a metabolic disorder (e.g. tyrosinaemia or progressive familial intrahepatic cholestasis syndromes).
- Typical presentation is with abdominal pain and an abdominal mass.
- AFP is often elevated, though not as much as in hepatoblastoma.
- CT and MRI can help to determine whether tumour resection is an option.
- Liver biopsy under USS guidance is indicated if no underlying liver pathology is present.
- Treatment consists of resection, chemotherapy or combined chemotherapy and resection, but the prognosis is very poor, with a reported 10–20% long-term survival.

Inflammatory pseudotumour

- Rare, benign lesion that can arise in different organs and tissues, with the liver being a relatively common site of origin.
- Histology consists of proliferation of spindle-shaped cells, myofibroblasts, mixed with inflammatory cells, consisting of plasma cells, lymphocytes, and occasional histiocytes.
- Since 1971, 15 paediatric cases have been reported in the literature, ranging in age from 10 months to 15 years.
- The lesion can be solitary or multiple.
- Presentation is commonly with non-specific symptoms such as fever jaundice and impaired growth with raised inflammatory markers on biochemistry.
- There are no specific laboratory or radiological findings and differential diagnosis with FNH can be difficult on imaging.
- A final diagnosis is made at the time of surgical resection, which is the most common form of treatment; prognosis is generally good.

Fibropolycystic liver disease

- Heterogeneous group of disorders.
- Often associated with fibrocystic anomalies in the kidneys and share the same genetic defect.
- Gene was localized to chromosome region 6p21 in 1994 and described as *PKHD1* in 2002; 119 different mutations have been reported so far.

Four types have been described:
- Congenital hepatic fibrosis:
  - associated with autosomal recessive polycystic kidney disease
  - presentation during childhood or adolescence with isolated hepatomegaly or variceal bleeding secondary to portal hypertension
  - can be associated with carbohydrate-deficient glycoprotein syndrome type Ib (CDGS Ib), characterized by congenital hepatic fibrosis associated with cyclical vomiting, protein-losing enteropathy and prothrombotic tendency, as well as neurological impairment; screening with transferrin iso-electrofocusing for a glycosylation defect
  - management is symptomatic treatment of portal hypertension.
- Caroli disease:
  - caused by malformation of the larger bile ducts; hepatic fibrosis is absent.
  - clinical presentation is often with recurrent episodes of cholangitis
  - management involves aggressive antibiotic therapy.
- Caroli syndrome
  - ductal plate malformation of larger bile ducts associated with hepatic fibrosis
  - complications of portal hypertension and recurrent cholangitis are common.
- Von Meyenburg complexes
  - known as biliary hamartomas, discrete foci of ductal plate malformation affecting the smallest bile ducts, commonly present as an incidental finding on liver histology.

Complications of chronic liver disease

Definition

The complications of chronic liver disease and cirrhosis are a consequence of the impaired metabolic and synthetic function and structural alteration of the parenchyma leading to elevated portal pressure (see box).

Complications of cirrhosis in children

- Growth faltering and malnutrition
- Hepatic encephalopathy
- Coagulopathy
- Hepatopulmonary syndrome
- Portal hypertension and variceal bleeding
- Ascites
- Spontaneous bacterial peritonitis
- Hepatorenal syndrome
- Pruritus
- Hepatic osteodystrophy
- Endocrine dysfunction
- Hepatocellular carcinoma

Growth failure and malnutrition

Epidemiology

Can occur in 50–80% of children with chronic liver disease.

Pathophysiology

There are combined disturbances of intake (anorexia), absorption, metabolism of nutrients, and increased energy expenditure.

- **Fat malabsorption** particularly of the LCTs and PUFAs may also impair absorption of fat-soluble vitamins by up to 50%, although 95% of water-soluble lipids (MCTs) are absorbed. In cholestatic liver disease it is due to reduced delivery of bile salts to the small bowel. Pancreatic exocrine function may also be affected. Hypercholesterolaemia and hypertriglyceridaemia are common as a result of altered lipoprotein synthesis and cholesterol excretion.
- **Carbohydrate metabolism** is abnormal due to peripheral insulin resistance, hyperinsulinaemia, and reduced hepatic glycogen stores.
- **Protein synthesis** is impaired as liver plays key role in the synthesis of albumin, transferrin, and clotting factors. The metabolism of aromatic amino acids is affected, leading to imbalance of branched-chain amino acids and aromatic amino acids. Inadequate detoxification of nitrogenous waste via urea cycle leads to rise in blood ammonia levels. There is also a resultant increase in muscle protein degradation causing a relatively reduced muscle mass despite nutritional support.
- **Impaired GH–IGF1 axis** occurs as significant proportion of IGF1 and IGFBP are synthesized in the liver.

- **Increased energy expenditure** up to 140% of normal is estimated.
- **Trace elements** may also be deficient as a result of reduced intake and increased losses.

Clinical features

- Severe deficiency of fat-soluble vitamins may produce clinical signs and symptoms. Increased bruising, epistaxis, coagulopathy due to vitamin K deficiency; osteopenia, rickets and fractures due to vitamin D deficiency; less commonly xerophthalmia and night blindness due to vitamin A deficiency; and peripheral neuropathy, ophthalmoplegia, and haemolysis due to vitamin E deficiency.
- Essential fatty acid deficiency may manifest as desquamation, thrombocytopenia and poor wound healing.
- Mineral deficiencies may occur (in particular anaemia due to iron deficiency and acrodermatitis due to zinc deficiency).
- In later stages of the disease protein energy malnutrition manifests with muscle wasting, stunting, peripheral oedema, and motor developmental delay.

Nutritional assessment and management

See Chapter 62.

Hepatic encephalopathy

Definition
This is defined as a reversible decrease in neurological function caused by liver disease. It is difficult to recognize in children.

Pathophysiology
Precise mechanisms are still not defined.
- Porto-systemic shunting leads to increased blood concentrations of nitrogenous by-products, which are implicated in the alteration of CNS function.
- Hepatocellular dysfunction with poor clearance of nitrogenous metabolites from the intestine.
- Nitrogen metabolites and short-chain fatty acids absorbed from the intestine have been implicated in directly altering CNS function.
- Altered neurotransmitter function leading to imbalance of excitatory and inhibitory functions in particular of the glutamine–nitric oxide system.

Diagnosis
- Requires high index of suspicion and appropriate clinical assessment.
- Commonest symptoms are irritability and lethargy; subtle presentation may be with neurodevelopmental delay, school problems, sleep pattern reversal, personality changes, delayed reaction times, impaired computation and concentration. Late signs are clouding of consciousness leading to stupor and coma.
- Signs that may be elicited particularly in older children are tremors, incoordination, and asterixis.
- EEG is non-specific.
- MRI may reveal high signal in globus pallidus on T1 weighted images.
- Arterial ammonia concentrations are difficult to interpret in isolation especially in children; serial monitoring may, however, be used as guide to the effectiveness of treatment.
- It is very important to rule out other causes such as hypoxia, hypoglycaemia, acidosis, drug toxicity, and metabolic insults.

Treatment
- Identify and treat precipitating factors.
- Lactulose only to achieve 2–3 semi-formed stools per day.
- Gut decontamination and IV antibiotics should be considered.
- Branched-chain amino acid enriched nutritional supplements have been used but without proven benefit.
- Over-zealous protein restriction in children can lead to nutritional depletion and exacerbate growth failure.
- Liver transplantation.

Coagulopathy

Definition
Increased risk of bleeding in chronic liver disease due to development of specific disorders of coagulation characterized by prolonged PT, INR, and reduced platelets.

Pathophysiology
- Vitamin K malabsorption leading to deficiency.
- Reduced synthesis of coagulation factors particularly II, VII, IX, X, proteins C and S, and inhibitors of coagulation.
- Thrombocytopenia may occur secondary to portal hypertension, hypersplenism and immunological destruction; platelet aggregation is also defective.
- Dysfibrinogenemia due to increase in levels of d-dimers and FDPs.

Diagnosis
- May present as epistaxis, GI bleeding, or bruising.
- Check platelet count, coagulation screen including INR, FDP, and d-dimers. NB: fibrinogen concentrations may be normal.
- Therapeutic administration of vitamin K distinguishes vitamin K deficiency from synthetic failure of the liver.

Management
- Vitamin K supplement oral or IV given as 1 mg/year of age or maximum of 5 mg/day.
- During bleeding episodes or invasive procedures FFP, cryoprecipitate, and platelets should be given.
- Persistent severe coagulation disturbances may require factor VII infusions and desmopressin.
- Evaluate and treat associated sepsis.

Portal hypertension and variceal bleeding

See Chapter 64.

Ascites

Definition

Accumulation of fluid in the abdominal cavity in a child with liver disease usually indicates worsening portal hypertension and hepatic insufficiency.

It is a common major complication of decompensated cirrhosis. Onset may be insidious or precipitated by events such as GI bleeding, infections, or development of hepatoma.

Pathophysiology

• The factors involved are portal venous pressure and plasma oncotic pressure secondary to hypoalbuminemia.

Diagnosis

• Clinical features include distended abdomen, bulging flanks, protrusion of umbilicus, and development of inguinal hernias and hydrocele; percussion of fluid level and shifting dullness may be elicited.
• USS is more sensitive and can detect small volumes of ascites or be employed when clinical examination is difficult.
• Abdominal paracentesis is a rapid and relatively safe procedure with added advantage of ruling out spontaneous bacterial peritonitis.

Management

• Nutritional support.
• Dietary restriction of sodium should be considered.
• Spironolactone at 2–3 mg/kg per day to 7 mg/kg per day.
• If there is inadequate response, furosemide can be added; chorothiazide is a preferred agent for long-term use.
• If the ascites is still resistant consider 20% human albumin infusion over 3–4 h with furosemide cover.
• Monitor weight, serum electrolytes, urea and creatinine closely. If significant hyponatraemia occurs, consider stopping diuretics and fluid restrict cautiously (50–75% of requirement).
• Therapeutic paracentesis should be considered in resistant ascites especially if compromising respiratory function. Concurrent infusion of albumin is recommended; replace 10% of the removed ascitic fluid volume with 20% albumin IV.
• Surgical intervention apart from liver transplantation is rarely necessary but may include LeVeen shunt (peritoneal to jugular) and transjugular intrahepatic portosystemic shunt (TIPS).

Spontaneous bacterial peritonitis

Definition
Bacterial infection of ascitic fluid in the absence of secondary causes such as bowel perforation or intra-abdominal abscess.

Clinical features
These may be subtle, with fever and irritability.

Diagnosis
- High index of suspicion in a child with ascites and non-specific deterioration is required.
- Abdominal paracentesis and ascitic fluid microscopy and culture is essential. Presence of polymorphonuclear cells (PMN) >250/mm^3 is diagnostic and usually the infection is mono-microbial.

Treatment
- IV antibiotics, usually third generation cephalosporins, are the first choice but should be guided by the microbiologist and the culture yield. The duration of treatment is 5–7 days.
- Recurrent episodes of SBP should lead to consideration for liver transplantation.

Hepatorenal syndrome

Definition
Functional renal failure in patients with severe liver disease.

Epidemiology
It occurs in up to 10% of adults with chronic liver disease; mortality rate of 70% without liver transplantation. It is much less common in children.

Pathophysiology
Characterized by intense renal vasoconstriction with co-existent systemic vasodilatation, thereby reducing the renal blood flow despite increased cardiac output and fall in blood pressure.

Diagnosis
- Exclusion of all other potential causes of renal impairment especially hypovolaemia, shock, nephrotoxic drugs, or kidney disease.
- Hereditary tyrosinaemia, Alagilles, and polycystic liver kidney disease are conditions where chronic liver disease and kidney disease occur concomitantly.
- Urine sodium <10 and urine: plasma creatinine ratio <10 help rule out ATN or glomerular disease.
- GFR is markedly reduced.

Treatment
- Haemofiltration may be used whilst awaiting transplant.
- Terlipressin has been used with some success in adults.
- Liver transplantation usually reverses the condition.

Pulmonary complications

Hepatopulmonary syndrome

Definition
- Triad of hypoxaemia (SaO_2 <90%), intrapulmonary vascular dilatation and liver disease.
- Arterial P_aO_2 <70% in room air with alveolar arterial gradient of >20 mmHg.

Epidemiology
The prevalence varies from 0.5% to 20% in adults; a similar prevalence may be expected in children.

Pathophysiology
- Multifactorial with development of intrapulmonary shunts, A-V shunts, V-Q mismatch and portopulmonary venous anastomosis.
- Extensive dilatation of pre-capillary circulation resulting in V-Q mismatch may be responsible for the milder disease where P_aO_2 can be increased with administration of 100% oxygen.
- In a smaller percentage anatomic A-V shunts may be formed within pulmonary circulation; these have poorer prognosis.

Diagnosis
- Requires high index of suspicion.
- Cyanosis, digital clubbing with or without spider naevi is suggestive. Typically, there may be dyspnoea on standing, improving on lying down (platypnoea) with associated change in P_aO_2 (orthodeoxia).
- Suggested diagnostic criteria are (1) presence of chronic liver disease; (2) absence of intrinsic cardiopulmonary disease; (3) pulmonary gas exchange abnormalities; (4) evidence of intrapulmonary vascular shunting.
- The intrapulmonary vascular shunts can be demonstrated by technetium 99m-labelled macroaggregated albumin study, or by contrast-enhanced echocardiography.

Management
Definitive treatment is by timely liver transplantation. Liver transplantation should be considered once the shunt on technetium 99m-labelled macro-aggregated albumin scan is >5%.

Portopulmonary hypertension

Definition
Pulmonary arterial vasoconstriction causing mean pulmonary artery pressures >25 mmHg with capillary wedge pressure of <15 mmHg in the absence of secondary causes of pulmonary hypertension.

Prevalence in children is unknown.

Pathophysiology
Concentric medial hypertrophy with intimal fibrosis in the pulmonary arteries is the hallmark.

Diagnosis
- ECG may show right ventricular hypertrophy, right axis deviation, and RBBB.
- Cardiac catheterization of right heart is essential for diagnosis.

Treatment
- No treatment guideline is available for children.
- Vasodilators such as NO and calcium channel blockers have been tried in adults.
- Early liver transplantation may reverse the process.

Pruritus

Definition

A complication of cholestatic liver disease (in particular PFIC); when intense, may affect sleep, feeding, and behaviour.

Management (see also Chapter 51)

- Antihistamines are used as first line but are usually ineffective.
- Phenobarbital and choleretics are helpful.
- Ursodeoxycholic acid may help by improving bile flow.
- Rifampicin may improve bile flow
- IV naloxone, plasmapheresis, acupuncture, and phototherapy may be used if itching is very intense.
- Partial biliary diversion has been found to be helpful in some children.

Hepatic osteodystrophy

Definition

Metabolic bone disease occurring in patients with chronic liver disease.

Epidemiology

Prevalence reported in adults is 20–100% depending on patient selection and diagnostic criteria.

Pathophysiology

- Aetiology is still unclear.
- Trabecular bone loss occurs to a much greater degree than cortical bone loss.
- Potential factors directly or indirectly associated are IGF1 deficiency, hyperbilirubinemia, hypogonadism (especially adults and adolescents), subnormal levels of vitamin D, and immunosuppressive and corticosteroid therapy.
- In general the degree of osteopenia correlates with severity of liver disease.

Diagnosis

- Often diagnosed when present with atraumatic fractures and on screening.
- DEXA scan to measure bone mass.
- Plain radiographs if there is a suspicion of fracture

Management

- General measures: avoid long-term use of corticosteroids and loop diuretics; encourage regular weight-bearing exercises.
- Nutritional therapy: early calcium supplementation in particular, together with vitamin D, may be useful.
- Hormone replacement therapy may be tried in adolescents especially with delayed puberty under guidance of paediatric endocrinologist.
- Bisphosphonates such as pamidronate prevent osteoclast-mediated resorption and may be administered 3–6 monthly.
- Calcitonin and sodium fluoride have been tried in adults with some benefit.

Endocrine dysfunction

Definition
The regulation and function of multiple endocrine systems is affected in chronic liver disease. These are more frequent and more severe with progression of liver disease and development of portal hypertension.

Pathophysiology
- Although there is an increased secretion of GH, there is reduced synthesis of IGF-1 and IGFBP-3 in the liver. There may therefore be increased GH resistance leading to poor growth and wasting.
- **Feminization and hypogonadism** in males has been studied in adults. There is impairment of hypothalamic–pituitary regulation of testicular function with decrease in serum testosterone and relative increase in oestrone and oestradiol.
- **Hypothyroidism** occurs with increase in TBG and total T_4 but reduced free T_3 and T_4.
- **Renin–angiotensin–aldosterone** activation occurs due to activation of hepatorenal reflex contributing to the hepatorenal syndrome.
- Increased **peripheral insulin resistance** has been described leading to glucose intolerance.

Diagnosis
- In adolescent boys the clinical features may include loss of muscle mass, testicular atrophy, palmar erythema, and spider naevi. Adolescent girls may have amenorrhoea or menstrual irregularities. The features of hypothyroidism may be non-specific.
- Total testosterone and free testosterone and oestrogen levels along with LH and FSH levels may be helpful in older adolescents but are difficult to interpret in early puberty.
- Low free T_3 and high TSH suggest hypothyroidism; when there is uncertainty in diagnosis TRH stimulation test may be required.

Management
- Hypothyroidism is treated with levothyroxine; monitoring of treatment should be based on clinical response and free T_4 and TSH levels.
- There is minimal data on treatment of feminization and hypogonadism in children and adolescents.
- The long- term affects of liver transplant on recovery of endocrine dysfunction are not fully defined.

Hepatocellular carcinoma

See Chapter 60.

Dietary interventions in liver disease

Potential causes of malnutrition

- Inadequate intake: anorexia, nausea, vomiting, early satiety as a result of ascites, organomegaly.
- Impaired nutrient digestion, absorption, and metabolism: bile salt deficiency, pancreatic exocrine insufficiency, portal hypertension, enteropathy.
- Increased nutritional requirements: accelerated protein breakdown, hypermetabolism during stress.

Chronic liver disease

Symptoms that necessitate nutritional intervention:
- Growth faltering
- Cholestasis/inadequate bile flow
- Ascites
- Hepatosplenomegaly
- Portal hypertension and malabsorption
- Encephalopathy (acute on chronic liver disease).

Infants (0–1 years)

Energy and protein daily requirements
- Energy: 100–150 kcal/kg depending on degree of malabsorption, hypermetabolism, disease state
- Protein: 2–4 g/kg.

Feed
- Aim for150–180 mL/kg formula via oral/nasogastric top up.
- If cholestatic, use formula containing at least 50% of fat content as medium-chain triglyceride (MCT) (see Table 62.1 for suitable formulas).
- Formulas with >75% MCT fat (e.g. Monogen® 90% MCT) should be used with caution, as essential fatty acid deficiency has been reported when higher MCT feeds are used.
- If breast-fed, give at least 100 mL/kg formula containing MCT in addition to breast milk.

Additional energy/protein
If inadequate growth despite adequate intake of MCT-based formula:
- Supplement formulas to provide 80–100 kcal, 2–2.6 g protein per 100 mL formula. This can be done by:
  - concentrating the MCT-based formula to 15–17% w/v as tolerated (caution: increased sodium content, renal solute load, osmolality and gut tolerance)
  - addition of energy and protein supplements to formula
  - high-energy formula if not cholestatic.
- NB: To achieve catch-up growth the protein:energy ratio of the formula should be kept between 9 and 12% when adding additional calories. It may therefore be necessary to add a protein supplement in addition to calorie supplements. See Table 62.2 for suitable energy and protein supplements.

Vitamin supplementation

Fat-soluble vitamins A, D, E, K. Ketovite® Liquid 5 ml and 3 tablets (see Table 62.2).

Preschool children

Energy and protein requirements

- Energy: 120–150% EAR depending on degree of malabsorption, hypermetabolism, disease state
- Protein: 3–6 g/kg per day.

Diet

- High-calorie, high-protein diet; frequent meals/snacks.
- To ensure an energy-dense diet, fats should not be restricted although if symptomatic steatorrhoea, adjust fat intake according to tolerance.

Nutritional supplements

Oral

- High calorie/high protein nutritional supplement (Table 62.3)
- It may be preferable to use one of the supplements containing MCT if there is cholestasis. An MCT emulsion can be given as an additional energy supplement e.g. Liquigen® (SHS) 10–30 mL per dose to tolerance.

Nasogastric

If the child is unable to achieve growth with above measures, then supplementary nasogastric (NG) feeding is required. This is best achieved by continuous pump overnight feeding, which may be tolerated better than bolus if hepatosplenomegaly, ascites, hypoglycaemia are problems. In the first instance aim to provide 50% of energy requirements overnight. See Table 62.4 for suitable NG feeds.

If tolerance of proproietary feeds is poor, a modular feed can be adapted to individual tolerance. Modular feeds include protein, carbohydrate, MCT, LCT, vitamin, mineral supplement and electrolyte sources. Modular feeds are time consuming to make, expensive, and run a greater risk of bacterial contamination and mistakes in preparation.

School-age children

Energy and protein requirements

- Energy 100–130% EAR
- Protein 3–5 g/kg per day.

Diet

High calorie, high protein. To ensure an energy-dense diet, fats should not be restricted. If symptomatic steatorrhoea, adjust fat intake according to tolerance.

Nutritional supplements

High calorie/high protein nutritional supplements. See Table 62.3.

Nasogastric feeding

See Table 62.4. It may be preferable to use one of the supplements containing a proportion of the fat as MCT if there is cholestasis; a peptide-based feed may be appropriate in portal hypertension.

Acute liver disease

Infants

Energy and protein requirements

- Energy: aim to meet RNI for energy for age and prevent catabolism.
- Protein: aim at least to meet minimum protein requirements.

Feed dependent on diagnosis/inborn error of metabolism(IEM) suspected

- If IEM suspected, e.g. fatty acid oxidation defect, tyrosinaemia, galacto-saemia, urea cycle disorder, initially opt for emergency regime (R) of glucose polymer solution. See Table 62.2.
  - the emergency regime should aim to meet glucose oxidation rates to prevent catabolism, as estimated in Table 62.5. A modular feed can then be developed (with addition of fat, protein, vitamin and mineral, electrolyte source), as possible metabolic diagnoses are excluded.
- Energivit® (SHS) protein-free formula—useful if IEM involving protein metabolism suspected.

Children

Energy and protein requirements

- Energy: aim to provide at least 100–120% RNI
- Protein: aim meet minimum protein requirements 0.8–1 g/kg and increase as tolerated. See Table 62.6.

Feeds

As above.

Encephalopathy/high ammonia

Protein may need to be restricted. Aim to meet minimum protein requirement (see Table 62.6) and provide at least RNI for energy (see Table 62.5) to prevent catabolism. Branched-chain amino acids (BCAA) are metabolized in skeletal muscle. and a formula containing a proportion of the protein as BCAA (e.g. Generaid plus®, SHS) may therefore allow a higher protein intake to be tolerated without causing a deterioration in encephalopathic state.

Hypoglycaemia

Infants

- Optimize feed volumes 150–180 mL/kg formula.
- Frequent feeds, 2–3 hourly day and night.
- Background continuous NG feeds plus oral feeds on top.
- Increase carbohydrate content of formula to 10% by addition of a glucose polymer (see Table 62.2) e.g. formula containing 7 g CHO/100 mL, add 3 g glucose polymer/100 mL.
- Caution: glucose polymer should be increased gradually up to 5% dilution. Rebound hypoglycaemia may potentially occur at higher glucose concentrations.

Children

- Meals/snacks 2–3 hourly (including bedtime snack) containing complex carbohydrate; uncooked cornstarch 2 g/kg per dose in yoghurt or milk, usually given at bedtime.
- Continuous NG feeds (see Table 62.4).

Nutritional assessment and monitoring of children with liver disease

It is essential to assess adequacy of nutritional intervention.

Nutritional assessment
- Feeding history, nutritional intake compared with estimated requirements.

Growth/anthropometry
- Weight: misleading if organomegaly and ascites.
- Length/height: indicator of chronic malnutrition.
- Mid upper arm muscle circumference; reference ranges available >1 year; serial measurements useful.
- Tricep skinfold thickness; reference ranges available >1 year; serial measurements useful.
- Head circumference.

Biochemical parameters
- Levels of e.g. albumin and prealbumin reflect their synthesis within the liver and thus liver function rather than nutritional status.
- Plasma concentration of vitamins A, D, E.

Extrahepatic biliary atresia

- Aggressive nutritional support is important in first year of life.
- Conjugated hyperbilirubinaemia likely to persist for several months after Kasai portenterostomy.

Feed
- Infant formula containing MCT required for the first year (see Table 62.1)
- 150–180 mL/kg
- Additional energy/protein often required (see section on chronic liver disease, p. 000).
- From 6 months of age a higher protein/energy feed may be required (see section on additional calories and protein in chronic liver disease, p. 000).

Essential fatty acid (EFA) supplementation
The EFAs linoleic and α-linolenic acid are present in LCT and therefore are absorbed in variable amounts in infants and children with cholestatic liver disease. The EFA requirement in children with liver disease is unknown. ESPGHAN recommendations are that all infant formulas should contain 4.5–10.8% linolenic acid and the ratio of linolenic to α-linoleic should be between 5 and 15. Formulas for infants with liver disease should therefore be based on the upper end of these levels.

If there are concerns about EFA deficiency then formulas/diet should be supplemented with walnut oil (0.2 mL/100 kcal of feed/diet).

Conjugated hyperbilirubinaemia

- Unknown cause, awaiting diagnosis: see flow diagram 1
- Lactose-free formula until galactosaemia excluded.
- Classical galactosaemia is diagnosed by measuring blood levels of galactose-1-phosphate in the infant. This measurement will not be valid if the infant has received a blood transfusion in the preceding 3 months.
- Reducing substances can be measured in the urine, although this is neither sensitive nor specific. NB: The infant must be taking a lactose-containing formula for several hours before testing the urine.

Fat-soluble vitamins/minerals

- Additional fat-soluble vitamins are required by all infants and children with cholestatic liver disease. See Table 62.8.
- Colestyramine (Questran) can impair absorption of fat-soluble vitamins and should be given separately.
- Monitoring of serum vitamin concentrations is required. IM fat-soluble vitamins may be necessary.

Table 62.1 Infant formula containing MCT

Product	Company	Protein source	Fat source	CHO Source	Osmolality mosm/kg	Kcal	6:3	Na mmol	Pro g	Fat g	Cho g	Lactose g
Caprilon®	SHS	Whey protein skimmed milk powder	MCT 75% Soya bean oil	Dried glucose syrup Lactose	233	66	7.5:1	0.9	1.5	3.6	7	0.82
Generaid plus at 22 % w/v®	SHS	Whey protein 32% as BCAA	MCT 33% Maize. Coconut, palm kernel oil	Glucose syrup.	287	102	4:1	0.7	2.4	4.2	13.6	< 0.1
Pepti-junior®	Cow & Gate	Whey hydrolysate suppl amino acids	MCT 50% maize, rape seed, soya bean oil)	Dried glucose syrup Tr. Lactose	190	67	7:1	0.9	1.8	3.6	6.8	<0.1
Pregestimil®	Mead Johnson	Casein hydrolysate suppl aa	MCT 55% corn, soya and safflower oils	Glucose syrup. Modified corn starch	330	68	14:1	1.26	1.9	3.8	6.9	<0.0005
MCT pepdite®	SHS	Hydrolysed Soya & pork proteins. Suppl aa	MCT 75% Coconut, walnut, maize, palm oil	Dried glucose syrup	290	68	6.9:1	1.5	2.0	2.7	10.3	Nil

Table 62.2 Energy & protein supplements/high energy formulas

Product	Company	Energy Source	Usual dose Per 100ml formula	Per g/mL			
				Kcal	Pro g	CHO g	Fat g
Duocal®	SHS	Fat/CHO	1–5 g	4.9	0	0.73	0.22
Polycose®	Abbott	Glucose polymer	1–5g	3.8	0	0.94	0
Maxijul®	SHS	Glucose polymer	1–5g	3.8	0	0.95	0
Polycal®	Nutricia	Glucose polymer	1–5g	3.8	0	0.96	0
Vitajoule®	Vitaflo Ltd	Glucose polymer	1–5 g	3.85	0	0.96	0
Calogen®	SHS	LCT	1–3mL	4.5	0	0	0.5
Liquigen®	SHS	MCT	1–3mL	4.5	0	0	0.5
Maxipro®	SHS	Whey Protein	1g	4	0.76	0.08	0.08
Infatrini®	Nutricia	Complete formula	Per 100mL	100	2.6	10.3	5.4
SMA high energy®	SMA	Complete formula	Per 100mL	91	2	9.8	4.9

Table 62.3 Vitamin supplementation

Vitamin	Ketovite® 5ml + 3 tablets	Vit K	Abidec® 0.3mL	Abidec® 0.6ml
A	750mcg 2500iu		667iu	1333iu
D	10mcg		5mcg	10mcg
E	15mg		-	-
K	1.5mg	1mg	-	-

Table 62.4 Nutritional sip feeds suitable for children over 1 year

Product	Company	Nutritionally Complete	Per 100mL standard w/v				
			Energy kcal	Pro g	CHO g	Fat g	% Fat MCT
Fortini®	Nutricia	Y	150	3.38	18.8	6.8	0
Paediasure plus®	Abbott	Y	151	4.2	16.7	7.47	0
Resource junior®	Novartis	Y	150	3	20.6	6.2	0
Peptamen junior®	Nestlé	Y in 1500 kcal	100–150	3–4.5	13.8–20.7	3.9–7.7	60
Frebini energy®	Fresenius Kabi	Y	150	3.75	18.75	6.7	19
Generaid plus + flavourings®	SHS	N- low Na	150–200	2.4–4.8	13.6–27.2	4.2–8.4	33

Table 62.5 Glucose oxidation rates

Age	Glucose mg/kg per min	Glucose g/kg per h
Infants	8–9	0.5
Children	5–7	0.3–0.4
Adolescents	2–4 (night)	0.2–0.25

Table 62.6 Tube feeds suitable for children over 1 with chronic liver disease

Product	Company	Nutritionally complete	Features	Per 100mL standard w/v				
				Energy kcal	Pro g	CHO g	Fat g	% Fat MCT
Frebini energy®	Fresenius kabi	Y	Ready-made	150	3.75	18.75	6.7	19
Generaid Plus®	SHS	N Low Sodium	Branched Chain AA. Can concentrate to 2 kcal/ml Low Na	100–200	2.4–4.8	13.6–27.2	4.2–8.2	33
Nutrini Energy®	Nutricia	Y	Ready-made	150	4.1	18.5	6.7	0
Paed'asure plus®	Abbott	Y	Ready-made	151	4.2	16.7	7.47	0
Pepdite 1+®	SHS	Y	Peptide based. milk protein & lactose free	100	3.1	13	3.9	35
Peptamen junior®	Nestlé		peptide based. Can concentrate to 1.5kcal/ml	100	3	13.8	3.85	60

Table 62.7 D.O.H. Dietary reference values for food energy & nutrients for the U.K. C.O.M.A 1991

Age	Weight kg	Fluid mL/kg	Energy (EAR)		Protein (RNI)	
			kcal/day	kcal/kg	g/day	g/kg/d
Male						
months						
0-3		150	545	100-115	12.5	2.1
4-6		130	690	95	12.7	1.6
7-9		120	825	95	13.7	1.5
10-12		110	920	95	14.9	1.5
years						
1-3		95	1230	95	14.5	1.1
4-6		85	1715	90	19.7	1.1
7-10		75	1970	-	28.3	-
11-14		55	2220	-	42.1	-
15-18		50	2755	-	55.2	-

Females

months					
0-3	150	515	100–115	12.5	2.1
4-6	130	645	95	12.7	1.6
7-9	120	765	95	13.7	1.5
10-12	110	865	95	14.9	1.5
years					
1-3	95	1165	95	14.5	1.1
4-6	85	1545	90	19.7	1.1
7-10	75	1740	-	28.3	-
11-14	55	1845	-	42.1	-
15-18	50	2110	-	45.4	-

Table 62.8 Mimimum safe levels of protein intake (g protein/kg/day)

Age (years)	FAO/WHO/UNU*	Dewey**
0–1 months	-	2.69
1–2 months	-	2.04
2–3	-	1.53
3–4 months	1.86	1.37
4–5 months	1.86	1.25
5–6 months	1.86	1.19
6–9 months	1.65	1.09
9–12 months	1.48	1.02
12–18 months	1.26	1.0
18–24 months	1.17	0.94
2–3 years	1.13	0.92
3–4 years	1.09	0.9
4–5 years	1.06	0.88
5–6 years	1.02	0.86
6–9 years	1.01	0.86
9–10 years	0.99	0.86
Girls		
10–11	1.0	0.87
11–12	0.98	0.86
12–13	0.96	0.85
13–14	0.9	0.84
14–15	0.9	0.81
15–16	0.87	0.81
16–17	0.83	0.78
17–18	0.8	0.7

Table 62.8 Mimimum safe levels of protein intake (g protein/kg/day)
(*Continued*)

Age (years)	FAO/WHO/UNU*	Dewey**
Boys		
10–11	0.99	0.86
11–12	0.98	0.86
12–13	1.0	0.88
13–14	0.97	0.86
14–15	0.96	0.86
15–16	0.92	0.84
16–17	0.9	0.83
17–18	0.86	0.81

* Energy & protein requirements. Report of a joint FAO/WHO/UNU expert consultation.
WHO Technical report no 724 Geneva 1985
**Dewey KG et al Protein Requirements of infants & children Eur J. Clin Nutr. 1996,
50 (suppl 1) 119–150

Acute liver failure

Definition

Acute liver failure (ALF) in children is defined as 'a rare multisystem disorder in which severe impairment of liver function, with or without encephalopathy, occurs in association with hepatocellular necrosis in a patient with no recognized underlying chronic liver disease'. Liver function is considered severely impaired if prothrombin time (PT) is >15 s or international normalized ratio (INR) is >1.5 and not corrected by vitamin K, in the presence of hepatic encephalopathy (HE) or a PT >20 s or INR >2.0 in the absence of HE.

Aetiology

The aetiology of ALF varies depending on the age of the child, with metabolic liver disease and infections being most common in those <1 year of age. The aetiology largely remains indeterminate in older children; however, of the known aetiologies viral infections, drug-induced hepatitis, autoimmune hepatitis, and Wilson's disease are the commonest causes (Table 63.1). The aetiology of ALF not only provides indication of prognosis but also dictates specific management options.

Table 63.1 Aetiologies of ALF in children in a tertiary referral unit (King's College Hospital, London)

Aetiology	
ALF due to indeterminate cause (non-A–E hepatitis)	45 (34%)
Infections	15 (11%)
Metabolic	37 (28%)
Paracetamol overdose	9 (7%)
Other drug/toxins	5 (4%)
Shock	4 (3%)
Miscellaneous	16 (12%)
Total	131 (100%)

Viral hepatitis

- Hepatotropic viruses are probably the most identifiable cause of ALF worldwide.
- Hepatitis A and hepatitis E are amongst the most common causes in Asia and Africa.
- Hepatitis B infection can lead to acute liver failure during acute infection or reactivation of chronic HBV infection in immunocompromised patients, co-infection or superinfection with hepatitis D virus or during the seroconversion from hepatitis e antigen positive state to hepatitis B e antibody positive state. Rarely infants born to HbeAb positive mothers can develop ALF around 6 weeks to 6 months of age.

- ALF of indeterminate aetiology encompasses viruses and metabolic disorders yet to be identified.
- Heterotropic viruses like herpes simplex virus, cytomegalovirus, Epstein–Barr virus, and varicella-zoster virus can cause severe hepatitis especially in immunocompromised state leading to ALF. HSV-induced ALF in the newborn carries a high mortality rate; it should be considered in every sick neonate with coagulopathy and raised transaminases even if there are no vesicular lesions on the skin. Treatment with IV aciclovir should begin immediately.
- Parvovirus B19 infection also causes severe hepatitis or ALF and bone marrow failure in children.
- Viruses such as echovirus, coxsackie virus and other enteroviruses can cause ALF.

Metabolic diseases

- Inherited disorders of metabolism are an important cause of ALF in the paediatric population, especially in the neonatal period; diagnosis requires a high degree of suspicion because overt signs and symptoms of liver disease are usually absent.
- Galactosaemia, which usually presents with conjugated hyperbilirubinaemia, hypoglycaemia, and Gram-negative septicaemia, can progress to liver failure; immediate exclusion of lactose from the diet and medications usually lead to recovery except in severe cases.
- Tyrosinaemia can present with severe coagulopathy, jaundice, and sometimes rickets; dietary management and the use of NTBC have improved the survival of these children.
- A history of administration of fructose as in fruit juice, honey, or sugar coinciding with the onset of symptoms suggests the diagnosis of hereditary fructose intolerance.
- Neonatal haemochromatosis (NH) is a disorder of iron handling during the antenatal period leading to excess iron deposition in the non-reticuloendothelial system. Liver disease is generally present at birth and progresses to liver failure in the first few days of life. Familial recurrence in children born from same mother but different father has been reported. Elevation of ferritin is a sensitive, but not specific, diagnostic test. Transferrin hypersaturation with relative hypotransferrinaemia is a valuable finding. MRI of the liver or pancreas to demonstrate iron deposition in the non-reticuloendothelial system is not usually rewarding, but a punch biopsy of buccal mucosa showing presence of iron in minor salivary glands is very suggestive of NH. Iron chelation and antioxidant cocktail therapy with N-acetylcysteine (100 mg/kg per day IV infusion), selenium (3 g/kg/d IV is g correct?), desferrioxamine (30 mg/kg per day IV infusion), alprostadil (0.4–0.6 g/kg/h IV) and vitamin E (25 U/kg per day IV/PO) has shown variable results. An alloimmune aetiology has been suggested and this has now led to usage of weekly IV immunoglobulin as prophylaxis (1 g/kg) from 18th week of gestation until term in mothers known to have given birth to babies with NH.
- Recently mitochondrial respiratory chain disorders like Pearson syndrome, mitochondrial DNA depletion syndrome, nuclear DNA defect, mitochondrial enzyme complex deficiency, etc. have been implicated

as an aetiological factor for ALF in children. They usually present with hypoglycaemia, vomiting, coagulopathy, acidosis, and raised lactate with or without neurological symptoms. However, usually not all the features are present, hence diagnosis should be considered in every child with ALF. Diagnosis is based on quantitative assessment of the respiratory chain enzyme complexes in muscle, liver, or skin fibroblasts.
- Rarely fatty acid oxidation defects and inborn errors of bile acid synthesis can present as ALF.

Wilson's disease (see Chapter 56)

- Wilson's disease, (WD) an autosomal recessive disorder, is an uncommon cause of ALF in older children.
- It can present acutely with Coomb's negative haemolytic anaemia, mixed hyperbilirubinaemia (both conjugated and unconjugated), and liver failure.
- Kayser–Fleischer rings, present in about 50% of cases of WD, are diagnostic in a patient presenting with ALF.
- Serum caeruloplasmin is typically low but may be normal in about 15% of cases, and serum free copper concentration may be normal or raised.
- Very low serum alkaline phosphatase or uric acid levels or a high bilirubin (μmol/dL) to alkaline phosphatase (IU/L) ratio of >2 are indirect indicators of WD as a cause of ALF.
- Treatment depends on the severity of illness. ALF in WD with encephalopathy is an indication for emergency liver transplantation. Children with ALF due to WD but without encephalopathy may respond to chelation treatment. The role of liver assist devices like MARS is unproven.

Drugs and toxins

- Drugs and toxins are the second most common cause of ALF.
- Since it is a diagnosis of exclusion a detailed history should be taken with name of all medications used, the time period of their use, and the quantities ingested.
- Drug-induced hepatotoxicity can be a dose-dependent response, an idiosyncratic or a synergistic reaction.
- Paracetamol, the most common over-the-counter medicine, is a dose-dependent hepatotoxic agent causing ALF. Commonly paracetamol hepatotoxicity is either due to intended suicidal overdose or the inadvertent use of a supratherapeutic dose. Serum paracetamol levels 4 h after ingestion are useful to identify high-risk patients but these levels may not be informative if toxicity is due to chronic administration. Activated charcoal may be useful for GI decontamination in suspected or known paracetamol overdose, specially if administered within 4–6 h of ingestion. The antidote for paracetamol overdose, N-acetylcysteine (NAC), has been shown to be quite effective and safe even if patients have presented quite late after the overdose. In acute paracetamol overdose the dose of NAC is 150 mg/kg in 5% glucose over 15 min followed by 50 mg/kg given over 4 h followed by 100 mg/kg over 16 h. If the patient has any evidence of coagulopathy then NAC should be continued at a dose of 100 mg/kg per day till the INR is <1.5.
- 'Mushroom' (*Amanita phalloides*) poisoning as a cause of ALF has been reported from Europe, USA, and South Africa. It usually presents with

severe diarrhoea with or without vomiting a few hours after ingestion and progresses to overt liver failure in 3–4 days. Penicillin G (300 000–1 million units/kg per day) and silibinin (30–40 mg/kg per day I/V or orally) have been used as an antidote.

- Sodium valproate can lead to ALF by unmasking an underlying mitochondrial cytopathy, hence detailed investigations should be carried out for the same.
- Other common hepatotoxic agents are antituberculous drugs, antiepileptics, or antibiotics (sulfonamides, erythromycin, augmentin, etc.).
- There are no specific antidotes for idiosyncratic drug reactions but corticosteroids have been used in suspected drug hypersensitivity reaction.

Autoimmune hepatitis

- Autoimmune hepatitis can rarely present with ALF; the diagnosis may be difficult since autoantibodies may be negative.
- Patients with fulminant hepatic failure due to autoimmune hepatitis need emergency liver transplantation.

Ischaemic injury

- Ischaemic injury due to aetiologies such as heart failure, hypotensive/hypovolaemic/septic shock can lead to ALF.
- Usually the typical features of ischaemia are over by the time the patient presents with ALF; hence a careful history is important.

Vascular causes

- Any conditions causing obstruction of hepatic venous outflow (Budd–Chiari syndrome, veno-occlusive disease, cardiomyopathies) can also present as ALF.
- Abdominal pain, ascites, and significant hepatomegaly are useful clinical clues.
- Doppler USS, CT, or MR venography is usually diagnostic.

Malignancies

- Hemophagocytic lymphohistiocytosis:
  - may be primary (familial) or secondary to infection
  - clinical presentations include fever, hepatosplenomegaly, and pancytopenia.
  - biochemical abnormalities include high serum triglycerides and low fibrinogen
  - usually these patients bleed disproportionately from venepuncture sites considering the degree of coagulation abnormalities present
  - bone marrow aspiration is usually diagnostic
  - treatment is immunosuppression followed by bone marrow transplantation.
- Leukaemia or lymphoma can present with ALF due to massive infiltration of the liver. Presence of high fever with hepatosplenomegaly, high alkaline phosphatase, high lactate dehydrogenase, and abnormalities on peripheral blood film are the diagnostic clues and bone marrow examination is confirmatory.

Table 63.2 lists disease-specific tests.

Therapy

General measures

- All patients with ALF should be nursed in a quiet environment.
- Vital parameters (heart rate, respiratory rate, and blood pressure), urine output, metabolic parameters (electrolytes, blood sugar) and neurological status (presence of encephalopathy) should be monitored each 4–6 h.
- Coagulation status, metabolic parameters, full blood count, and arterial blood gases in ventilated patients should be checked each 4–6 h.
- Controlled trials in adults have failed to substantiate any beneficial effect of corticosteroids, interferon, insulin and glucose, prostaglandin E1, bowel decontamination, and charcoal haemoperfusion in patients with ALF.
- Maintenance of nutrition is crucial and hypoglycemia should be avoided; a protein intake of 1 g/kg is well tolerated and should be provided.
- Total fluid intake is usually restricted to 2/3 of the maintenance.
- Routine surveillance and treatment of infection is essential. Use of prophylactic broad-spectrum antibiotics and antifungals have decreased the incidence of infection significantly and improved survival.

Complications

Neurological

- The most serious complications of ALF are cerebral oedema with resultant intracranial hypertension and hepatic encephalopathy. It is rarely present with grade I–II encephalopathy but the risk increases to 25–35% in grade III and 65–75% or more in grade IV encephalopathy.
- Patients in grade I–II encephalopathy can be safely managed with skilful nursing in a quiet environment with frequent monitoring of their neurological status.
- Sedation is contraindicated, but if it is required then patient should be electively ventilated.
- Grade II encephalopathic but agitated patient and grade III–IV encephalopathic patients should be electively intubated and transferred to a liver transplantation centre.
- Intracranial pressure monitoring with intracranial bolts:
  - Helps in accurate monitoring of ICP during interventions such as central line insertion, tracheal suctioning, and haemodialysis or haemodiafiltration but overall survival is not affected; there is a risk of intracranial bleeding
  - aim of ICP monitoring is to maintain ICP <20–25 mmHg and cerebral perfusion pressure (mean arterial blood pressure—ICP) at >50 mmHg.
  - if the cerebral perfusion pressure falls below 50 mmHg, the adequacy of sedation and paralysis should be checked first followed by P_aCO_2 levels (in ventilated patients, P_aCO_2 should be kept between 4 and 4.5 kPa). If the P_aCO_2 is >4.5 kPa, then hyperventilation may be helpful. Excessive hyperventilation should be avoided because

it may paradoxically compromise the cerebral perfusion pressure. Sometimes vasopressor agents are needed to increase the blood pressure to keep the desired CPP.

* Mannitol:
  * mainstay of treatment for increased ICP because of osmotic diuretic effect
  * a rapid bolus of 0.5 g/kg as a 20% solution over a 15 min period is recommended, and the dose can be repeated if the serum osmolarity is <320 mOsm/L. In anuric patients, a diuresis is simulated by ultrafiltrating three times the administered volume over the next 30 min.
* A recent controlled trial of administration of 3% hypertonic saline to maintain serum sodium concentrations of 145–155 mmol/L in adults with ALF suggests that induction and maintenance of hypernatraemia may be used to prevent the rise in ICP, but a larger study will be required to prove its role as a prophylactic measure.
* Other measures include sodium thiopental infusion, hypothermia (core body temperature of 32 °C), phenytoin infusion for subclinical seizure activity.
* Corticosteroids have been shown to be ineffective in patients with ALF with respect to controlling oedema or improving survival.

Infection

* Infection can lead to development and progression of multiorgan failure; about 60% of deaths in ALF have been attributed to sepsis.
* Active uncontrolled infection is a relative contraindication for liver transplantation.
* Most common bacterial infections are due to *Staphylococcus aureus*, but streptococci or Gram-negative organisms such as coliforms are also isolated.
* Prophylactic IV antibiotics have been shown to reduce the incidence of culture-positive bacterial infection from 61.3% to 32.1%.
* *Candida* spp. are the most common fungal infections and often unrecognized; fluconazole is the preferred prophylactic agent.
* Deterioration of HE after initial improvement, a markedly raised leucocyte count, pyrexia unresponsive to antibiotics, and established renal failure are strong indicators of fungal infection.

Coagulopathy

* ALF is characterized by decreased synthesis of clotting factors (factors II, V, VII, IX, X), accelerated fibrinolysis, and impaired hepatic clearance of activated clotting factors and fibrin degradation products.
* The PT expressed as an INR is markedly elevated and is used as an indicator of the severity of the liver damage.
* Significant disseminated intravascular coagulation is unusual in ALF.
* Clinically, bleeding tends to be less severe than might be expected from the degree of INR prolongation, although the risk of haemorrhage correlates with thrombocytopenia (platelet count <450 × 10^9/L).
* Common sites of haemorrhage include the GI tract, nasopharynx, lungs, and retroperitoneum; intracranial haemorrhage is uncommon.

- The presence of significant disseminated intravascular coagulation usually indicates sepsis or secondary haemophagocytic lymphohistio-cytosis.
- Since coagulopathy is a very good tool for assessment of prognosis and monitoring of disease progression, correction of coagulopathy is indicated only if the patient is already listed for transplant, in premature babies, or before an invasive procedure such as insertion of a central venous catheter or ICP monitor (please discuss with the tertiary referral centre before correcting coagulopathy)
- Prophylactic ranitidine (histamine 2 blocker) or proton pump inhibitors have been shown to decrease the incidence of gastric bleeding.

Haemodynamic changes

- In ALF, there is a state of hyperdynamic circulation with decreased systemic peripheral vascular resistance and increased cardiac output (similar to SIRS).
- Circulatory failure is a common mode of death in patients with ALF, often complicating sepsis or multiorgan failure.
- Invasive haemodynamic monitoring is recommended to determine the adequacy of intravascular volume and optimize the fluid management.
- In the presence of persistent hypotension despite normal filling pressure, vasopressors such as adrenaline are the inotropic agents of choice.
- Newer monitoring devices such as pulse contour cardiac output (PiCCO) and lithium dilutional cardiac output (LiDCO) monitoring, which can measure various body water compartments, are good devices to rationalize fluid management and the choice of vasopressors.
- Cardiac arrhythmias of most types may occur in the later stages and are usually caused by electrolyte disturbances (e.g. hypo- or hyperkalemia, acidosis, hypoxia, or cardiac irritation by a central venous catheter).

Renal failure

- In the paediatric population, the incidence of renal failure is lower (10–15%) than in the adult population.
- Renal failure could be due either to the direct toxic effect on kidneys, as in paracetamol overdose, or to a complex mechanism such as hepa-torenal syndrome or acute tubular necrosis secondary to complications of ALF (sepsis, bleeding, and/or hypotension).
- Blood urea estimation is unreliable as a marker of renal dysfunction because GI haemorrhage may increase urea disproportionately.
- Serum creatinine is a better indicator of kidney function.
- Intravascular hypovolaemia, if present, needs correction.
- Low-dose dopamine is not only ineffective but can have deleterious effects especially in the setting of profound vasodilatation, which is seen typically in ALF.
- Renal replacement therapy:
  - haemodiafiltration and haemodialysis should be instituted when the urine output is less than 1 ml/kg per hour
  - continuous filtration or dialysis systems are associated with less haemo-dynamic instability and consequently less risk of aggravating latent or established encephalopathy than intermittent haemodialysis

- epoprostenol infusion at a rate of 5 ng/kg per minute has been found to be superior to heparin anticoagulation with respect to functional duration of the filters and the haemorrhagic complications.

Metabolic derangements

- Hypoglycaemia in ALF can be present in 40% of patients.
- Classic signs and symptoms of hypoglycaemia are often masked specially in the presence of encephalopathy, hence regular blood glucose monitoring is important.
- Metabolic acidosis is associated with poor outcome; 50% of patients with grade III or IV encephalopathy can have lactic acidosis due to inadequate tissue perfusion.
- Other metabolic disturbances include respiratory alkalosis, hypokalaemia, hyponatraemia, hypophosphataemia, hypocalcaemia, and hypomagnesaemia.

Others

- Acute pancreatitis:
  - rare in ALF but mild elevation of serum amylase may be present
  - should be suspected if patient has abdominal pain and hypocalcaemia
  - precipitating factors are sodium valproate, shock, causative virus, etc.
  - treatment is supportive.
- Adrenal suppression:
  - seen in about 60% of adults with ALF
  - should be investigated with short tetracosactide test
  - corticosteroid replacement should be considered in patients with poor tetracosactide response or intractable hypotension.

Transplantation

- Liver transplantation is the only definitive treatment available.
- Contraindications are permanently fixed and dilated pupils, uncontrolled active sepsis, and severe respiratory failure (ARDS). Relative contraindications are accelerating inotropic requirements, infection under treatment, cerebral perfusion pressure of <40 mmHg for >2 h, and a history of progressive or severe neurological problems in which the ultimate neurological outcome may not be acceptable.
- In very unstable patients, a two-stage procedure with hepatectomy followed by liver transplant has been tried with some success.
- Auxiliary liver transplantation:
  - because of the potential of regeneration of native liver if given sufficient time to recover, auxiliary liver transplantation has been used to provide liver function while the native liver regenerates
  - the advantage of this procedure is that once the native liver shows signs of recovery, immunosuppression can be weaned and eventually stopped.
  - 60% of children who had auxiliary liver transplantation in our institution (King's College Hospital, London) have shown regeneration of their own liver and have stopped immunosuppression.
- Hepatocyte transplantation:
  - to provide a functioning hepatic mass while the native liver regenerates; has shown some encouraging results as a bridge to transplantation and in one child, liver transplant was avoided; however, the technique remains experimental.

Liver support system

- Liver support devices are either cleansing devices or a bioartificial liver support system.
- Cleansing devices perform only the detoxifying function of the liver, whereas bioartificial liver support systems have a theoretical advantage of providing the synthetic and detoxifying properties.
- A recent meta-analysis, considering all forms of devices together, demonstrated no efficacy for bioartificial liver devices for the treatment of ALF.

Prognosis

- The prognosis of ALF varies greatly with the underlying aetiology.
- PT is the best predictor of survival.
- Factor V concentration has been used as a prognostic marker, especially in association with encephalopathy (Clichy criteria). In children, a factor V concentration of <25% of normal suggests a poor outcome.
- Liver biopsy is rarely helpful in ALF and is usually contraindicated because of the presence of coagulopathy. Hepatic parenchymal necrosis of >50% is associated with a reduced survival but the potential for sampling error is considerable.
- A small liver, or more particularly a rapidly shrinking liver, is an indicator of a poor prognosis. CT volumetry of the liver has been used to assess both the size of the liver and its functional reserve.
- Fulminant Wilson's disease is invariably fatal, and emergency liver transplantation is the only effective treatment.
- There is no single criterion that can predict the outcome with absolute certainty and be universally applicable for all patients with ALF with different aetiologies. However, prediction of a low chance of survival (<20%) is clinically useful in deciding whether to list the patient for orthotopic liver transplant (OLT), which has a 1-year survival rate of 75%.

Table 63.2 Diagnostic tests

Cause	Test
Infections	
Hepatitis A infection	Anti-HAV antibody (IgM)
Hepatitis B infection	
Acute infection/seroconversion	Anti–core antibody (IgM)/HBV profile
Increased replication	Full HBV profile
Hepatitis D infection	Anti-HDV antibody (IgM)
Parvovirus, adenovirus, EBV, HSV	Viral serology/antigen tests, PCR
ALF of indeterminate cause (NANE hepatitis, seronegative hepatitis)	Diagnosis of exclusion (all tests)
Metabolic disorders	
Galactosemia	Galactose-1-phosphate uridyl transferase level in blood
Tyrosinemia	Urinary succinylacetone
Neonatal hemochromatosis	Buccal mucosal biopsy, high ferritin, high transferrin saturation
Hemophagocytic lymphohistiocytosis	Bone marrow aspiration (typical cells)
Mitochondrial hepatopathies	Muscle and liver biopsies for quantitative assay of respiratory chain enzyme
Wilson's disease	Urinary copper, Kayser–Fleischer rings, Coombs-negative hemolytic anemia
Drugs and toxins	
Paracetamol (acetaminophen)	History, drug level in blood
Idiosyncratic drug reactions	History, eosinophil count
Mushroom poisoning	History, diarrhea
Autoimmune hepatitis	Autoantibodies, immunoglobulins
Vascular causes	
Veno-occlusive disease	Doppler ultrasonography/venography
Budd–Chiari syndrome	Doppler USS/ CT scan/MR venography
Malignancies	
HLH	Bone marrow aspiration, Perforin expression
Leukemia/Lymphoma	Bone marrow aspiration

Portal hypertension

Definition

Portal hypertension is increased blood pressure within the portal venous system and defined as an increase in the pressure gradient between the portal veins and the hepatic veins (>5 mmHg).

Pathophysiology

The portal vein carries nutrient-rich blood to the liver from the GI tract and spleen. At the hilum of the liver it divides into the major right and left portal veins. Within the liver these veins undergo further divisions to supply each segment, and terminate in small branches, which pierce the limiting plate of the portal tract and enter the hepatic sinusoids through small channels (Fig. 64.1).

Portal pressure depends upon portal blood flow and vascular resistance. A rise in portal pressure leads to the development of collaterals to carry blood from the portal system to the systemic circulation. These portosystemic collaterals occur in specific sites: the distal oesophagus (oesophageal and gastric varices), the anal canal (anorectal varices) the falciform ligament (umbilical varices) and the abdominal wall and retroperitoneum. Dilated cutaneous collateral veins are a sign of established portal hypertension and carry blood from the umbilicus towards tributaries of the vena cava. Portal hypertension also causes splenomegaly, the development of ascites, and may cause small intestine mucosal oedema leading to malabsorption and consequent failure to thrive.

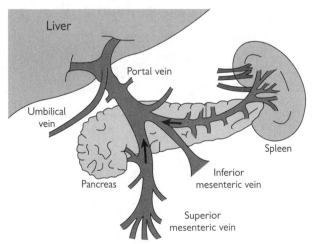

Fig. 64.1 Portal venous system.

Clinical features

The major cause of morbidity and mortality is bleeding varices. This is the commonest cause of serious GI haemorrhage in children. It presents with haematemesis and/or melaena, and is usually from distal oesophageal varices. Other significant problems include ascites and nutritional disturbance. Splenomegaly and hypersplenism rarely require specific intervention.

Causes

Intrinsic liver disease

Cirrhosis and fibrosis from chronic liver disease are the commonest causes of portal hypertension and have many underlying aetiologies including:
- Extrahepatic biliary atresia
- Choledochal cyst
- Alagille syndrome
- Autoimmune hepatitis
- Infectious hepatitis
- Progressive familial intrahepatic cholestasis
- Drugs
- Genetic and metabolic defects such as cystic fibrosis, α_1-antitrypsin deficiency and Wilson's disease.

The aetiologies of portal hypertension can be classified as prehepatic, intrahepatic, and posthepatic.

Prehepatic

Portal vein occlusion (accounts for 30% of children with bleeding oesophageal varices). Most commonly idiopathic, there are also many potentially identifiable causes. The portal vein becomes replaced by multiple venous collaterals forming a portal vein cavernoma.

Causes of portal vein occlusion
- Developmental/structural malformations (portal vein web, hypoplasia)
- Sepsis (septicaemia, umbilical, intra-abdominal, cholangitis)
- Thrombophilia
- Myeloproliferative disorders
- Protein C/S, antithrombin III, factor V Leiden, antiphospholipid antibodies
- Umbilical catheterization/infusion of irritant fluid
- Abdominal trauma/surgery
- Pancreatitis.

Intrahepatic

Usually caused by intrinsic liver disease but some conditions predominantly affect the venous circulation of the liver. Veno-occlusive disease (sinusoidal obstruction syndrome) involves injury to the sinusoidal endothelium leading to occlusion of the centrilobular veins, sinusoidal congestion, and hepatocyte necrosis. Features are rapid onset, painful hepatomegaly, and ascites, with later-onset cirrhosis and portal hypertension. In developed countries the cause is usually irradiation and/or cytotoxic drug injury to the liver. It is also seen in graft versus host disease after haematopoietic stem cell transplantation. Treatment is supportive, puls, or together with, diuretics, N-acetyl cysteine, and the thrombolytic defibrotide.

Posthepatic (hepatic vein occlusion)

Budd–Chiari syndrome results from hepatic venous thrombosis, usually secondary to a myeloproliferative disorder or thrombophilia. Features are hepatomegaly, ascites, and portal hypertension, and the onset may be acute or chronic. The caudate lobe of the liver may be spared because of its separate drainage into the IVC, then subsequent caudate lobe hypertrophy may compress the IVC leading to lower limb oedema.

Other cases of hepatic vein occlusion include trauma and malignancy.

Investigations

Haematology

- FBC—anaemia, leucopaenia, thrombocytopaenia in hypersplenism
- PT/INR—prolonged in intrinsic liver disease
- Thrombophilia screen (sometimes to include bone marrow aspirate) must be performed to investigate underlying causes of portal vein occlusion or Budd–Chiari syndrome.

Biochemistry

Biochemical liver function may be deranged in intrinsic liver disease, with raised bilirubin, transaminases and low albumin. Sodium may be low in ascites, and renal function may become deranged in severe disease.

Radiology

- Abdominal USS—splenomegaly, collateral veins, reduced portal vein flow, raised hepatic artery resistance index may be seen in portal hypertension and heterogenous hepatic echotexture with underlying intrinsic liver disease.
- MRI—to evaluate focal liver lesions.
- MR angiography—to delineate vasculature of the portomesenteric system. Useful before shunt surgery, or to examine portal vein before liver transplantation.

Gastrointestinal endoscopy

- To evaluate varices and mucosal features of portal hypertension.

Liver biopsy

- May be diagnostic of underlying liver disease, used to assess liver architecture, fibrosis, or cirrhosis.

Management

Emergency management of variceal bleeding

- Resuscitation:
  - AIRWAY—secure
  - BREATHING—O_2 if shocked
  - CIRCULATION—two large-bore cannulae, IV fluids.
- Investigation:
  - FBC, clotting, U&E, LFT, blood culture, cross-match (at least 2 units)
  - Monitor and maintain blood glucose
  - Monitor and stabilize fluid balance and cardiorespiratory status
  - Watch for encephalopathy.
- Treatment:
  - Nil by mouth
  - Ranitidine 1 mg/kg IV tds and sucralfate PO
  - Antibiotics IV if evidence of sepsis
  - Vitamin K 1–5 mg IV
  - FFP and/or platelets if coagulopathy
  - Octreotide infusion 25 mcg/h (continue until after bleeding ceases for 24 h and wean slowly)
  - Blood transfusion to 10 g/dL (avoid overtransfusion)
  - Upper GI endoscopy to confirm source of bleeding and treat varices
  - Balloon tamponade with a Sengstaken tube is rarely required and should only be used by an experienced clinician.

Octreotide is a somatostatin analogue; somatostatin reduces splanchnic blood flow and therefore portal pressure.

Endoscopic treatment of oesophageal varices

- Variceal banding is an endoscopic ligation technique whereby the varix is aspirated into a plastic tube placed on the distal end of the endoscope. An elastic band is then released from the plastic tube to around the varix, thus strangulating the varix which then thromboses and sloughs off.
- Injection sclerotherapy involves injecting a sclerosant via the endoscope into the variceal columns.

Other varices

Gastric varices are usually contiguous with oesophageal varices and are therefore eradicated by treating oesophageal varices. Ectopic varices are much less likely to bleed, but rarely may require evaluation by endoscopy or angiography and occasionally resection. If bleeding is persistent or recurrent, liver transplantation or portosystemic shunting may be required.

Surgery

Surgical portosystemic shunting is indicated in children with portal vein occlusion or those with chronic liver disease and reasonable liver function if:

- uncontrolled variceal bleeding unresponsive to banding/sclerotherapy
- severe hypersplenism

Many types of shunt are possible, but mesocaval and splenorenal are the most commonly used. Shunt thrombosis is a major complication and may be manifest by recurrent variceal bleeding.

- Rex shunt (mesenterico–left portal) is the insertion of a vein graft to bypass portal vein occlusion and restore hepatic portal blood flow.
- Transjugular intrahepatic portosystemic stent shunt (TIPSS). Used in refractory variceal bleeding as a bridge to transplantation. In this technique a wire is passed into a hepatic vein and a needle advanced into a portal vein. Balloon catheter dilatation of this tract is followed by stent insertion.

Encephalopathy is a complication of shunting in those with cirrhotic liver disease

Liver transplantation

The treatment of choice in portal hypertension and variceal bleeding complicating end stage liver disease.

Primary prophylaxis

Beta-blockers reduce portal pressure by causing splanchnic vasoconstriction and reducing cardiac output. They are effectively used in adults, but in children the benefits must be weighed against the side-effects.

Prophylactic sclerotherapy and/or banding is being investigated in controlled trials.

Paediatric liver transplantation

Liver transplantation is now a standard treatment for:
- Acute liver failure
- Chronic liver failure
- Selected metabolic disorders
- Selected hepatic malignancies.

Indications and contraindications

Indications
- The likelihood of death secondary to liver disease in 18 months or less.
- Unacceptable quality of life secondary to liver disease.
- Growth failure or impairment, due to liver disease, that is not responsive to maximal medical therapy.
- Reversible neurodevelopmental impairment due to liver disease.
- Likelihood of irreversible other end-organ damage that is remediable by liver transplantation.

Contraindications
- The only generally accepted contraindication for liver transplantation is expected patient survival of <50% at 5 years post transplant (see Table 65.1).

Relative contraindications
- Mitochondrial and other disorders with progressive extrahepatic organ involvement.
- Uncontrolled sepsis at the time of transplantation.
- Irreversible severe neurological damage.

Timing of transplantation

The timing of transplantation must balance the risks involved with the additional surgical morbidity in the very unwell child, and the risk of death on the waiting list. The clinical features that inform this decision making process include:

- Synthetic liver dysfunction (prolonged INR, low serum albumin, ascites)
- Disordered metabolism (jaundice, encephalopathy, loss of muscle mass, osteoporosis, intractable pruritus)
- Portal hypertension (variceal bleeding, intractable ascites)
- Profound lethargy
- Spontaneous bacterial peritonitis, recurrent cholangitis
- Hepatorenal or hepatopulmonary syndrome.

Table 65.1 Liver transplantation: survival

	1 year	5 years	10 years
Graft survival	85–90%	70–80%	70–80%
Patient survival	85–95%	75–85%	75–85%

Pre-transplant assessment

Before transplantation, patients require rigorous assessment to identify pre-existing co-morbidities that may preclude transplantation or may impact on management after transplantation.

Cardiac
- 12 lead ECG
- Selected patients may require echocardiogram or cardiac pressure.

Pulmonary
- Pulse oximetry to detect intrapulmonary shunts, if oxygen saturation in room air <95%, macroaggregated albumin scan or contrast echocardiography is performed.
- Chest radiograph
- Formal pulmonary functional assessment is required in patient with cystic fibrosis.

Renal
- EDTA GFR is required to assess for pre-existing renal dysfunction. After transplant calcineurin inhibitor may be minimized by the use of adjuvant immunosuppressants (mycophenolate mofitil or sirolimus).

Nutritional
- Height, weight, skin fold thickness, and mid arm circumference
  - aggressive nutritional support is required before transplantation as nutritional status has important implications for the morbidity and mortality after transplantation.

Vascular
- Pre-transplantation assessment by Doppler USS to detect anomalous vascular anatomy.

Viral immune status (IgG)
- Hepatitis A, B, C, adenovirus, parvovirus, B19, cytomegalovirus, measles, varicella zoster, herpes simplex, Epstein–Barr virus.

Immunization
- It is important that all routine vaccinations are given before transplantation. In addition varicella, hepatitis A and B should be given.
- Live vaccines are usually not given after transplantation.

Dental
- Patients on long-term immunosuppression need excellent dental hygiene.

Social
- Significant social, financial and medical burdens are placed on transplant families. It is important that issues that may impact on the ability of the family to comply fully with the care of a transplanted child are identified and resolved before transplantation.

Education

- The care of a child with a liver transplant requires a high level of understanding from the family. This is important for compliance with medication and follow-up, recognition of complications. Education is a multidisciplinary issue that is led by the transplant coordinators.

Types of liver transplantation

Whole graft transplantation

The diseased liver is removed and is replaced by a donor liver. The hepatic artery, portal vein, and hepatic vein are then anastamosed to their corresponding structure. Bile duct is usually anastomosed to a Roux-en-Y loop created from small bowel.

Reduced liver transplantation

Patients who are small are disadvantaged in organ allocation because of the relative rarity of size-matched organ donors. For this reason surgical techniques have been developed to reduce the size of an adult liver to fit within the morphological restrictions of a paediatric recipient. Patients as small as 2.5 kg may be transplanted with the use of a monosegment graft.

Split graft

The donor liver is divided and shared between two recipients. The smaller left lobe usually goes to a paediatric recipient and the larger right lobe to an adult. Although technically more difficult, the outcomes compare favourably with whole graft transplantation.

Living related

The mortality of patients on waiting lists has led to the expansion of the donor pool to include family members of patients. Potential donors are rigorously screened to assess their suitability for donation. Donation of a portion of the liver carries with it a risk of both morbidity and mortality.

Auxiliary

In this operation a recipient partial hepatectomy is performed and a reduced donor graft is transplanted into the resulting space. The recipient then has
* A residual portion of their own liver
* A donor graft.

The two indications for this are:
* Acute fulminant hepatic failure
* Metabolic liver disease.

Hepatocyte transplantation

Hepatocyte transplantation occurs by the vascular injection of hepatocytes derived from cadaveric liver into the spleen or liver. The donated cells are maintained by the use of immunosuppression. Although this method of treatment remains experimental, it has been successfully used in conditions requiring a small amount of functional hepatocyte mass, i.e. factor VII deficiency, urea cycle defects, and Crigler–Najjar syndrome, as bridge to transplantation.

Choice of an appropriate graft

* ABO blood group compatibility is the principal requirement for matching donor to recipient.
* HLA typing has not been shown to have a role in liver transplantation.

Immediately after transplantation

Postoperative management

Ventilation
Patients return from the operating theatre ventilated. Extubation can be considered after Doppler USS demonstrates patent portal vein and hepatic vessels. Patients with significant malnutrition, systemic unwellness, or encephalopathy before transplantation may require a longer period of ventilation.

Fluid management
The goal of post-transplantation fluid management is to maintain a normal intravascular circulating volume. Intravascular sufficiency is measured by central venous pressure (5–6 mmHg) and urine output (>1 mL/kg per hour).

Infection
Sepsis is a major problem in paediatric liver transplantation.
- All patients receive broad-spectrum antibiotics (cefuroxime and amoxicillin) and antifungal prophylaxis (oral nystatin and systemic fluconazole).
- Selected high-risk patients (acute liver failure, renal dysfunction, prolonged ventilation and patients requiring repeat laparotomy) should receive prophylactic antifungals.
- Patients who are cytomegalovirus (CMV) naive who receive a CMV-positive liver are treated with IV ganciclovir (5 mg/kg twice a day) for 14 days.

Immunosuppression (Table 65.2)
To reduce the risk of rejection:
- Methylprednisolone 2 mg/kg per day (max. dose 60 mg) is given for 3–5 days and then a reducing course of prednisolone is started.
- Doses are rapidly weaned to a maintenance dose which is 0.1 mg/kg per day.
- Calcineurin inhibitors (tacrolimus or ciclosporin) are started as soon as it is clear that the patient has maintained renal function. This is usually day 1 after transplantation. Tacrolimus is the first choice of calcineurin inhibitor as it has a lower level of steroid resistant rejection and chronic rejection compared with ciclosporin. The dose is started at 0.15 mg/kg per day, q12 h. (Table 65.3)

Complications

Primary non-function of the graft (2%)
- Failure of graft functions, marked by haemodynamic instability, metabolic acidosis, synthetic dysfunction, and elevation of liver transaminases.
- Treatment is emergency re-transplantation.

Hepatic artery thrombosis (5–10%)
- Early thrombosis of the hepatic artery may result in ischaemia of the graft.
- Patients should be screened for an underlying pro-coagulant status.

Portal vein thrombosis (PVT) (5%)
- Presents with graft dysfunction or splenic enlargement.

Treatment options include surgical re-anastamosis, interventional radiological dilatation and splint insertion or portal decompression shunt surgery, i.e. splenorenal shunt.

Biliary complication
- Perforation
- Stricture.

Biliary stricture occurs in 10–15% of paediatric liver transplants. Strictures are often anastomotic or may be ischaemic in origin, relating to hepatic artery compromise.

Intestinal
- Perforation
- Bleeding.

Acute cellular rejection
- 50–75% of patients have an episode of acute cellular rejection in the first 3 months after transplantation. The rate is lower in infants.
- Acute cellular rejection (ACR) is detected by a rise in the blood levels of aspartate and alanine transaminases (AST, ALT).
- Doppler USS is performed and diagnosis is confirmed on liver biopsy.
- Treatment is with 3 days of methylprednisolone (10 mg/kg per day) followed by a decreasing course of oral prednisolone (2 mg/kg per day).

Table 65.2 Immunosuppressants: mechanism and possible complications

Drug	Mechanism	Complications
Prednisolone	Multiple	Acute: Hypertension Hyperglycaemia Psychosis
Ciclosporin/tacrolimus	Calcineurin inhibitor IL-2 gene transcription inhibitor	Hypertension Hyperglycaemia PTLD Renal impairment Neurotoxicity
Ciclosporin		Hirsutism Gingival hyperplasia
Sirolimus	IL-2 post receptor signal transduction inhibition	Hyperlipidaemia Leucopenia Thrombocytopenia Poor wound healing Hepatic artery thrombosis
Basiliximab/daclizumab	Anti-IL-2 antibody	Infections PTLD
Mycophenolate mofetil	Purine synthesis inhibitor	Bone marrow suppression Gastrointestinal
Anti-thymoglobulin (ATG)	Anti-T-cell antibody	Allergic reaction Infections, PTLD

Table 65.3 Tacrolimus levels

Time post transplant	Trough level of tacrolimus (ng/L)
0–3 months	10–12
3 months to 1 year	5–8
1 year on	5

- Failure to respond to steroid treatment requires repeat USS and biopsy.
- Additional agents that may be used include:
  - monoclonal antibodies
  - anti-thymocyte globulin or OKT 3.

Chronic rejection

- Chronic rejection presents as cholestatic liver disease.
- Histological features include loss of bile ducts and graft arteriopathy.
- Treatment is currently undefined and may require re-transplantation in time.
- Some grafts could be rescued with newer immunosuppressive agents such as sirolimus.

Hypertension

Elevated blood pressure occurs in 10–20% of patients after transplantation. It is often multifactorial:
- Corticosteroids
- Calcineurin inhibition
- Renal impairment.

Treatment
- Nifedipine
- Atenolol.

De novo autoimmune liver disease

- 2–5% of liver transplant recipients, irrespective of initial diagnosis, develop autoimmune liver disease.
- It is characterized by elevations in liver transaminases and anti-nuclear antibody, smooth muscle antibody, and rarely liver kidney mitochondrial antibody positivity.
- It is treated by long-term prednisolone administration.

Post-transplant lymphoproliferative disorder (PTLD)

- Dysregulation of the immune system leads to an increased risk of virally (usually EBV) mediated malignancy. It occurs in 5% of patients at 1 year.
- PTLD represents a spectrum of disorders, ranging from EBV viraemia to high-grade lymphoma.

Detection
Requires routine assessment for:
- Lymphadenopathy
- Unexplained anaemia
- Unexplained fever
- Microscopic or macroscopic blood in stool
- EBV viral load.

Diagnosis/staging
- EBV viral load
- Liver biopsy
- Radiological assessment of lymphadenopathy (CT chest, abdomen)
- Biopsy of affected lymph nodes
- Cerebrospinal fluid
- Upper and lower GI endoscopy with mucosal biopsies.

Treatment
Treatment is dependent upon the grade of illness.
- Viraemia may improve with a decrease in immunosuppression.
- Lymphoma requires withdrawal of calcineurin inhibitors and adminis-tration of corticosteroids with-
  - anti-CD20 monoclonal antibody (rituximab) is the first line therapy.
  - chemotherapy is used in recalcitrant cases.

Skin cancer

- The risk of all types of cutaneous malignancy is increased. This may be minimized by the use of skin protection, hat, long-sleeved garments, and sun-screen.
- In addition, adult series report an increase of many types of malignancy above the expected rate for age.

Infection

Patients who are receiving immunosuppression are at increased risk of infection.

- CMV is the most common early transplant viral infection. The highest risk patients are those who are CMV naive at the time of transplantation and receive a CMV-positive graft. These patients are treated with prophylactic ganciclovir for 14 days.
- EBV infection and post transplant lymphoproliferative disease: See Post-transplant lymphoproliferative disorder (PTLD).
- Varicella: Patients who are varicella IgG negative and who have a significant contact with primary or secondary varicella infection should receive IV immunoglobulin within 3 days of contact. Oral aciclovir has also been shown to be effective as prophylactic agent.
- Patients who develop a clinical illness should receive IV aciclovir or valaciclovir until the disease is resolved.
- Herpes simplex.

Renal function

Renal dysfunction is common and multifactorial in liver transplantation. Risk factors include:

- Calcineurin inhibitors
- Pre-existing renal dysfunction
- Hypertension.

Management includes careful monitoring of renal function through nuclear medicine scan—radioisotope labelled clearance.

If decreased renal function is detected, calcineurin inhibitors exposure may be decreased by the use of adjuvant immunosuppressants like mycophenolate mofetil and sirolimus.

Growth

- Most patients achieve normal height after liver transplantation. 90% of patients are >3% height for age. The exceptions are patients with syndromes associated with decreased growth, i.e. Alagille's syndrome and PFIC1 disease.
- Successful liver transplantation is not associated with pubertal delay.

Quality of life

- The majority of patients have good general health after liver transplantation, and most are found to have a good quality of life on objective measure.
- The burden of lifelong immunosuppression, uncertainty about the future, and the requirement for regular medical follow-up all impact negatively on quality of life in some patients.

Immunosuppressants

Standard
- Corticosteroids
- Calcineurin inhibitors

Renal sparing
- Sirolimus
- Mycophenolate mofetil

Rescue therapy
- Anti-thymoglobulin
- Basilixumab and daclizumab

Useful websites

Nutritional information

- American Dietetic Association www.eatright.org
- American Academy of Allergy, Asthma and Immunology www. aaaai.org
- Bandolier (independent evidence based health care) www.jr2. oc.ac.uk/bandolier
- British Association for Parenteral and Enteral Nutrition www. bapen.org.uk
- British Dietetic Association www.bda.org.uk
- British Nutrition Foundation www.nutrition.org.uk/home. asp?siteId=43&sectionId=305&which=7
- British Society of Paediatric Gastroenterology, Hepatology and Nutrition www.bspghan.org.uk
- Coeliac UK www.coeliac.co.uk
- Department of Health www.dh.gov.uk;
- European Academy of Allergy and Clinical Immunology www. eaaci.net
- European Society for Paediatric Gastroenterology, Hepatology and Nutrition www.espghan
- Food in schools programme www.teachernet.gov.uk; www. wiredforhealth.gov.uk
- Food Standards Agency www.food.gov.uk; www.eatwell.gov.uk; www.salt.gov.uk
- Food and Nutrition Information Centre. National Agricultural Library of the United States Department of Agriculture http:// fnic.nal.usda.gov
- Infant and Dietetic Foods Association. Infant feeding in the UK. May 2005. www.isdfa.org.uk/inform
- Medicines and Healthcare Products Regulatory Agency www. mhra.gov.uk
- Royal College of Paediatrics and Child Health www.rcpch.ac.uk
- Scientific Advisory Committee on Nutrition www.sacn.gov.uk

Infant feeding

- www.babyfriendly.org.uk/commun.asp#plan
- www.breastfeeding.nhs.uk;
- www.nctpregnancyandbabycare.com; www.surestart.gov.uk;
- www.laleche.org.uk; www.bliss.org.uk
- breast-feeding: www.dh.gov.uk/en/Policyandguidance/index.htm
- Summary and comparison of recommendations for nutrient content of low-birth-weigh infant formulas. Life Sciences Research Office http://www.lsro.org/articles/lowbirthweight_ rpt.pdf

Guidelines

- The Resuscitation Council (UK) guideline entitled: 'The Emergency Medical Treatment of Anaphylactic Reactions for First Medical Responders and for Community Nurses' www.resus.org.uk/pages/reaction.htm
- Cochrane Reviews on Gastroesophageal Reflux, Inflammatory Bowel Disease, www.cochrane.org/reviews
- Guidelines on Gastroesophageal Reflux, Helicobacter Infection in Children, Coeliac disease www.naspghan.org
- Guidelines on Coeliac disease, Inflammatory bowel disease, Chronic disease www.bsg.org
- Guideline on Inflammatory bowel disease, Coeliac disease www.bspghan.org
- Cyclical Vomiting Syndrome (includes treatment guidelines)
- www.cvsa.org.uk/treatmentframe.html

Anthropometry and growth assessment

- http://www.cdc.gov/nchs/data/nhanes/nhanes3/cdrom/nchs/manuals/anthro.pdf
- Scientific Advisory Committee on Nutrition. Application of WHO Growth Standards in the UK. www.sacn.gov.uk/pdfs/report_growth_standards_2007_08_10.pdf
- Growth and its measurement. Factsheet and interactive tutorial available from: www.infantandtoddlerforum.org
- Use of skinfold callipers
- http://healthsciences.qmuc.ac.uk/labweb/Equipment/skin_fold_calipers.htm
- Child Growth Foundation (growth charts) www.childgrowthfoundation.org
- NHANES III reference manuals and reports. U.S. Department of Health and Human Services, Centers for Disease Control and Prevention, National Center for Health Statistics www.cdc.gov/nchs/data/nhanes/bc.pdf

Enteral nutrition

- ESPEN Guidelines on adult enteral nutrition. Clinical Nutrition 2006;25:177-360 http://www.espen.org/education/guidelines.htm
- NICE guidelines: Nutritional support in adults. http://guidance.nice.org.uk/CG32
- British National Formulary for Children: http://bnfc.org/bnfc/bnfc/current/129132.htm
- Stroud M, Duncan H, Nightingale J. Guidelines for enteral feeding in adult hospital patients. Gut 2003;52:1-12 http://gut.bmj.com/cgi/reprint/52/suppl_7/vii1

Useful contacts

- The Anaphylaxis Campaign, PO Box 275, Farnborough GU14 6SX; tel: 01252 373793, helpline: 01252 377140; fax: 01252 377140; email: info@anaphylaxis.org.uk
- Patients on Intravenous and Nasogastric Nutrition Therapy (PINNT) PO Box 3126, Christchurch, Dorset, BH23 2XS.Tel: 01202 481 625 Fax: 01202 481 625; www.pinnt.com
- Children's Liver Disease Foundation 36, Great Charles Street, Birmingham B33JY UK; http://www.childliverdisease.org
- Coeliac UK, www.coeliac.co.uk
- Crohn's in Childhood Research Association (CICRA), www.cicra.org
- National Association of Colitis and Crohn's disease (NACC), www.nacc.org.uk

Index